D1245728

Instant Work-Ups:
A Clinical Guide to Medicine

Instant Work-Ups:
A Clinical Guide to Medicine

Second Edition

Theodore X. O'Connell, M.D.

ELSEVIER

ELSEVIER

1600 John F. Kennedy Blvd.
Ste 1800
Philadelphia, PA 19103-2899

Instant Work-Ups: A Clinical Guide to Medicine, second edition.
ISBN: 978-0-323-37641-9

Notices

Knowledge and best practice in this field are constantly changing. As new research and experience broaden our understanding, changes in research methods, professional practices, or medical treatment may become necessary.

Practitioners and researchers must always rely on their own experience and knowledge in evaluating and using any information, methods, compounds, or experiments described herein. In using such information or methods they should be mindful of their own safety and the safety of others, including parties for whom they have a professional responsibility.

With respect to any drug or pharmaceutical products identified, readers are advised to check the most current information provided (i) on procedures featured or (ii) by the manufacturer of each product to be administered, to verify the recommended dose or formula, the method and duration of administration, and contraindications. It is the responsibility of practitioners, relying on their own experience and knowledge of their patients, to make diagnoses, to determine dosages and the best treatment for each individual patient, and to take all appropriate safety precautions.

To the fullest extent of the law, neither the Publisher nor the authors, contributors, or editors, assume any liability for any injury and/or damage to persons or property as a matter of products liability, negligence or otherwise, or from any use or operation of any methods, products, instructions, or ideas contained in the material herein.

Library of Congress Cataloging-in-Publication Data
Names: O'Connell, Theodore X., author.
Title: Instant work-ups : a clinical guide to medicine / Theodore X.
  O'Connell.
Description: Second. | Philadelphia, PA : Elsevier, [2017] | Preceded by
  Instant work-ups / Theodore X. O'Connell. c2008. | Includes bibliographical
  references and index.
Identifiers: LCCN 2016003317 | ISBN 9780323376419 (paperback : alk. paper)
Subjects: | MESH: Clinical Medicine | Handbooks
Classification: LCC RC55 | NLM WB 39 | DDC 616—dc23 LC record available at
http://lccn.loc.gov/2016003317

Content Strategist: Lauren Willis
Content Development Specialist: Angie Breckon
Publishing Services Manager: Patricia Tannian
Project Manager: Ted Rodgers
Design Direction: Paula Catalano

Printed in United States of America

Last digit is the print number: 9 8 7 6 5 4 3 2 1

Working together
to grow libraries in
developing countries

www.elsevier.com • www.bookaid.org

About the Author

Theodore X. O'Connell, M.D., is the Founding Program Director of the Kaiser Permanente Napa-Solano Family Medicine Residency Program. Dr. O'Connell is an assistant clinical professor in the Department of Family and Community Medicine at the University of California, San Francisco School of Medicine and is an assistant clinical professor in the Department of Family Medicine at the David Geffen School of Medicine at UCLA. He is the recipient of numerous clinical, teaching, and research awards. He has been published widely as the author of medical textbooks, textbook chapters, journal articles, and editorials. He received his medical degree from the University of California, Los Angeles School of Medicine and completed a residency and chief residency at Santa Monica-UCLA Medical Center in Santa Monica, California.

Contributing Authors

Aakash Agarwal, D.O.
Gallbladder Polyp and Elevated Amylase chapters
Clinical Faculty
Kaiser Permanente Napa-Solano
Family Medicine Residency Program
Clinical Instructor
Department of Family and Community Medicine
University of California, San Francisco School of Medicine

Michael Mason, M.D.
Memory Loss and Dementia chapter
Clinical Faculty
Kaiser Permanente Napa-Solano
Family Medicine Residency Program
Clinical Instructor
Department of Family Medicine
David Geffen School of Medicine at UCLA

Candace Y. Pau, M.D.
Visual Disturbances chapter
Resident Physician, Department of Family Medicine
Kaiser Permanente Napa-Solano
Graduate of the Stanford University School of Medicine

For Nichole, Ryan, Sean, and Claire

Preface

Most medical textbooks are oriented on the basis of a known diagnosis. If one wants to learn more about congestive heart failure, hepatitis C, or bronchogenic carcinoma, traditional textbooks and online resources can be great sources of information. However, patients do not come to the clinician labeled with a diagnosis, except for those problems that have been previously identified. Patients instead come with symptoms such as fatigue, edema, dyspnea, or memory loss. They may also present with laboratory abnormalities such as transaminase elevation, hyponatremia, leukocytosis, or hypercalcemia. It is the role of the busy clinician to utilize the history, physical examination, and selected laboratory or imaging studies to sort out the patient's present symptoms or laboratory abnormality and provide a diagnosis.

This text is directed to primary care physicians but may be beneficial for physicians in almost all specialties. The work-ups outlined in each chapter are suggested courses of action based upon the current medical literature. However, they are not a replacement for clinical judgment and may not be uniformly applied to all patients. Every patient is different, and the history and physical examination may indicate need for more or less evaluation than the work-ups suggest. These work-ups should be viewed as general guidelines to help the busy clinician be exacting and thorough while also being efficient. At the same time, deviating from these work-ups on the basis of clinical judgment is encouraged and expected.

The purpose of this book is not to discuss treatment options, as this would make the text unwieldy and many excellent resources are available to help guide treatment decisions once a diagnosis has been made.

I hope that this text eases your practice of medicine while helping you provide the highest quality care to your patients.

Contents

1 ACUTE KIDNEY INJURY

General Discussion

Acute kidney injury (AKI) is defined as an abrupt (within 48 hours) reduction in kidney function based on an elevation in serum creatinine (Cr), reduction in urine output, the need for dialysis, or a combination of these factors. Although the definition includes the 48-hour window, in the outpatient setting, it may be difficult to determine when the rise in Cr actually occurred. The term *acute kidney injury* replaces previously used terms such as *acute renal failure* and *acute renal insufficiency*.

False elevations of serum Cr can be seen with medications (e.g., trimethoprim-sulfamethoxazole, cimetidine, and cephalosporins) because these agents can inhibit the tubular secretion of Cr without causing actual damage to the kidneys. However, these medications can also cause renal failure as a result of interstitial nephritis.

The causes of AKI can be broadly divided into three categories. The first is prerenal AKI, which is a reversible increase in serum Cr and blood urea nitrogen (BUN) that results from decreased renal perfusion, leading to a reduction in the glomerular filtration rate (GFR). The second category is intrinsic AKI, in which the structures of the nephron are affected. This second category can be further subdivided based on the structure that is affected: the glomeruli, tubules, interstitium, or vasculature. The third category is postrenal AKI, which is caused by an obstruction of the urinary collection system by either intrinsic or extrinsic masses.

Prerenal AKI accounts for 60% to 70% of cases of acute renal failure. Decreased renal perfusion associated with intravascular volume depletion or decreased arterial pressure results in a reduced GFR. In patients with preexisting chronic kidney disease, the susceptibility to develop acute-on-chronic renal failure is higher.

The most common cause of intrinsic AKI is acute tubular necrosis (ATN), which is caused by an ischemic or nephrotoxic injury to the kidney. In contrast to a prerenal etiology, AKI caused by ATN does not improve with adequate repletion of intravascular volume and perfusion to the kidneys. However, it may resolve over time, depending on the degree of renal injury. Glomerular causes of AKI are the result of acute inflammation of blood vessels and glomeruli, usually as a manifestation of a systemic illness or pulmonary renal syndromes. Renal biopsy is often required to confirm the diagnosis before initiating immunosuppressive therapy. Acute interstitial nephritis (AIN) is most commonly related to medication use. In approximately one-third of cases, there is a history of maculopapular erythematous rash, fever, and/or arthralgias. Renal atheroembolic disease is the most common vascular cause of AKI.

It is always important to exclude a postrenal obstructive cause (e.g., prostatic hyperplasia) in a patient presenting with AKI because prompt intervention may result in improvement or complete recovery of renal function. Bladder catheterization may be considered, especially in elderly men with unexplained AKI. Renal ultrasonography can be used to diagnose obstruction by assessing for hydronephrosis.

Probable causes of AKI may be identified from the history and physical examination. Urine collected before the initiation of intravenous fluid or diuretic treatment can be used to calculate the fractional excretion of sodium (FE_{Na}) using the following equation:

$$FE_{Na} = \frac{\text{Urine sodium/plasma sodium}}{\text{Urine creatinine/plasma creatinine}} \times 100$$

Figure 1-1. From Rahman M, Shad F, Smith MC. Acute kidney injury: a guide to diagnosis and management. *American Family Physician* 2012;86(7):631–639.

An FE_{Na} less than 1% suggests a prerenal cause of AKI. An FE_{Na} greater than 1% suggests an intrinsic cause of AKI, most commonly ATN. The FE_{Na} is often greater than 3% in intrinsic causes of acute renal failure. It should be noted that a prerenal FE_{Na} of greater than 1% can occur in patients receiving long-term diuretic therapy or in patients with AKI superimposed on chronic renal failure. Conversely, an intrinsic FE_{Na} of less than 1% can occur with radiocontrast nephropathy and rhabdomyolysis.

Medications Associated with Acute Kidney Injury

Prerenal Acute Kidney Injury

- Angiotensin-converting enzyme inhibitors
- Angiotensin receptor blockers
- Aspirin
- Cyclosporine
- Nonsteroidal anti-inflammatory drugs (NSAIDs)
- Tacrolimus
- Prostaglandin inhibitors

Intrinsic Acute Kidney Injury

Interstitial Injury
- Acyclovir
- Allopurinol
- Cephalosporins
- Cimetidine
- Ciprofloxacin
- Furosemide
- Interferon

- NSAIDs
- Penicillins
- Phenytoin
- Proton pump inhibitors
- Rifampin
- Sulfonamides
- Thiazide diuretics
- Trimethoprim-sulfamethoxazole

Tubular Injury
- Acyclovir
- Aminoglycosides
- Amphotericin B
- Angiotensin-converting enzyme inhibitors
- Cisplatin
- Cyclosporine
- Foscarnet
- Ifosfamide
- Methotrexate
- NSAIDs
- Oxalic acid
- Pentamidine
- Radiographic contrast agents

Causes of Acute Kidney Injury

Prerenal Acute Kidney Injury

Dissection
Embolus
Heart failure
Hemorrhage
Intravascular volume depletion
- Diarrhea
- Diuretics
- Fever
- Insufficient fluid intake
- Sweating
- Third-space losses
- Vomiting

Liver failure
Massive pulmonary embolism
Medications
Nephrotic syndrome
Pericardial effusion with tamponade
Thrombosis

Intrinsic Acute Kidney Injury

Glomerular Injury
- Churg-Strauss
- Endocarditis
- Goodpasture syndrome
- Henoch-Schönlein purpura
- Idiopathic crescentic glomerulonephritis
- Immunoglobulin-A nephropathy
- Lupus nephritis
- Membranoproliferative glomerulonephritis
- Polyarteritis nodosa
- Postinfectious glomerulonephritis
- Rapidly progressive glomerulonephritis
- Wegener granulomatosis

Interstitial
- Acute interstitial nephritis due to the previously listed medications
- Bacterial pyelonephritis

Tubular
- Acute falciparum malaria
- Cocaine
- Ethylene glycol ingestion
- Heavy metals
- Hemoglobin and myoglobin
- Incompatible blood transfusion
- Ischemia due to sepsis, shock, hemorrhage, trauma, or pancreatitis
- Medications
- Myeloma light chains
- Radiocontrast media
- Rhabdomyolysis
- Uric acid

Vascular
- Aortic disease
- Aortic dissection
- Atheroembolism secondary to atrial fibrillation
- Atheroembolism after procedures (e.g., aortic catheterization, arteriography, or vascular surgery)
- Atheroembolism after abdominal trauma
- Hemolysis, elevated liver enzymes, low platelets (HELLP) syndrome
- Hemolytic uremic syndrome
- Malignant hypertension
- Postpartum acute renal failure
- Renal artery stenosis or thrombosis
- Scleroderma renal crisis
- Small vessel thrombosis
- Thrombotic thrombocytopenic purpura

Postrenal Acute Kidney Injury

- Autonomic neuropathy
- Blood clots
- Catheter
- Crystals
- Prostatic hyperplasia
- Retroperitoneal fibrosis
- Stones
- Stricture
- Tumors (prostate cancer, lymphoma, carcinoma of the bladder, cervix, uterus, ovaries, or rectum)
- Valves

Key Historical Features

✓ Symptoms of heart failure (shortness of breath, fatigue, dyspnea on exertion, paroxysmal nocturnal dyspnea, orthopnea) that may cause decreased renal perfusion
✓ Pulmonary symptoms that may suggest pulmonary–renal syndrome or vasculitis
✓ Diarrhea or vomiting that predisposes to hypovolemia
✓ Abdominal pain suggestive of nephrolithiasis
✓ Benign prostatic hypertrophy symptoms
✓ Sinus symptoms that may suggest pulmonary–renal syndrome or vasculitis
✓ Bone pain suggestive of multiple myeloma or metastatic malignancy
✓ Trauma that may cause rhabdomyolysis
✓ Prolonged immobilization that may cause rhabdomyolysis
✓ Constitutional symptoms (e.g., fever, weight loss, or anorexia) that may suggest malignancy or vasculitis
✓ Medical history, especially diabetes, multiple sclerosis, or cerebrovascular accident, which may lead to neurogenic bladder
✓ Prosthetic heart valve or valvular disease as a risk factor for endocarditis
✓ Surgical history, especially recent surgery and procedures that may increase the risk for atheroembolism, ischemia, or endocarditis
✓ Recent administration of contrast agent
✓ Medications
✓ History of intravenous drug as a risk factor for endocarditis

Key Physical Findings

✓ Temperature for evidence of fever/infection
✓ Blood pressure for hypertension or hypotension
✓ Head and neck examination for oral and/or nasal ulcers or evidence of dehydration

- ✓ Cardiovascular examination for evidence of heart failure, heart murmur, or jugular venous distention
- ✓ Pulmonary examination for evidence of heart failure
- ✓ Abdominal examination, especially for abdominal bruits or evidence of bladder distention
- ✓ Skin examination for rash that may be a sign of interstitial nephritis, lupus erythematosus, vasculitis, thrombotic thrombocytopenic purpura, or atheroembolic disease; splinter hemorrhages or Osler nodes suggestive of endocarditis
- ✓ Extremity examination for edema
- ✓ Pelvic examination for masses
- ✓ Rectal examination for prostate enlargement or nodules

Suggested Work-Up

Renal ultrasonography	To evaluate for hydronephrosis as a marker for obstruction
BUN and Cr	To evaluate renal function and compare with previous levels to determine the duration and acuity of the disease BUN/Cr ratio >20:1 in prerenal causes BUN/Cr ratio 10:1 to 20:1 in intrinsic causes
Serum electrolytes	To evaluate for hyperkalemia Serum sodium used to calculate the FE_{Na}
Serum glucose	Used to calculate serum osmolality
Calcium	To evaluate for malignancy
Phosphorus	To evaluate for phosphorus imbalance and possibly chronic renal failure
Albumin	To evaluate for liver disease or nephrotic syndrome
Complete blood count with differential	To evaluate for infection, hemolysis, or thrombocytopenia
Serum osmolality	Used to calculate the osmolar gap
Urine dipstick and microscopy	Prerenal acute kidney injury may show hyaline casts. Postrenal acute kidney injury may show few hyaline casts or few red blood cells.

	Acute tubular necrosis may show epithelial cells, muddy brown, coarsely granular casts, white blood cells, or low-grade proteinuria. Allergic interstitial nephritis may show white blood cells, red blood cells, epithelial cells, eosinophils, white blood cell casts, or low to moderate proteinuria. Glomerulonephritis may show red blood cell casts, dysmorphic red cells, or moderate to severe proteinuria.
Urine sodium level	<10 in prerenal causes of acute renal failure >20 in intrinsic causes of acute renal failure
Urine Cr level	Used to calculate the FE_{Na}
Urine osmolality	>500 in prerenal causes of acute renal failure 300–500 in intrinsic causes of acute renal failure

Additional Work-Up

Creatine kinase and myoglobin	If rhabdomyolysis is suspected
Uric acid	If gouty nephropathy, malignancy, or tumor lysis is suspected
Prostate-specific antigen	If prostate cancer is suspected
Serum protein electrophoresis	If multiple myeloma is suspected
Complement levels	If lupus erythematosus, postinfectious glomerulonephritis, or subacute bacterial endocarditis is suspected (levels would be decreased in these conditions)
Antinuclear antibody	If autoimmune disease is suspected
Double-stranded DNA antibody	Elevated in systemic lupus erythematosus
Antineutrophilic cytoplasmic antibody	If Wegener granulomatosis or polyarteritis nodosa is suspected
Antibasement membrane antibody	Elevated in Goodpasture syndrome
Antineutrophil cytoplasmic antibody	Elevated in in vasculitis and Wegener granulomatosis

HIV	If HIV nephropathy is suspected
Antistreptolysin-O titer	Elevated in poststreptococcal glomerulonephritis
Serum haptoglobin (decreased), indirect bilirubin (elevated), lactate dehydrogenase (elevated)	To evaluate for hemolysis if thrombotic thrombocytopenic purpura, hemolytic uremic syndrome, systemic lupus erythematosus, or other autoimmune diseases are suspected; thrombocytopenia and schistocytes on peripheral smear are also seen.
Hemoglobin electrophoresis	If sickle cell nephropathy is suspected
Urine eosinophils	If allergic interstitial nephritis is suspected
Blood cultures	If endocarditis is suspected
Abdominal plain-film radiograph	If nephrolithiasis or ureterolithiasis is suspected
Abdominal/pelvic computed tomographic scan	If malignancy, nephrolithiasis, or ureterolithiasis is suspected
Renal biopsy	May be necessary to establish the diagnosis, determine the prognosis, or guide therapy

Further Reading

Agrawal M, Swartz R. Acute renal failure. *Am Fam Physician.* 2000;61:2077–2088.

Albright Jr RC. Acute renal failure: a practical update. *Mayo Clin Proc.* 2001;76:67–74.

Dursun B, Edelstein CL. Acute renal failure. *Am J Kidney Dis.* 2005;45:614–618.

Holley JL. Clinical approach to the diagnosis of acute renal failure. In: Greenberg A, Cheung AK, eds. *Primer on Kidney Diseases.* 5th ed. Philadelphia: National Kidney Foundation; 2009:278.

Lameire N. The pathophysiology of acute renal failure. *Crit Care Clin.* 2005;1:197–200.

Needham E. Management of acute renal failure. *Am Fam Physician.* 2005;72:1739–1746.

Pascual J, Liano F, Ortuno J. The elderly patient with acute renal failure. *J Am Soc Nephrol.* 1995;6:144–153.

Rahman M, Shad F, Smith MC. Acute kidney injury: a guide to diagnosis and management. *Am Fam Physician.* 2012;86:631–639.

Thadhani R, Pascual M, Bonventre JV. Acute renal failure. *N Engl J Med.* 1996;334:1448–1460.

General Discussion

An adrenal "incidentaloma" is an adrenal mass, generally 1 cm or more in diameter, that is discovered incidentally on radiological examination performed for indications other than an evaluation for adrenal disease. The majority of adrenal incidentalomas are clinically nonhypersecreting, benign adrenocortical adenomas. Other adrenal incidentalomas that may be encountered include cortisol-secreting adrenocortical adenoma, cyst, myelolipoma, hemorrhage, pheochromocytoma, metastatic carcinoma, and adrenocortical carcinoma.

A lesion measuring at least 1 cm is normally considered large enough for further hormonal and imaging evaluation. There are no data for determining the accuracy of imaging for masses measuring less than 1 cm. The purpose of further imaging and clinical workup is to determine whether the lesion is benign or malignant and whether the lesion is functioning or nonfunctioning. The two most important factors in the diagnostic evaluation are the lesion's size and functional status. In general, the larger the mass, the greater the likelihood of malignancy. Because of the high mortality rate associated with adrenal carcinoma, most centers recommend excision of lesions 4 cm or more in diameter. However, if computed tomography (CT) characteristics point to a myelolipoma or cyst, and the patient is asymptomatic, nonsurgical management is appropriate, regardless of the size of the mass.

To determine the functional status of an adrenal mass, the patient should be assessed for signs and symptoms of Cushing syndrome, pheochromocytoma, and hyperaldosteronism. These signs and symptoms are outlined in the following.

If the adrenal mass has a benign appearance on imaging, the patient has no signs or symptoms, and the screening laboratory tests outlined in the following are normal, the patient should have repeat imaging (contrast-enhanced CT) at 6, 12, and 24 months, as well as repeat hormonal testing annually for 4 years. If the patient has signs or symptoms, or the laboratory tests are not normal, referral to a surgeon is indicated.

If the adrenal mass has a suspicious appearance on imaging and the screening laboratory tests outlined in the following are normal, the patient should have fine-needle aspiration biopsy if metastatic disease or infection is suspected. Surgical consultation and close follow-up (imaging at 3 months) are indicated.

Any patient with a history of malignancy who is found to have an adrenal mass should probably have a needle biopsy of the adrenal lesions, because metastatic disease is the most likely cause of the adrenal lesion in this situation.

Signs and Symptoms of Systemic Disease

Cushing Syndrome

- Abdominal striae
- Buffalo hump
- Diabetes
- Diaphoresis
- Easy bruising
- Emotional and cognitive changes
- Hirsutism
- Hyperglycemia
- Hyperlipidemia
- Hypertension
- Hypoglycemia
- Menstrual abnormalities
- Moon-shaped facies
- Obesity, especially central
- Osteoporosis
- Proximal muscle weakness
- Thin skin

Pheochromocytoma

- Diaphoresis
- Fever
- Headache
- Hypertension
- Orthostatic hypotension
- Pallor
- Palpitations
- Paroxysmal hypertension
- Sweating
- Tremor

Hyperaldosteronism

- Hypernatremia
- Hypertension
- Hypokalemia (may be accompanied by polyuria, nocturia, muscle cramps, and palpitations)

Suggested Work-Up

Overnight 1-mg dexamethasone suppression test	To evaluate for Cushing syndrome
24-h urinary fractionated	To evaluate for pheochromocytoma metanephrines, and catecholamines
Morning plasma aldosterone concentration and plasma renin activity	If hypertension is present, to evaluate for hyperaldosteronism

Additional Evaluation

Serum corticotropin, cortisol in a blood specimen, and 24-h urine specimen, midnight salivary measurement of cortisol, and 2-day high-dose dexamethasone suppression test	Confirmatory tests for Cushing syndrome
Iodine-123 metaiodobenzylguanidine scintigraphy, magnetic resonance imaging, subspecialty consultation	Confirmatory tests for pheochromocytoma
Aldosterone suppression testing with either a saline infusion test or 24-h urinary aldosterone secretion test	Confirmatory tests for primary aldosteronism

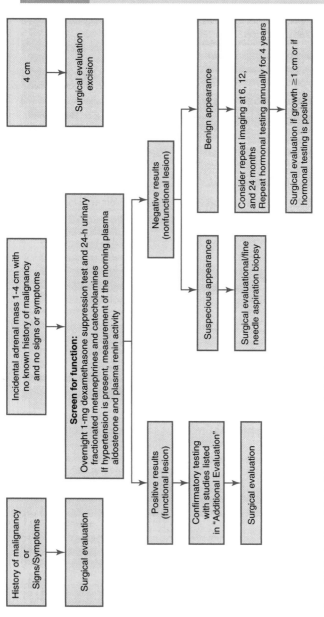

Figure 2-I. Evaluation of the incidentally discovered adrenal mass.

Further Reading

Cook DM, Loriaux DL. The incidental adrenal mass. *Am J Med.* 1996;101:88–94.

Copeland PM. The incidentally discovered adrenal mass. *Ann Surg.* 1984;199:116–122.

Higgins JC, Fitzgerald JM. Evaluation of incidental renal and adrenal masses. *Am Fam Physician.* 2001;63:288–291.

Nieman LK. Approach to the patient with an adrenal incidentaloma. *J Clin Endocrinol Metab.* 2010;95:4106–4113.

Prinz RA, Brooks MH, Churchill R, et al. Incidental asymptomatic adrenal masses detected by computed tomographic scanning. Is operation required? *JAMA.* 1982;248:701–704.

Ross NS, Aron DC. Hormonal evaluation of the patient with an incidentally discovered adrenal mass. *N Engl J Med.* 1990;323:1401–1405.

Scott Jr HW, ed. *Surgery of the Adrenal Glands.* Philadelphia: JB Lippincott; 1990.

Vaughan ED. Diseases of the adrenal gland. *Med Clin North Am.* 2004;88:443–466.

Willatt JM, Francis IR. Radiologic evaluation of incidentally discovered adrenal masses. *Am Fam Physician.* 2010;81:1361–1366.

Young WF. The incidentally discovered adrenal mass. *New Engl J Med.* 2007;356:601–610.

General Discussion

Primary amenorrhea is defined as the failure to reach menarche and should be evaluated if there is no pubertal development by 13 years of age, if menarche has not occurred 5 years after initial breast development, or if the patient is 15 years or older. Secondary amenorrhea is the cessation of previously regular menses for 3 months or previously irregular menses for 6 months. Secondary amenorrhea is more common than primary amenorrhea.

Primary amenorrhea is often the result of chromosomal irregularities that lead to primary ovarian insufficiency or anatomic abnormalities. The most common cause of secondary amenorrhea is pregnancy. Other common causes of secondary amenorrhea are polycystic ovary syndrome (PCOS), thyroid disease, hyperprolactinemia hypothalamic amenorrhea, and primary ovarian insufficiency.

In all cases of amenorrhea, pregnancy must be ruled out. The patient then can be evaluated for thyroid disease and hyperprolactinemia. Luteinizing hormone (LH), follicle stimulating hormone (FSH), and pelvic ultrasonography, as clinically indicated, allow the categorization of amenorrhea as follows: (1) anatomic defects in the outflow tract; (2) primary dysfunction of the ovary; (3) disruption of hypothalamic or pituitary function; (4) systemic disease affecting the hypothalamic–pituitary axis; (5) or pathology of other endocrine glands. The major difference in the evaluation of primary and secondary amenorrhea is the need to determine the presence or absence of the uterus in patients with primary amenorrhea.

Medications and Substances Associated with Amenorrhea

Antidepressants
Antihistamines
Antihypertensives
Antipsychotics
Butyrophenones
Cocaine
Contraceptive medications
Domperidone
Exogenous androgens
Haloperidol
H_2 blockers
Methyldopa
Metoclopramide
Opiates

Phenothiazine
Reserpine
Risperdone
Sulpiride
Valproic acid
Verapamil

Causes of Secondary Amenorrhea

Anatomic Defects (Outflow Tract)

- Cervical agenesis
- Cervical stenosis
- Complete androgen resistance (testicular feminization)
- Endometrial hypoplasia or aplasia
- Imperforate hymen
- Intrauterine synechiae (Asherman syndrome)
- Müllerian agenesis
- Transverse vaginal septum
- Vaginal agenesis

Hypothalamic Causes

- Dysfunctional
  - Exercise
  - Nutrition-related
    - Eating disorders (anorexia nervosa, bulimia)
    - Weight loss, diet, malnutrition, malabsorption
  - Pseudocyesis
  - Stress
- Other disorders
  - Chronic debilitating disease
  - Infection
    - Encephalitis
    - Meningitis
    - Sarcoidosis
    - Syphilis
    - Tuberculosis
  - Isolated gonadotropin deficiency
    - Idiopathic hypogonadotropic hypogonadism
    - Kallmann syndrome
  - Tumors
    - Craniopharyngioma
    - Endodermal sinus tumor
    - Germinoma
    - Hamartoma

- Langerhans cell histiocytosis
- Metastatic carcinoma
- Teratoma

Pituitary Causes

- Autoimmune disease
- Galactosemia
- Tumors
- Prolactinoma
- Other hormone-secreting pituitary tumor (e.g., adrenocorticotropic hormone, growth hormone)

Primary Hypogonadism

- Enzymatic deficiency
  - 17α-hydroxylase deficiency
  - 17,20-lyase deficiency
  - Aromatase deficiency
- Gonadal agenesis
- Gonadal dysgenesis
  - Abnormal karyotype
    - Mosaicism
    - Turner syndrome 45,X
  - Normal karyotype
    - 46,XX
    - 46,XY (Swyer syndrome)
- Premature ovarian failure
  - Idiopathic
  - Injury
    - Chemotherapy
    - Mumps oophoritis
    - Radiation
  - Resistant ovary
    - Idiopathic

Other Endocrine Gland Disorders

- Adrenal disease
  - Adult-onset adrenal hyperplasia
  - Cushing syndrome
- Gonadotropin mutations (FSH)
- Inflammatory/infiltrative
  - Hemochromatosis
  - Lymphocytic hypophysitis
  - Sarcoidosis

- Necrosis
  - Panhypopituitarism
  - Sheehan syndrome
- Ovarian tumors
  - Brenner tumors
  - Cystic teratomas
  - Granulosa-theca cell tumors
  - Krukenberg tumors
  - Metastatic carcinoma
  - Mucinous/serous cystadenomas
  - Nonfunctional tumors (craniopharyngioma)
- Space-occupying lesions
  - Arterial aneurysm
  - Empty sella
- Thyroid disease
  - Hyperthyroidism
  - Hypothyroidism

Multifactorial Causes

- PCOS

Key Historical Features

✓ Menarche and menstrual history
✓ Sexual history
✓ Diet history
✓ Exercise patterns
✓ Changes in weight
✓ Galactorrhea
✓ Symptoms of hyperthyroidism or hypothyroidism
✓ Acne or hirsutism
✓ Headache or visual disturbances
✓ Anosmia or galactorrhea
✓ Cyclic abdominal pain
✓ Breast changes
✓ Easy bruising
✓ Medical history, including chronic illness or history of chemotherapy or radiation
✓ Surgical history
✓ Medications
✓ Supplement use
✓ Family history, especially of infertility, genetic defects, and menstrual disorders

Key Physical Findings

✓ Vital signs
✓ Height and weight compared against normative data
✓ Body mass index
✓ Evaluation of breast development
✓ Tanner staging to assess pubertal development
✓ Signs of an eating disorder (e.g., parotid gland enlargement, Russell sign, or dental erosions)
✓ Thyroid examination
✓ Abdominal examination for masses
✓ Pelvic examination for imperforate hymen, transverse vaginal septum, clitoral hypertrophy, or undescended testes
✓ Rectal examination for skin tags, fissures, or occult blood that may indicate inflammatory bowel disease
✓ Skin examination for acne or hirsutism
✓ Evaluation for striae, buffalo hump, central obesity, or proximal muscle weakness, suggesting Cushing syndrome
✓ Dysmorphic features (e.g., webbed neck or low hairline), suggesting Turner syndrome

Suggested Work-Up of Primary Amenorrhea

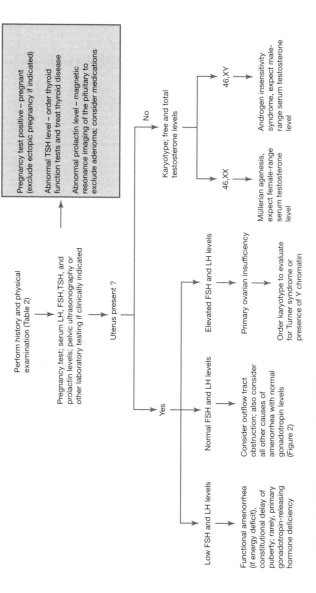

Perform history and physical examination (Table 2)

↓

Pregnancy test; serum LH, FSH, TSH, and prolactin levels; pelvic ultrasonography or other laboratory testing if clinically indicated

↓

Uterus present ?

Pregnancy test positive – pregnant (exclude ectopic pregnancy if indicated)

Abnormal TSH level – order thyroid function tests and treat thyroid disease

Abnormal prolactin level – magnetic resonance imaging of the pituitary to exclude adenoma; consider medications

Yes

Low FSH and LH levels → Functional amenorrhea (if energy deficit), constitutional delay of puberty; rarely, primary gonadotropin-releasing hormone deficiency

Normal FSH and LH levels → Consider outflow tract obstruction; also consider all other causes of amenorrhea with normal gonadotropin levels (Figure 2)

Elevated FSH and LH levels → Primary ovarian insufficiency → Order karyotype to evaluate for Turner syndrome or presence of Y chromatin

No

Karyotype; free and total testosterone levels

46,XX → Müllerian agenesis, expect female-range serum testosterone level

46,XY → Androgen insensitivity syndrome, expect male-range serum testosterone level

Figure 3-1. Diagnosis of Primary Amenorrhea. *FSH,* Follicle-stimulating hormone; *LH,* luteinizing hormone; *TSH,* thyroid-stimulating hormone. From Klein DA, Poth MA. Amenorrhea: an approach to diagnosis and management. *American Family Physician* 2013;87:781–788.

Suggested Work-Up of Secondary Amenorrhea

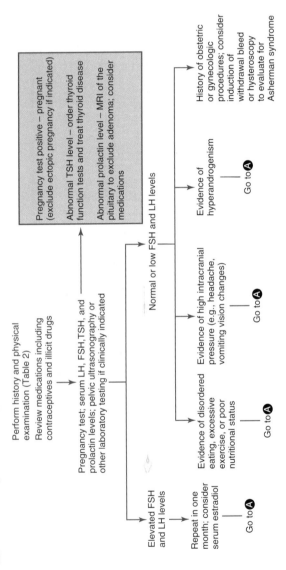

Perform history and physical examination (Table 2)

Review medications including contraceptives and illicit drugs

Pregnancy test; serum LH, FSH, TSH, and prolactin levels; pelvic ultrasonography or other laboratory testing if clinically indicated

Pregnancy test positive – pregnant (exclude ectopic pregnancy if indicated)

Abnormal TSH level – order thyroid function tests and treat thyroid disease

Abnormal prolactin level – MRI of the pituitary to exclude adenoma; consider medications

Elevated FSH and LH levels

Repeat in one month; consider serum estradiol

Go to Ⓐ

Normal or low FSH and LH levels

Evidence of disordered eating, excessive exercise, or poor nutritional status

Go to Ⓐ

Evidence of high intracranial pressure (e.g., headache, vomiting vision changes)

Go to Ⓐ

Evidence of hyperandrogenism

Go to Ⓐ

History of obstetric or gynecologic procedures; consider induction of withdrawal bleed or hysteroscopy to evaluate for Asherman syndrome

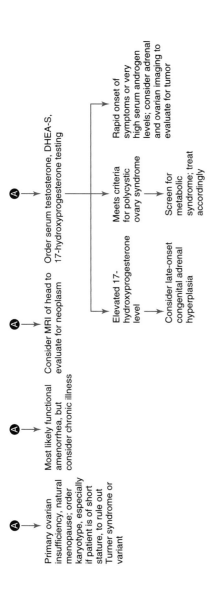

Figure 3-2. Diagnosis of Secondary Amenorrhea. *DHEA-S,* Dehydroepiandrosterone sulfate; *FSH,* follicle-stimulating hormone; *LH,* luteinizing hormone; *MRI,* magnetic resonance imaging; *TSH,* thyroid-stimulating hormone. From Klein DA, Poth MA. Amenorrhea: an approach to diagnosis and management. *American Family Physician* 2013;87:781–788.

The following text appears within the figure:

A → Primary ovarian insufficiency, natural menopause; order karyotype, especially if patient is of short stature, to rule out Turner syndrome or variant

A → Most likely functional amenorrhea, but consider chronic illness

A → Consider MRI of head to evaluate for neoplasm

A → Order serum testosterone, DHEA-S, 17-hydroxyprogesterone testing

Elevated 17-hydroxyprogesterone level → Consider late-onset congenital adrenal hyperplasia

Meets criteria for polycystic ovary syndrome → Screen for metabolic syndrome; treat accordingly

Rapid onset of symptoms or very high serum androgen levels; consider adrenal and ovarian imaging to evaluate for tumor

Further Reading

Adams-Hillard PJ, Deitch HR. Menstrual disorders in the college age female. *Pediatr Clin North Am.* 2005;52:179–197.

Kazis K, Iglesias E. The female athlete triad. *Adolesc Med.* 2003;14:87–95.

Klein DA, Poth MA. Amenorrhea: an approach to diagnosis and management. *Am Fam Physician.* 2013;87:781–788.

Master-Hunter T, Heiman DL. Amenorrhea: evaluation and treatment. *Am Fam Physician.* 2006;73:1374–1382.

Pickett CA. Diagnosis and management of pituitary tumors: recent advances. *Prim Care.* 2003;30:765–789.

Pletcher JR, Slap GB. Menstrual disorders: amenorrhea. *Pediatr Clin North Am.* 1999;46:505–518.

Practice Committee of the American Society for Reproductive Medicine. Current evaluation of amenorrhea. *Fertil Steril.* 2008;90(5 suppl):S219–S225.

Speroff L, Fritz MA. Amenorrhea. In: *Clinical Gynecologic Endocrinology and Infertility.* 7th ed. Philadelphia: Lippincott Williams & Wilkins; 2005:401–464.

General Discussion

Anemia is defined as a decrease in hemoglobin or hematocrit level from an individual's baseline value. In general, normal hemoglobin levels are 1 to 2 g/dL lower in women and African American men than in white men.

The initial laboratory evaluation of anemia should include a complete blood count, red blood cell indexes, a reticulocyte count, and peripheral blood smear. The mean corpuscular volume (MCV) is used first to classify the anemic process as microcytic, normocytic, or macrocytic.

Microcytic Anemia

The evaluation of microcytic anemia begins by ruling out iron deficiency anemia. The definitive test for iron deficiency anemia is the serum ferritin, because a low serum ferritin level is diagnostic of an iron-depleted state. Other iron studies such as serum iron, total iron-binding capacity, and transferring saturation do not accurately distinguish iron deficiency anemia from the anemia of chronic disease. In equivocal cases, a finite treatment trial with iron supplementation may help distinguish the two.

Other clues may help diagnose iron deficiency anemia. Microcytic anemia associated with increased red blood cell distribution width favors a diagnosis of iron deficiency anemia over anemia of chronic disease. The peripheral blood smear in iron deficiency anemia usually shows anisocytosis and poikilocytosis. Iron deficiency anemia may be associated with reactive thrombocytosis. In contrast, microcytic anemia associated with an increased red blood cell count is characteristic of the thalassemia trait. Polychromasia, basophilic stippling, and target cells are absent in iron deficiency anemia, but these are characteristic features of the peripheral blood smear in thalassemia.

If the serum ferritin level is normal, the physician should determine if microcytic anemia is preexisting or new. If microcytosis is preexisting, a diagnosis of thalassemia should be considered. If microcytosis is new, the differential diagnosis includes anemia of chronic disease and hereditary or acquired sideroblastic anemia. Anemia of chronic disease is usually normocytic but may be microcytic in some systemic diseases, such as temporal arteritis, rheumatoid arthritis, polymyalgia rheumatica, diabetes mellitus, connective tissue disease, chronic infection, Hodgkin lymphoma, and renal cell carcinoma. The diagnosis is made on clinical grounds, and microcytic anemia is often accompanied by systemic signs and symptoms.

Normocytic Anemia

The evaluation of normocytic anemia begins by identifying treatable causes, such as nutritional anemias, anemia of renal insufficiency, bleeding, and hemolytic anemia. The initial investigation should include a fecal occult blood test and determination of serum ferritin, serum vitamin B_{12}, serum folate levels, and serum creatinine. The diagnosis of renal insufficiency anemia may be made on the basis of an elevated serum creatinine. Mild to moderate anemia may be seen when the serum creatinine level is 1.5 to 3 mg/dL, whereas more severe anemia is found with more advanced renal disease. Renal insufficiency anemia is associated with an unremarkable peripheral blood smear.

If hemolysis is suspected, this diagnosis may be supported by a low haptoglobin level and increased lactate dehydrogenase, indirect bilirubin, and reticulocyte count. These tests are nonspecific and do not distinguish among the various causes of hemolytic anemia. The peripheral blood smear guides the evaluation of suspected hemolytic anemia and is outlined in further detail in the following.

If normocytic anemia is not linked to bleeding, nutrition, renal insufficiency, or hemolysis, the differential diagnosis includes a primary bone marrow disorder or normocytic anemia of chronic disease. The patients' history and peripheral blood smear may help to differentiate these two diagnoses, and hematology consultation should be considered. Other possible causes of normocytic anemia are alcohol abuse, drug effects, radiation therapy, chemical exposure, and recent trauma or surgery.

Macrocytic Anemia

The evaluation of macrocytic anemia begins by excluding alcohol or drug use associated with macrocytosis. Drugs associated with macrocytosis include hydroxyurea, methotrexate, trimethoprim, zidovudine, and 5-fluorouracil.

Vitamin B_{12} and folate deficiencies must be ruled out. In vitamin B_{12} deficiency, the serum vitamin B_{12} levels are usually low but may be falsely low in elderly patients, in patients with low white blood cell counts, and in pregnant patients. The serum methylmalonic acid (MMA) level is a more sensitive and highly specific test. (The MMA level is increased in vitamin B_{12} deficiency.) A normal level makes the diagnosis of vitamin B_{12} deficiency very unlikely. In folate deficiency, serum folate levels are usually low but may be affected by recent dietary changes. The serum homocysteine level is increased during folate deficiency and may be used instead to evaluate for folate deficiency.

If vitamin B_{12} deficiency is confirmed, intrinsic factor antibodies should be ordered. If they are present, a working diagnosis of pernicious anemia is made. If intrinsic factor antibodies are not present, the Schilling test can help differentiate pernicious anemia from primary intestinal malabsorptive disorders (although this test is now infrequently performed; proceeding to vitamin B_{12} replacement is often preferred).

If vitamin deficiency, alcohol abuse, or drug exposure cannot be implicated as the cause of macrocytic anemia, the process should be classified into mild (MCV 100–100 fL) or marked (MCV >110 fL) macrocytosis. Marked macrocytosis that is not due to nutritional deficiency, alcohol, or drug exposure is usually associated with primary bone marrow disease, such as myelodysplastic syndrome, aplastic anemia, or pure red cell aplasia. A bone marrow biopsy should be considered if the hematologic diagnosis affects management decisions. For mild macrocytosis, the peripheral blood smear should be examined for evidence of an association with diseases such as liver disease or hypothyroidism. Bone marrow biopsy may be necessary to clarify the diagnosis.

Causes of Anemia

Microcytic Anemia

- Anemia of chronic disease
- Iron deficiency anemia
- Sideroblastic anemia
- Thalassemia

Normocytic Anemia

- Acute blood loss
- Anemia of chronic disease
- Autoimmune hemolytic anemias (warm-reactive anemias, cold-reactive anemias, drug-induced anemias)
- Chronic renal failure
- Endocrine deficiency states (hypothyroidism, adrenal insufficiency, pituitary deficiency, hypogonadism)
- Glucose-6-phosphate dehydrogenase deficiency
- Hemoglobinopathies (sickle cell disease and sickle hemoglobin C disease)
- Hereditary elliptocytosis
- Hereditary spherocytocis
- Hypersplenism
- Hyperthyroidism
- Liver disease
- Macrovascular disorders
- Marrow hypoplasia or aplasia
- Microangiopathic disorders (disseminated intravascular coagulopathy, hemolytic-uremic syndrome, thrombotic thrombocytopenic purpura)
- Myelopathies
- Myeloproliferative diseases
- Over-hydration
- Paroxysmal nocturnal hemoglobinuria
- Pregnancy
- Pure red blood cell aplasia
- Pyruvate kinase deficiency
- Sideroblastic anemias

Macrocytic Anemia

- Alcohol abuse
- Aplastic anemia
- Clonal hematologic disorder
- Drug-induced
- Hemolytic anemia
- Large granular lymphocyte disorder
- Liver disease
- Myelodysplastic syndrome
- Nutritional
- Spurious

Key Historical Features

✓ Fever
✓ Fatigue
✓ Weakness
✓ Dyspnea
✓ Dizziness
✓ Apathy
✓ Cognitive impairment
✓ Worsening congestive heart failure
✓ Pruritis
✓ Dark urine
✓ Hematuria
✓ Back pain
✓ Recent blood loss
✓ History of anemia
✓ Medical history
✓ Surgical history
✓ Family history
✓ Medications and supplement use
✓ Illicit drug use

Key Physical Findings

✓ Vital signs
✓ Evidence of conjunctival pallor
✓ Skin examination for jaundice or pallor
✓ Cardiac examination for tachycardia or flow murmur
✓ Lymphadenopathy
✓ Abdominal examination for hepatosplenomegaly
✓ Extremity examination for leg ulcers

Initial Evaluation of Anemia

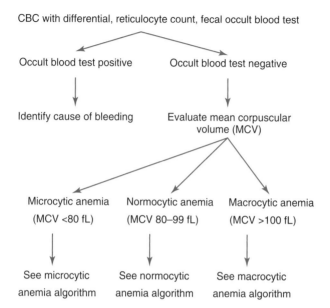

Figure 4-1. Initial evaluation of anemia. *CBC*, Complete blood count.

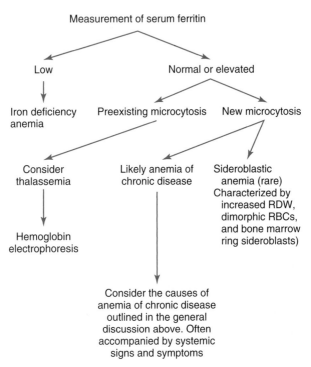

Figure 4-2. Evaluation of microcytic anemia. *RBC*, Red blood cells; *RDW*, red blood cell distribution width.

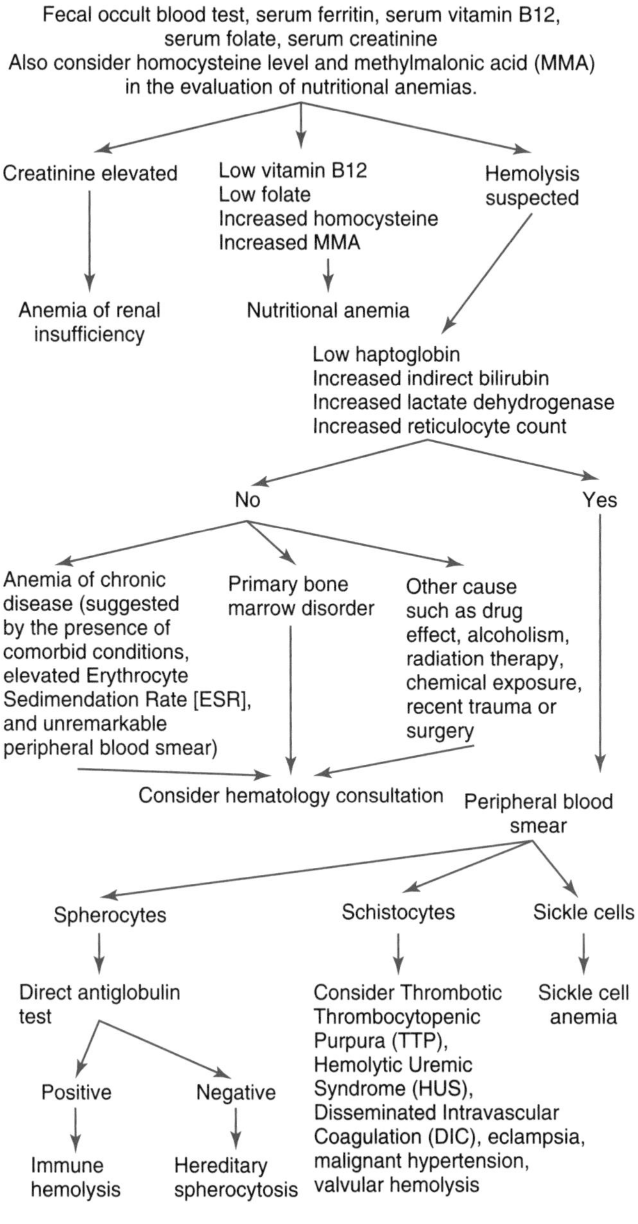

Figure 4-3. Evaluation of normocytic anemia.

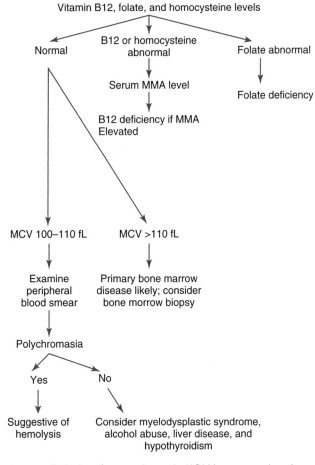

Figure 4-4. Evaluation of macrocytic anemia. *MCV,* Mean corpuscular volume; *MMA,* methylmalonic acid.

Further Reading

Abramson SD, Abramson N. "Common" uncommon anemias *Am Fam Physician*.
    1999;59:851–858.

Brill JR, Baumgardner DJ. Normocytic anemia. *Am Fam Physician*. 2000;62:2255–2263.

Dhaliwal G, Cornett PA, Tierney Jr LM. Hemolytic anemia. *Am Fam Physician*.
    2004;69:2599–2606.

Smith DL. Anemia in the elderly. *Am Fam Physician*. 2000;62:1565–1572.

Tefferi A. Anemia in adults: a contemporary approach to diagnosis. *Mayo Clin Proc*.
    2003;78:1274–1280.

Tefferi A, Hanson CA, Inwards DJ. How to interpret and pursue an abnormal complete blood
    cell count in adults. *Mayo Clin Proc*. 2005;80:923–936.

General Discussion

Several different terms are often used to describe joint disorders that result in joint pain. *Arthralgia* means joint pain. *Arthritis* implies the presence of an inflammatory component to the disorder. *Arthropathy* is a general term meaning joint disease, but it usually means that there is some degree of cartilage damage. Rheumatologic disease (e.g., rheumatoid arthritis, ankylosing spondylitis, psoriatic arthritis), infection, and crystal deposition are examples of conditions that produce an inflammatory response and a resultant loss of cartilage. Osteoarthritis, or degenerative joint disease, occurs primarily as a result of cartilage breakdown, but it often has a component of secondary inflammation. This chapter focuses on arthritis; however, some of the medications and conditions listed in the following may cause arthralgia without an inflammatory process.

Before attributing a patient's pain to arthritis, the physician must consider other potential causes of pain. These potential diagnoses include intra-articular processes that are distinct from arthritis (impingement, neoplasm) and periarticular sources of pain (bursitis, tendonitis). Patients may also have referred pain from an adjacent site or a distant site, which occurs with radiculopathy and spinal stenosis.

The 2010 American College of Rheumatology and European League Against Rheumatism classification criteria for rheumatoid arthritis provides a tool to diagnose rheumatoid arthritis earlier and distinguish it from other types of inflammatory synovitis. The 2010 criteria (Table 5-1) differ from the 1987 criteria because the new criteria no longer include the presence of rheumatoid nodules or radiographic erosive changes, which are less likely in early rheumatoid arthritis. Symmetric arthritis is also not included in the 2010 criteria.

Criteria	Score

Target population (who should be tested?): patients who:
   1) have at least one joint with definite clinical synovitis (swelling)*
   2) with the synovitis not better explained by another disease†	

Classification criteria for RA (score-based algorithm: add score of categories A through D; a score of ≥6 of 10 is needed for classification of a patient as having definite RA)‡	

A. Joint involvement§
   One large joint‖
   Two to 10 large joints
   One to three small joints (with or without involvement of large joints)¶
   Four to 10 small joints (with or without involvement of large joints)
   >10 joints (at least one small joint)#
	0
	 1
	 2
	 3
	 5

B. Serology (at least one test result is needed for classification)**
   Negative RF and negative ACPA
   Low-positive RF or low-positive ACPA
   High-positive RF or high-positive ACPA
	0
	 2
	 3

Table 5-1. The 2010 American College of Rheumatology/European League Against Rheumatism Classification Criteria for Rheumatoid Arthritis—cont'd

Criteria	Score
C. Acute phase reactants (at least one test result is needed for classification)[††] ,	
Normal CRP and normal ESR	0
Abnormal CRP or normal ESR	1
D. Duration of symptoms[‡‡]	
<6 wks	0
≥6 wks	1

ACPA, Anticitrullinated protein antibody; *CRP*, C-reactive protein; *ESR*, erythrocyte sedimentation rate; *RA*, rheumatoid arthritis.

[*]The criteria are aimed at classification of newly presenting patients. In addition, patients with erosive disease typical of RA with a history compatible with previous fulfillment of the 2010 criteria should be classified as having RA. Patients with chronic disease, including those whose disease is inactive (with or without treatment), who, based on retrospectively available data, have previously fulfilled the 2010 criteria should be classified as having RA.

[†]Differential diagnoses differ in patients with different presentations, but may include conditions such as systemic lupus erythematosus, psoriatic arthritis, and gout. If it is unclear about the relevant differential diagnoses to consider, an expert rheumatologist should be consulted.

[‡]Although patients with a score of less than 6 of 10 are not classifiable as having RA, their status can be reassessed, and the criteria might be fulfilled cumulatively over time.

[§]Joint involvement refers to any swollen or tender joint on examination, which may be confirmed by imaging evidence of synovitis. Distal interphalangeal joints, first carpometacarpal joints, and first metatarsophalangeal joints are excluded from assessment. Categories of joint distribution are classified according to the location and number of involved joints, with placement into the highest category possible based on the pattern of joint involvement.

[‖]"Large joints" refers to shoulders, elbows, hips, knees, and ankles.

[¶]"Small joints" refers to the metacarpophalangeal joints, proximal interphalangeal joints, second to fifth metatarsophalangeal joints, thumb interphalangeal joints, and wrists.

[#]In this category, at least one of the involved joints must be a small joint; the other joints can include any combination of large and additional small joints, as well as other joints not specifically listed elsewhere (e.g., temporomandibular, acromioclavicular, sternoclavicular).

[**]Negative refers to international unit values that are less than or equal to the upper limit of normal for the laboratory and assay; low positive refers to international unit values that are higher than the upper limit of normal but three or less times the upper limit of normal for the laboratory and assay; high positive refers to international unit values that are more than three times the upper limit of normal for the laboratory and assay. When rheumatoid factor information is only available as positive or negative, a positive result should be scored as low positive for the rheumatoid factor.

[††]Normal and/or abnormal is determined by local laboratory standards.

[‡‡]Duration of symptoms refers to patient self-report of the duration of signs or symptoms of synovitis (e.g., pain, swelling, tenderness) of joints that are clinically involved at the time of assessment, regardless of treatment status.

Adapted with permission from Aletaha D, Neogi T, Silman AJ, et al. 2010 rheumatoid arthritis classification criteria: an American College of Rheumatology/European League Against Rheumatism collaborative initiative. Ann Rheum Dis 2010;69:1583 [published correction appears in Ann Rheum Dis. 2010;69:1892].

Table 5-1. The 2010 American College of Rheumatology/European League Against Rheumatism Classification Criteria for Rheumatoid Arthritis

Medications Associated with Arthritis/Arthralgia

Acyclovir
Adalimumab
Amiodarone
Amphotericin
Atorvastatin
Beta-blockers
Bacillus Calmette-Guerin (BCG)
Carbamazepine
Chlorpromazine
Cyclosporine
Diuretics
Erythropoetin
Estrogens
Etanercept
Ethambutol
Fibrates
Fluoride
Granulocyte colony-stimulating factor
Gold salts
Griseofulvin
Hydralazine
Infliximab
Interferons
Interleukin-2 and interleukin-6
Isoniazid
Letrozole
Levodopa
Lithium
Methimazole
Methyldopa
Minocycline
Nicardipine
Nicotinic acid
Para-aminosalicylic acid
Penicillin
Penicillamine
Phenytoin
Procainamide
Propylthiouracil
Pyrazinamide
Quinidine
Quinolones
Raloxifene
Reserpine

Simvastatin
Steroids (systemic)
Sulfasalazine
Tacrolimus
Tamoxifen
Terbinafine
Tetracycline
Ticlopidine
Vitamin A excess

Causes of Arthritis

Ankylosing spondylitis
Degenerative joint disease (osteoarthritis)
Giant cell arteritis
Gout
Hemochromatosis
Hemophilia
Infection
- Atypical mycobacteria
- Bacterial (*Staphylococcus aureus, Streptococcus, Salmonella, Neisseria gonorrhoeae, Haemophilus influenzae, Escherichia coli, Pseudomonas*)
- Fungi (*Coccidioides immitis, Histoplasma capsulatum, Blastomyces dermatitidis*)
- Gonorrhea
- HIV arthritis
- Lyme disease
- Tuberculosis
- Viral (HIV, hepatitis B, hepatitis C, parvovirus B19, rubella, coxackieviruses, alphaviruses, Human T-Lymphocytic Virus [HTLV]-1)

Immune reconstitution syndrome following highly active antiretroviral therapy
Infectious endocarditis
Inflammatory bowel disease
Medications
Polymyalgia rheumatica
Pseudogout (calcium pyrophosphate dehydrate crystal deposition disease)
Psoriatic arthritis
Reactive arthritis (immunologic reaction to a previous infection)
Referred pain or pain from intra-articular disease other than arthritis
- Bursitis
- Impingement syndromes
- Neoplasm
- Spinal stenosis
- Radiculopathy
- Tendinitis

Rheumatoid arthritis
Scleroderma
Seronegative spondyloarthropathies
Sickle cell anemia
Still disease
Systemic lupus erythematosus
Trauma
Whipple disease

Key Historical Features

✓ Distribution/location of pain
✓ Quantification of pain
✓ Description of pain
✓ Radiation
✓ Duration and timing of symptoms
✓ Swelling
✓ Morning stiffness
✓ Degree of functional impairment
✓ Pain that wakes the patient
✓ Effect of treatment modalities
✓ Mechanical symptoms, such as catching, locking, or joint instability
✓ Systemic symptoms, such as fever, weight loss, night sweats, or fatigue
✓ Medical history, especially previous trauma to the affected joint
✓ Surgical history, especially surgery on the affected joint
✓ Medications
✓ Family history of arthritis or rheumatologic disease
✓ Social history, including smoking, alcohol use, illicit drug use
✓ Occupational history, especially jobs associated with repetitive trauma
✓ Review of systems for constitutional symptoms, urethritis, conjunctivitis, or skin lesions

Key Physical Findings

✓ Inspection
  • Posture
  • Body habitus
  • Use of mobility aids
  • Gait
  • Leg length discrepancy
  • Scars from previous trauma or surgery
  • Swelling
  • Erythema
  • Muscle atrophy
  • Deformity of shape or alignment
  • Skin lesions

✓ Palpation
  • Warmth
  • Effusion
  • Tenderness to palpation over individual structures
✓ Range of motion
  • Active and passive range of motion testing
  • Presence of crepitus
✓ Muscle testing
✓ Ligament testing for laxity and joint instability

Suggested Work-Up

Radiographs of the affected joint	For most patients presenting with chronic, progressive joint pain, recent joint trauma, history of childhood joint problems, or night pain. Suggested radiographic views are outlined in the following.
Anticitrullinated protein antibody, rheumatoid factor (RF), antinuclear antibodies (ANA), C-reactive protein, erythrocyte sedimentation rate (ESR), complete blood count (CBC), renal function, and hepatic function	Screening for any patient in whom rheumatoid and seronegative arthropathies are in the differential diagnosis.
Serum uric acid level	For any patient with an inflammatory arthropathy in the absence of infection to evaluate for gouty arthritis
CBC and ESR	If septic arthritis is in the differential diagnosis
Joint aspiration and synovial fluid analysis	For any patient with suspected infection or suspected crystal-induced arthritis (see Chapter 70, "Synovial Fluid Analysis")

Additional Work-Up

Bone scan	If plain radiographs show a lesion suggestive of metastatic tumor, a total bone scan of the body can evaluate for metastatic tumor, except for multiple myeloma.

Magnetic resonance imaging of the affected area, serum protein electrophoresis, and urine protein electrophoresis	If multiple myeloma is suspected
CBC, ESR, uric acid, rheumatoid factor, urethral swab for chlamydia, stool culture, synovial fluid gram stain, culture, and crystal analysis	If reactive arthritis is suspected

Suggested Radiographic Views

Anterior hip (groin)	Anteroposterior (AP) pelvis Lateral view of affected hip
Posterior hip/buttock	AP pelvis (sacroiliac joints) AP/lateral lumbar spine
Knee	Standing AP both knees Lateral of affected knee Merchant view
Ankle	AP, lateral, and mortise views
Foot	Standing AP, lateral, and oblique views
Low back	AP/lateral lumbar spine Obliques (facet joints) Fergusson view (L5–S1 upshot)
Neck	AP/lateral C-spine Obliques (foraminal stenosis) Flexion/extension in rheumatoids
Shoulder	True AP of scapula Axillary lateral
Systemic arthritis	Views of primarily affected joints AP/lateral of hands and wrists

Further Reading

Aletaha D, Neogi T, Silman AJ, et al. 2010 rheumatoid arthritis classification criteria: an American College of Rheumatology/European League Against Rheumatism collaborative initiative. *Ann Rheum Dis.* 2010;69:1583 [published correction appears in Ann Rheum Dis. 2010;69:1892].

Calabrese LH, Naides SJ. Viral arthritis. *Infect Dis Clin North Am.* 2005;19:963–980.

Dearborn JT, Jergesen HE. The evaluation and initial management of arthritis. *Prim Care Clin Office Pract.* 1996;23:215–240.

Harrington L, Schneider JI. Atraumatic joint and limb pain in the elderly. *Emerg Med Clin North Am.* 2006;24:389–412.

Petersel DL, Sigal LH. Reactive arthritis. *Infect Dis Clin North Am.* 2005;19:863–883.

Quiceno GA, Cush JJ. Iatrogenic rheumatic syndromes in the elderly. *Clin Geriatr Med.* 2005;21:577–588.

Raj JM, Sudhakar S, Sems K, Carlson RW. Arthritis in the intensive care unit. *Crit Care Clin.* 2002;18:767–780.

Wasserman AM. Diagnosis and management of rheumatoid arthritis. *Am Fam Physician.* 2011;84:1245–1252.

6 ASCITES

General Discussion

In the United States, approximately 85% of ascites is caused by cirrhosis, whereas nonhepatic causes account for the remaining 15%. The main factor contributing to the development of ascites in patients with cirrhosis is portal hypertension, which results from increased intrahepatic resistance to blood flow and is compounded by splanchnic vasodilatation.

Paracentesis should be performed on all patients with new-onset clinically apparent ascites. The goals of the diagnostic assessment of a patient with ascites are to establish the presence of ascites, determine its severity, determine its cause, and to detect for the presence of complications of ascites. Complications include spontaneous bacterial peritonitis and renal failure.

The incidence of ascitic fluid infection (spontaneous bacterial peritonitis [SBP]) is 10% to 27% at the time of hospital admission. Patients with ascitic fluid infection may present with subtle symptoms, and early detection of infection with treatment at an early stage reduces morbidity and mortality. Diagnostic paracentesis should be repeated if a patient with ascites develops fever, abdominal pain, hypotension, abdominal tenderness, renal failure, encephalopathy, peripheral leukocytosis, or acidosis.

The serum ascites albumin gradient (SAAG) is useful in determining the cause of ascites and guiding management. Calculation of SAAG is performed by measuring same-day albumin concentrations of serum and ascitic fluid and then subtracting the ascitic fluid albumin value from the serum albumin value. When the SAAG is ≥ 1.1 g/dL, the patient has portal hypertension as the cause of ascites. The differential diagnosis includes cirrhosis, alcoholic hepatitis, hepatocellular carcinoma, massive liver metastases, fulminant hepatic failure, cardiac ascites, myxedema, Budd-Chiari syndrome, portal vein thrombosis, veno-occlusive disease of the liver, acute fatty liver of pregnancy, and mixed ascites.

When the SAAG is less than 1.1 g/dL, portal hypertension is not the cause of ascites. The differential diagnosis includes peritoneal carcinomatosis, tuberculous peritonitis, *Chlamydia* peritonitis, pancreatic ascites, biliary ascites, peritonitis from connective tissue disease (e.g., lupus), bowel infarction, bowel perforation, and postoperative lymphatic leakage. Peritoneal carcinomatosis is the most common cause of ascites in patients with a low SAAG.

Ascitic fluid polymorphonuclear (PMN) leukocyte count is a more reliable indicator for infection than the ascitic fluid white blood cell count. In calculating the PMN count, one PMN is subtracted from the absolute ascitic fluid PMN count for every 250 red blood cells. A corrected ascetic fluid PMN count greater than 250 cells/mm^3 should be treated as an ascitic fluid infection (SBP) until proven otherwise.

Causes of Ascites

Acute fatty liver of pregnancy
AIDS
Biliary tree leakage
Bowel infarction
Chemical burn to the peritoneum, causing biliary or pancreatic ascites
Chlamydia peritonitis (Fitz-Hugh-Curtis syndrome)
Cirrhosis
Coccidiomycosis
Congestive heart failure
Constrictive pericarditis
Endometriosis
Eosinophilic gastroenteritis
Familial Mediterranean fever
Glove starch (talc) peritonitis
Hepatic vein thrombosis (Budd-Chiari syndrome)
Hepatocellular cancer
Hereditary angioedema
Histoplasmosis
Intrahepatic portal hypertension
Lymphoma
Meig syndrome
Mesenteric lymphatic leakage
Mesothelioma
Metastatic cancer
Mixed ascites from two causes of fluid retention
Myxedema
Nephrogenic ascites in patients receiving hemodialysis
Nephrotic syndrome
Ovarian cancer
Ovarian hyperstimulation syndrome
Pancreatic duct or pseudocyst leakage
Peritoneal carcinomatosis
Pneumatosis cystoides intestinalis
Portal vein thrombosis
Systemic lupus erythematosus
Thoracic duct obstruction
Tuberculosis
Vasculitis
Vitamin A toxicity
Whipple disease

Key Historical Features

✓ Presence of fever
✓ Presence of abdominal pain
✓ Medical history, especially metabolic syndrome or autoimmune disease
✓ Surgical history
✓ Medications
✓ Family history of liver disease
✓ Risk factors for liver disease
   • Blood transfusions
   • Sexual practices
   • Alcohol use
   • Drug use
   • Tattoos
   • Accupuncture
   • Body piercings
✓ Country of origin
✓ Tuberculosis exposures
✓ Review of systems with focus on potential for congestive heart failure or cancer

Key Physical Findings

✓ Vital signs
✓ Cardiac examination for signs suggestive of right heart failure, such as abnormal jugular venous distention and systolic pulsation of the jugular veins or liver; examination for signs of constrictive pericarditis, such as pulsus paradoxus or Kussmaul sign
✓ Abdominal examination for shifting dullness to percussion, tympany, a fluid wave, hepatomegaly, or splenomegaly
✓ Back examination for venous distention
✓ Extremity examination for edema
✓ Evidence of chronic liver disease, such as vascular spiders, splenomegaly, or distended abdominal collateral veins
✓ Evidence of malignancy, such as an umbilical nodule or enlarged left supraclavicular lymph node

Suggested Work-Up

Serum albumin	Used to calculate the SAAG
Ascitic fluid albumin level	Used to calculate the SAAG
Ascitic fluid cell count	PMN count is usually more than 70% of the ascitic fluid white blood count (WBC) count in the setting of spontaneous bacterial peritonitis.

	Elevated WBC with lymphocytic predominance suggests tuberculous peritonitis or peritoneal carcinomatosis.
Ascitic fluid total protein and albumin levels	High ascitic fluid total protein level may suggest peritoneal carcinomatosis, tuberculous peritonitis, cardiac ascites, Budd-Chiari syndrome, myxedema, lymphatic rupture, intestinal perforation, biliary ascites, or pancreatic ascites
Ascitic fluid Gram stain and culture (aerobic and anaerobic)	To evaluate for infection
Serum and ascitic fluid glucose	Used to evaluate for infection. Ascitic fluid glucose is lower than serum levels in the presence of infection.
Serum and ascitic fluid lactic acid dehydrogenase (LDH)	Used to evaluate for infection. LDH levels may rise above that in the serum during infection.
Ascitic fluid amylase	Amylase level in uncomplicated ascites is approximately 44% that in serum but rises significantly with pancreatitis and gut perforation.
Serum bilirubin, albumin, aspartate aminotransferase, alanine aminotransferase, alkaline phosphatase, international normalized ratio	To assess for the presence of liver disease
Serum creatinine	To establish a baseline and determine if renal insufficiency is present

Additional Work-Up

Ascitic fluid triglycerides	Should be obtained if the ascitic fluid is opalescent or milky, because chylous ascitic fluid has a triglyceride level of at least 200 mg/dL. Chylous ascites is caused by lymphatic rupture, usually due to cirrhosis or lymphoma.

Ascitic fluid bilirubin	Should be tested if the ascitic fluid is dark brown. An ascitic fluid bilirubin level >6 mg/dL and greater than the serum level suggests biliary or upper gut perforation.
Ascitic fluid cytology	If malignancy is a potential diagnosis. However, positive cytologic results are expected only in peritoneal carcinomatosis. Hepatocellular carcinoma, liver metastases, and lymphoma usually do not produce positive cytology results unless there are metastases to the peritoneum.
Hepatitis B surface antigen and hepatitis C antibody	To determine the cause if liver disease is present
Peritoneal biopsy by laparoscopy (sent for acid-fast bacilli [AFB] stains and cultures)	If tuberculosis is suspected
Abdominal ultrasound, computed tomography, or magnetic resonance imaging plus serum-α fetoprotein	To screen for hepatocellular cancer, portal vein thrombosis, and hepatic vein thrombosis
Liver biopsy	If ascites and liver disease of unknown etiology are present

Further Reading

Cardenas A, Bataller R, Arroyo V. Mechanisms of ascites formation. *Clin Liver Dis.* 2000;4:447–465.

Hou W, Sanyal AJ. Ascites: diagnosis and management. *Med Clin N Am.* 2009;93:801–817.

Midha NK, Stratton CW. Laboratory tests in critical care. *Crit Care Clin.* 1998;14:15–34.

Reynolds TB. Ascites. *Clin Liver Dis.* 2000;4:151–168.

Yu AS, Hu KQ. Management of ascites. *Clin Liver Dis.* 2001;5:541–568.

General Discussion

Atrial fibrillation is the most common cardiac arrhythmia. The incidence of atrial fibrillation increases with age and approximately doubles with each decade of life. The incidence of atrial fibrillation is further affected by the presence of both chronic medical illnesses and acute precipitating factors, which are outlined in the following. Myocardial infarction can be complicated by atrial fibrillation. However, patients presenting with atrial fibrillation who do not have chest pain, anginal equivalent, or electrocardiographic changes suggestive of ischemia are unlikely to have silent heart disease. The general consensus is that these patients do not need to be worked up for ischemia. No apparent cause is identified in approximately 30% of patients with atrial fibrillation.

When atrial fibrillation is identified, the decision must be made whether the patient should be hospitalized. Indications for hospitalization include hemodynamic or cardiovascular instability, difficulty achieving rate control, or significant symptoms related to the arrhythmia. Hospitalization may also be indicated for patients who are candidates for early cardioversion.

Conditions Associated with Atrial Fibrillation

Cardiac disease
- Atrial amyloidosis
- Cardiac arrhythmias
- Cardiac tumor
- Cardiomyopathy
- Congenital heart disease
- Coronary artery disease
- Left ventricular hypertrophy and/or heart failure
- Myocardial infarction
- Myocarditis
- Pericarditis
- Rheumatic heart disease
- Valvular disease
- Wolff-Parkinson-White syndrome

Cerebrovascular accident

Diabetes mellitus

Exertion-induced

Hypertension

Increased sympathetic activity
- Anxiety
- Caffeine
- Drugs

- Hyperthyroidism
- Pheochromocytoma

Intoxicants
- Alcohol
- Amphetamines
- Carbon monoxide
- Cocaine
- Poison gas

Postoperative states
Pulmonary disease
- Chronic obstructive pulmonary disease
- Cor pulmonale
- Pneumonia
- Pulmonary embolism
- Pulmonary hypertension

Sleep apnea
Subarachnoid hemorrhage

Key Historical Features

✓ Precipitating factors for arrhythmia
✓ Symptoms associated with the arrhythmia
- Angina
- Change in exertional capacity
- Diaphoresis
- Dizziness
- Fatigue
- Palpitations
- Shortness of breath
- Syncope

✓ Medical history
✓ Surgical history, especially recent surgery
✓ Use of illicit substances

Key Physical Findings

✓ Vital signs for evidence of hemodynamic instability
✓ Cardiac examination
✓ Pulmonary examination
✓ Signs of atherosclerosis
- Arterial bruits
- Signs of heart failure
- Jugular venous distention

Suggested Work-Up

Electrocardiogram	To identify rhythm, signs of left ventricular hypertrophy, myocardial infarction, and preexcitation
Chest x-ray	To evaluate for pulmonary disease
Echocardiogram	To identify valvular heart disease, left ventricular hypertrophy, atrial size, left ventricular size and function, peak right ventricular pressure, and pericardial disease. May identify left atrial thrombus.
Thyroid-stimulating hormone	To evaluate for hyperthyroidism
Complete blood count	To evaluate for anemia or infection
Electrolytes	To evaluate for electrolyte abnormalities
Blood urea nitrogen and creatinine	To evaluate kidney function
Liver function tests	To evaluate liver function
Glucose	To evaluate for hyper- or hypoglycemia

Additional Work-Up

Troponin	If there is suspicion of myocardial ischemia
Exercise testing	To rule out coronary artery disease in patients suspected of having ischemia or who are at increased risk for coronary artery disease
Urinary metanephrines	If pheochromocytoma is suspected based on the history and physical examination

Further Reading

Gutierrez C, Blanchard DG. Atrial fibrillation: diagnosis and treatment. *Am Fam Physician.* 2011;83:61–68.

Jahangir A, et al. Atrial fibrillation. *Cardiac Arrhythmias; Mechanism, Diagnosis, and Management.* Philadelphia: Lippincott Williams & Wilkins; 2001:457–499.

Kannel WB, Abbott RD, Savage DD, et al. Epidemiological features of chronic atrial fibrillation; the Framingham Study. *N Engl J Med.* 1982;306:1018–1022.

Pelosi F, Morady F. Evaluation and management of atrial fibrillation. *Med Clin North Am.* 2001;85:225–244.

Podrid PJ. Atrial fibrillation in the elderly. *Cardiol Clin.* 1999;17:173–188.

Ziv O, Coudhary G. Atrial fibrillation. *Prim Care Clin Office Pract.* 2005;32:1083–1107.

8 BLEEDING AND BRUISING

General Discussion

Abnormal bleeding or bruising may cause significant anxiety for the patient and may be a sign of a serious inherited or acquired disorder. Numerous disorders can cause abnormal bleeding and bruising, including platelet function disorders, quantitative platelet disorders, factor deficiencies, and factor inhibitors. Diseases that affect connective tissue and the integrity of the blood vessel also may lead to bruising and bleeding.

A history of bleeding following dental extraction, minor surgery, or childbirth suggests an underlying hemostatic disorder. Bleeding that is severe enough to require a blood transfusion merits particular attention. A family history of bleeding abnormalities suggests an inherited systemic disorder (e.g., von Willebrand disease). Bleeding from a platelet disorder typically is localized to superficial sites such as the skin or mucous membranes and usually is easily controlled. However, bleeding from hemostatic or plasma coagulation defects may occur hours or days after injury and is difficult to control with local measures. This type of bleeding often occurs in the muscles, joints, or body cavities.

A thorough history is the most important step in establishing the presence of a hemostatic disorder and in guiding initial laboratory testing.

Medications and Supplements Associated with Bleeding

Abciximab
Aspirin
Cephalosporins
Chemotherapeutic agents
Clopidogrel
Dalteparin
Enoxaparin
Eptifibatide
Ginkgo biloba
Gold
Heparin
Interferon
Metaxalone
Nonsteroidal anti-inflammatory drugs
Penicillins
Phenytoin
Propylthiouracil
Quinine
Recombinant t-Pas
Selective serotonin reuptake inhibitors

Testosterone replacement
Ticlopidine
Tinzaparin
Tirofiban
Tricyclic antidepressants
Urokinase
Valproic acid
Warfarin

Causes of Bleeding and Bruising

Abuse
Acquired factor VIII inhibitors
Acute leukemia
Adenocarcinoma
Alcohol abuse
Alpha$_2$-antiplasmin deficiency
Amyloidosis
Aplastic anemia
Bernard-Soulier syndrome
Bone marrow failure
Chronic renal failure
Connective tissue diseases
Cryoglobulinemia
Cushing disease
Disseminated intravascular coagulation
Drug-related thrombocytopenia
Ehlers-Danlos syndrome
Factor inhibitors
Fat embolism
Glanzmann thrombasthenia
Hemolysis, elevated liver enzymes, and low platelet syndrome
Hemolytic uremic syndrome
Hemophilia type A or B
Heparin-induced thrombocytopenia
Hereditary hemorrhagic telangiectasia
HIV infection
Idiopathic thrombocytopenic purpura
Leukemia
Liver disease
Lyme disease
Lymphoma
Malignancy
Marfan syndrome
May-Hegglin anomaly

Medications
Paraproteinemias
Postprostatectomy hemorrhage
Post-transfusion purpura syndrome
Purpura simplex
Rat poison ingestion
Senile purpura
Scott syndrome
Storage pool disease
Systemic lupus erythematosus
Thrombotic thrombocytopenic purpura
Viral infections
Vitamin C deficiency
Vitamin K deficiency
Vasculitis
von Willebrand disease
Wiskott-Aldrich syndrome

Key Historical Features

✓ Duration and onset of the symptoms
✓ Mucous membrane bleeding (menorrhagia, epistaxis, gum bleeding)
✓ Bleeding into soft tissues, such as muscles and joints
✓ Excessive bleeding during surgical procedures, fractures, or serious injuries
✓ Medical history
✓ Surgical history
✓ Family history of bleeding
✓ Medications

Key Physical Findings

✓ Epistaxis or bleeding from the gums
✓ Evaluation of the skin for purpura, ecchymoses, or hematomas
✓ Hepatomegaly
✓ Splenomegaly
✓ Evidence of bleeding into muscles or joints

Suggested Work-Up

Complete blood count	To evaluate for aplastic anemia
Platelet count	To evaluate for thrombocytopenia
Peripheral blood smear	To evaluate the cell lines

Prothrombin time (PT)	To evaluate plasma coagulation function
Activated partial thromboplastin time (aPTT)	To evaluate plasma coagulation function
Platelet function analyzer-100 or bleeding time	To evaluate platelet function in patients suspected of having von Willebrand disease or other platelet function disorders
Thrombin time	Increased in hereditary or acquired deficiencies or dysfunctions of fibrinogen
Fibrinogen concentration	To evaluate the time for fibrin clot formation

Additional Work-Up

Blood urea nitrogen and creatinine	If renal disease is suspected
Liver function tests	If liver disease is suspected
Thyroid-stimulating hormone	If thyroid disease is suspected
Ferritin	To assess iron stores
Vitamin K level	If vitamin K deficiency is suspected (abnormal PT and normal aPTT)
Partial thromboplastin time mixing study	If PT is normal and aPTT is abnormal. If partial thromboplastin time corrects (normalizes), check factors VIII, IX, and XI assays. If factor VIII is low, evaluate for von Willebrand disease (see below). If partial thromboplastin time does not correct, screen for inhibitors (lupus anticoagulant and factor VIII inhibitor)
Factor VIII, von Willebrand factor antigen, von Willebrand factor activity (ristocetin cofactor assay), and template bleeding time	If von Willebrand disease is suspected
PT, aPTT, thrombin time, platelet count, factor VIII assay, factor V assay, fibrinogen, and D-dimer	If disseminated intravascular coagulation is suspected

PT	aPTT	TT	Fibrinogen	Interpretation
N	N	N	N	Normal profile, which can be seen with mild factor deficiencies, mild VWD, platelet function defects (PFD), FXIII deficiency, plasminogen activator inhibitor-1 (PAI-1) deficiency, α_2-antiplasmin deficiency and connective tissue disorders
↑	N	N	N	FVII deficiency, warfarin therapy, early liver failure, early DIC
N	↑	N	N	Deficiencies of FVIII, IX, XI, XII VWD if FVIII is significantly decreased
↑	↑	N	N	Deficiencies of FII, FV, FX Supratherapeutic warfarin
↑	↑	↑	↓	Dysfibrinogenemia or afibrinogenemia Late DIC or liver failure
↑	↑	↑	N	Large amounts of heparin (reptilase time is normal)
N	N	↑	↓	Mild cases of dysfibrinogenemia or hypofibrinogenemia
N	↑	↑	N	Heparin (reptilase time is normal)

aPTT, Activated partial prothrombin time; *DIC,* disseminated intravascular coagulation; *N,* within normal range; *PT,* prothrombin time; *VWD,* von Willebrand disease.
From Rydz N, James PD. Why is my patient bleeding or bruising? *Hematol Oncol Clin N Am* 2012;26:321–344; Table 6.

Table 8-1. Differential Diagnosis of Abnormal Screening Coagulation Tests and Further Investigations

Further Reading

Ballas M, Kraut EH. Bleeding and bruising: a diagnostic work-up. *Am Fam Physician.* 2008;77:1117–1124.

Ewenstein BM. The pathophysiology of bleeding disorders presenting as abnormal uterine bleeding. *Am J Obstet Gynecol.* 1996;175:770–777.

Handin RI. Bleeding and thrombosis. In: Isselbacher KJ, Braunwald E, Wilson JD, eds. *Harrison's Textbook of Internal Medicine.* 13th ed. New York: McGraw-Hill; 1994:317–322.

Lusher JM. Screening and diagnosis of coagulation disorders. *Am J Obstet Gynecol.* 1996;175:778–783.

McKenna R. Abnormal coagulation in the postoperative period contributing to excessive bleeding. *Med Clin North Am.* 2001;85:1277–1310.

Rydz N, James PD. Why is my patient bleeding or bruising? *Hematol Oncol Clin North Am.* 2012;26:321–344.

General Discussion

The central nervous system (CNS) is susceptible to bacterial, viral, and fungal infections, as well as to prion diseases and numerous local and systemic diseases. Examination of the cerebrospinal fluid (CSF) is crucial in helping to diagnose infections and other diseases. Although not definitive, certain CSF findings are suggestive of bacterial, viral, fungal, or tuberculous meningitis. These findings are outlined in Table 9-1.

These typical findings, in combination with specific antigen, antibody, and polymerase chain reaction (PCR) tests may help to reveal the origin of a CNS infection or disease. Tests that are ordered on the CSF should be guided by the suspected underlying cause of the patient's illness. Recommended CSF studies based upon specific disorders are outlined in Table 9-2.

In patients who have bacterial meningitis and who receive antibiotics before lumbar puncture is performed, CSF abnormalities, such as an elevated white blood cell (WBC) count, elevated protein concentration, and depressed glucose, may persist for 1 to 3 days, whereas results of Gram stain and culture of the CSF can become negative within hours after the antibiotics are administered. A mononuclear pleocytosis is usually present in patients who have viral meningitis, but it can be preceded by a transient predominance of polymorphonucleocytes (PMNs) for 8 to 48 hours. Elevated levels of CSF adenosine deaminase have a high sensitivity and specificity for tuberculous meningitis in adults.

A CSF Gram stain and culture are the diagnostic tests of choice for bacterial meningitis. Blood culture may also help identify the causative organism. CSF viral culture is able to detect 14% to 24% of cases of viral meningitis. Nucleic acid amplification testing has become a standard part of the diagnostic evaluation of viral meningitis and has superior sensitivity for the detection of herpes simplex virus and enterovirus. Tuberculous and fungal meningitis may be difficult to diagnose by routine CSF smear or culture. CSF culture is positive in 52% to 83% of cases of tuberculous meningitis.

CSF cell counts with differentials should be performed on every specimen. Typically, the CSF contains no red blood cells (RBC) per microliter and 0 to 1 WBC/μL. A traumatic lumbar puncture causes elevations of RBCs and WBCs, but these elevations are differentiated from subarachnoid hemorrhage, because in a traumatic lumbar puncture the elevations are high in the first tube but clear in the later tubes. In subarachnoid hemorrhage, the elevations persist in each test tube. To determine whether an elevated CSF WBC is due to blood from a traumatic tap or other causes, an expected ratio may be used. If the elevated WBC is due to blood in the CSF, 1 WBC/μL for every 700 RBC/μL is found. If the WBC exceeds this ratio, its origin must be accounted for from other etiologies (e.g., infection or inflammation).

The CSF glucose concentration is normally 60% of the plasma glucose concentration. It is important to obtain a serum glucose level at the time of the CSF sample. An elevated CSF glucose level results from an elevated plasma glucose level. A decreased CSF glucose concentration may be due to hypoglycemia, bacterial meningitis, fungal meningitis, certain viral meningitides, subarachnoid hemorrhage, meningeal carcinomatosis, chemical meningitis, and parasitic meningitis.

Elevation in CSF protein is a nonspecific but sensitive indicator of CNS disease. A CSF protein concentration greater than 500 mg/dL is an infrequent finding, but it can occur with bacterial meningitis, subarachnoid hemorrhage, or spinal–subarachnoid block. When a significant amount of blood is present in the CSF, the total protein concentration can be corrected by reducing the protein by 1 mg/dL for every 1000 RBCs in the CSF. Protein concentrations of 100 mg/dL or greater have a sensitivity and a specificity for bacterial meningitis of 82% and 98%, respectively. If the concentration is 200 mg/dL, the sensitivity is 86%, and the specificity is 100%.

The finding of oligoclonal bands in the CSF implies that a single clonal population of plasma cells is responsible for each band seen on gel electrophoresis. More than one oligoclonal band rarely occurs in normal CSF. A serum sample should be obtained simultaneously with a CSF sample to determine whether oligoclonal bands are unique to the CSF. Oligoclonal bands are present in 83% to 94% of patients with multiple sclerosis and are also present in disorders such as subacute sclerosing panencephalitis, CNS lupus, neurosarcoidosis, cysticercosis, Behçet syndrome, Guillain-Barré syndrome, some brain tumors, and viral, fungal, and bacterial infections.

CSF Parameter	Bacterial Meningitis	Viral Meningitis	Fungal Meningitis	Tuberculous Meningitis
Opening pressure (mm H$_2$O)	>180	Often normal	Variable	>180
WBC count (cells/mm^3)	1000–10,000 (range: <100–20,000)	<300 (range: 100–1000)	20–500 Variable, dependent upon fungus	50–500 (range: <50–4000)
Neutrophils (%)	>80	<20	Usually <50	20
Protein (mg/dL)	100–500	Often normal	Elevated	150–200
Glucose (mg/dL)	<40	>40	Usually <4	<40
Gram stain (% positive)	60–90	Negative	Negative	37–87 (acid-fast bacilli [AFB] smear)
Culture (% positive)	70–85	50	25–50	52–83

From Zunt JR, Marra CM. Cerebrospinal fluid testing for the diagnosis of central nervous system infection. *Neurologic Clinics* 1999;17:675–689.

Table 9-1. Typical Cerebrospinal Fluid Findings in Bacterial and Viral Meningitides

Domain	Disorder	Useful CSF Studies	Expected Results	Comments
Cerebral dysfunction				
Infectious	Meningitis (purulent)	pr, gl, cell cts, gs, cx, op	↑ pr, ↓ gl, ↑ CSF PMNs, + gs and cx, + bacterial ags, ↑ op	+ cryptococcal ag and India ink in cryptococcal meningitis
			↑ LA	Mononuclear cells possible in partially rx'd bacterial meningitis
	Meningitis (aseptic)	pr, gl, cell cts	↑ pr, nl gl, ↑ CSF WBC (10–1000 mononuc cells/mm³)	PMNs possible in early aseptic meningitis
	Encephalitis	pr, gl, cell cts, gs, cx	Mildly ↑ pr (50 to 100 mg/dL), nl gl, ↑ CSF WBC 50–100/mm³ (mononuc)	Herpes simplex encephalitis
			↑ RBC/xanthochromia, + CSF PCR	
	HIV encephalopathy	pr, gl, cell cts	Mildly ↑ pr, nl gl, nl or few WBC	
	Neurosyphilis (acute)	VDRL, pr, gl	↑ pr (>45 mg/dL), ↑ WBC (5–500 mononuc/mm³), + VDRL	CSF parameters may be normal
	Neuroborreliosis	pr, gl, cell cts, OCB, ab's	↑ pr (~100 mg/dL), nl or ↓ gl, ↑ WBC (~100 mononuc/mm³), + OCB, + Lyme ab's	CSF normalizes in stage III
	Tuberculous meningitis	pr, gl, cell cts, op, acid-fast stain, cx	↑ pr (100–200 mg/dL), ↓ gl (<45 mg/dL), ↑ WBC (25–100 mononuc/mm³), ↑ op	May be spinal block; stain and culture require large amounts of CSF
	Abscess	Not recommended		May be dangerous to perform LP in the face of abscess; risk of herniation or ventricular rupture
	Creutzfeldt-Jakob disease	pr, gl, cell cts	Normal	14-3-3 protein in CSF (not readily available)
	Progressive multifocal leukoencephalopathy	JC virus PCR	+ JC virus PCR	CSF o/w normal
	Cysticercosis	pr, gl, cell cts, op	↑ pr, ↓ gl, ↑ WBC (mixed w/eosinophilia), ↑ op	CSF eosinophils constitute 20%–75%

Table 9-2. Selected Disorders and Associated Cerebrospinal Fluid Studies—Cont'd

Domain	Disorder	Useful CSF Studies	Expected Results	Comments
Cerebrovascular	Stroke	pr, cell cts	Mildly ↑ pr and WBC	Not routinely performed; ↑ LDH, AST, and CK-BB in cortical CVA
	Subarachnoid hemorrhage	pr, gl, cell cts, color	↑↑ pr, ↓ gl, ↑↑ RBC, ↑ WBC, xanth	pr can be normal or significantly ↑, gl can be normal or slightly ↓
	Venous thrombosis	cell cts, op	↑ RBC, ↑ op	WBC may be ↑ if 2° to septic thrombosis
	Anoxic brain			Not routinely performed; CK-BB, NSE, MBP may be useful
Dementia	Alzheimer disease (AD)	pr, gl, cell cts	normal parameters	Abnormal CSF helps r/o AD
Degenerative	Huntington disease	pr, gl, cell cts	Normal	Abnormal CSF helps r/o Huntington disease
	Wilson disease	pr, gl, cell cts	Normal	Abnormal CSF helps r/o Wilson disease
Neoplastic	Meningeal carcinomatosis	pr, gl, cell cts, cyt, op	↑ pr (24 to 1200 mg/dL), ↓ gl, ↑ WBC (PMN), + cyt, mildly ↑ op	Large volumes of CSF and multiple LPs increase cytology yield
	Craniopharyngioma	cell cts	↑ WBC (mononuc)	A cause of chronic chemical meningitis
Metabolic	Hepatic encephalopathy	pr, color	↑ pr possible xanth	Not routinely performed; op may be ↑; CSF glutamine ↑
	Uremic encephalopathy	pr, cell cts, urea	Mildly ↑ pr and WBC, ↑ urea	Not routinely performed
	Myxedema coma	Pr	↑ pr (100–300 mg/dL)	
	Mitochondrial encephalopathies	pyruvate, lactate	↑ pyruvate, lactate	Mitochondrial encephalopathy, lactic acidosis, and stroke-like episodes (MELAS)
Demyelinating	Multiple sclerosis	pr, gl, cell cts, OCB, MBP, IgG index	↑ pr, mildly ↑ WBC, nl gl, + OCB, + MBP, ↑ IgG index	Abnormal CSF in 90% of cases; pr and cell cts nl in 2/3
	Acute disseminated encephalomyelitis	pr, gl, cell cts, OCB	Mildly ↑ pr and WBC, nl gl, + OCB	OCBs may disappear after resolution

Autoimmune	Sarcoid	pr, gl, cell cts	↑ pr (50 to 200 mg/dL), mildly ↓ gl (30 to 40 mg/dL); ↑ WBC (10 to 100 mononuc/mm³)	ACE ↑ in 50%, but not specific
	Behçet disease	pr, cell cts	↑ pr; ↑ WBC (mixed response) 10–200 cell/mm²	CSF results quite varied
	Angiitis	pr, gl, cell cts, op	↑ pr; ↓ gl; ↑ WBC (mononuc), ↑ op	Abnormal CSF in 80%–90%
Other disorders	Normal pressure hydrocephalus	Diagnostic high-volume LP, op	Gait and mental status improvement after LP, nl op	High-volume LP (40–50 mL of CSF)
	Pseudotumor cerebri	pr, cell cts, op	↓ pr, nl cell cts, ↑ op (250–600 mm H₂O)	CSF removal may be therapeutic in some cases
	Migraine	See comments		Little available data. May have ↑ pr and cell cts in severe complicated migraine
	Generalized seizure	pr, cell cts	nl ↑ pr; mild ↑ WBC	Postictal
	Reye syndrome	pr, gl, cell cts, op	pr and gl nl, <10 cell/mm²; ↑ op	
Cranial nerve dysfunction				
	Miller-Fisher variant of GBS	See GBS	See GBS/comments	Pr more commonly nl than in GBS
	Optic neuritis	pr, cell cts, OCB	Mild ↑ pr (45–60 mg/dL), 50%↑ with mild ↑ WBC (mononuc), + OCB	+ OCB increase risk of MS
	Lyme disease	cell cts	Mild ↑ WBC (mononuc)	
	Bell palsy	pr, gl, cell cts	nl CSF	Abnormal CSF helps r/o Bell palsy
	Trigeminal neuralgia			Not routinely performed; may have ↑ substance P and ↓ monoamines
	Kearns-Sayre syndrome	Pr	↑ pr (70–400 mg/dL)	

Table 9-2. Selected Disorders and Associated Cerebrospinal Fluid Studies—Cont'd

Domain	Disorder	Useful CSF Studies	Expected Results	Comments
Motor dysfunction				
CNS	Parkinson disease			Not routinely performed. Abnormal CSF helps r/o Parkinson disease
	Huntington disease	See above		Abnormal CSF helps r/o Huntington disease
	Wilson disease	See above		Abnormal CSF helps r/o Wilson disease
	Neurosyphilis (paretic)	VDRL, pr, cell cts,	+ + VDRL, pr: 50–100 mg/dL, cell cts: 25–75 leukocytes/mm^2	CSF abnormalities increase with duration of disease
	HTLV-I	pr, gl, IgG, OCB	Mild ↑ pr, nl gl, ↑ IgG, + OCB	Serum + HTLV-I ag
	Poliomyelitis	pr, gl, cell cts	Mild ↑ pr (50–200 mg/dL), nl gl, mild ↑ CSF WBC (mononuc)	CSF WBC ↓ with time
	Spinal cord tumor	pr, gl, cell cts, cytology	May be ↑↑ pr, nl gl, ↑ WBC (mononuc), + cyt	Froin syndrome (spinal cord block) may sig ↑
	Tetanus	pr, gl, cell cts	↑ pr (90–150 mg/dL), nl gl, nl cell cts	Care must be taken not to induce tetany. Normal cell cts differentiate from meningitis
	Stiff man syndrome	pr, cell cts, IgG, OCB	nl pr, nl cell cts, ↑ IgG,? + OCB	
Motor neuron	ALS	pr, cell cts	Mild ↑ pr and cell cts	Nondiagnostic
	GBS	pr, cell cts	↑ pr, nl cell cts	Pr peaks between 1 and 3 wks. Cell cts >>5 should prompt search for another cause
Nerve	Brachial plexopathy	pr, cell cts	Mild ↑ pr (50–60 mg/dL), nl cell cts	
	Chronic inflammatory demyelinating polyradiculopathy (CIDP)	pr, gl, cell cts	↑ pr (100–200 mg/dL), nl gl, mild ↑ WBC (5–50 cell/mm^3)	Similar to GBS; pr elevation correlates with severity; + WBC in 10%
	Inherited neuropathy	pr, gl, cell cts	Mod ↑ pr (−200 mg/dL), nl cell cts	
Muscle	Myopathy or myositis			Not routinely performed

Cerebellar dysfunction

| Cerebellum | Cerebellitis | pr; gl; cell cts | Mildly ↑ pr; nl gl; cell cts usually < 100/mm² (mononuc) | Usually secondary to varicella zoster |
| | Paraneoplastic cerebellar disease | pr; cell cts; abs | Mild ↑ pr; mild ↑ WBC (8–20 cells/mm³) + anti-Yo or anti-Hu ab | Anti-Yo in ovarian, uterine, or breast CA. Anti-Hu seen in lung CA |

Sensory dysfunction

Neuropathy	Diabetic	pr; gl; cell cts	↑ pr (50–400 mg/dL); nl cell cts; ↑ gl (secondary diabetes)	
	CIDP	See above		
	Inherited neuropathies	See above		
	Neurosyphilis (tabes dorsalis)	VDRL; pr; gl; cell cts	3/4 w/+ VDRL; CSF freq o/w WNL	CSF may resemble paretic form, but parameters improve w/progression

abs, Antibodies; *ACE*, angiotensin-converting enzyme; *AD*, Alzheimer dementia; *ag*, antigen; *ALS*, amyotrophic lateral sclerosis; *AST*, aspartate aminotransferase; *bact*, bacteria; *CA*, cancer; *cell cts*, cell counts; *cerebrovasc*, cerebrovascular; *CK-BB*, creatinine kinase BB isoenzyme; *CSF*, cerebrospinal fluid; *CVA*, cerebrovascular accident (stroke); *cyt*, cytology; *degen*, degenerative; *GBS*, Guillain-Barré syndrome; *gl*, glucose; *gs*, Gram stain; *IgG*, immunoglobulin-G; *LA*, lactic acid; *LDH*, lactate dehydrogenase; *MBP*, myelin basic protein; *mononuc*, mononuclear cells; *nl*, normal; *NPH*, normal pressure hydrocephalus; *NSE*, neuron-specific-enolase; *OCB*, oligoclonal bands; *OP*, opening; *o/w*, otherwise; *PCR*, polymerase chain reaction; *pr*, protein; *r/o*, rule out; *rx'd*, treated; *sig*, significantly; *VDRL*, Venereal Disease Research Laboratory test; *WBC*, white blood cell count; *WNL*, within normal limits; *xanth*, xanthochromia. From Goetz. Textbook of Clinical Neurology. 2nd ed. Philadelphia: Saunders; 2003:511–524.

Table 9-2.   Selected Disorders and Associated Cerebrospinal Fluid Studies

Further Reading

Coyle PK. Overview of acute and chronic meningitis. *Neurol Clin.* 1999;17:691–710.

Goetz CG. *Textbook of Clinical Neurology.* 2nd ed. Philadelphia: Saunders; 2003:511–524.

Huhn GD, Sejvar JJ, Montgomery SP, Dworkin MS. West Nile virus in the United States: an update on an emerging infectious disease. *Am Fam Physician.* 2003;68:653–660.

Plage CR, Petti CA. Assessment of the utility of viral culture of cerebrospinal fluid. *Clin Infect Dis.* 2006;43:1578–1579.

Re VL, Gluckman SJ. Eosinophilic meningitis. *Am J Med.* 2003;114:217–223.

Teunissen CE, Dijkstra C, Polman C. Biologic markers in CSF and blood for axonal degeneration in multiple sclerosis. *Lancet Neurol.* 2005;4:32–41.

Thomson RB, Bertram H. Laboratory diagnosis of central nervous system infections. *Infect Dis Clin North Am.* 2001;15:1047–1071.

Zunt JR, Marra CM. Cerebrospinal fluid testing for the diagnosis of central nervous system infection. *Neurol Clin.* 1999;17:675–689.

General Discussion

The cough reflex is complex, but cough generally results from an irritant stimulation of one or more receptors in the respiratory system. Estimating the duration of cough is the first step in narrowing the list of possible diagnoses. Cough may be classified as acute (less than 3 weeks), subacute (3–8 weeks), or chronic (more than 8 weeks). If the cough is productive of blood, the patient should be evaluated according to guidelines for hemoptysis.

In nonsmokers who do not take an angiotensin-converting enzyme (ACE) inhibitor and whose chest x-ray is normal, the most likely causes of chronic cough are asthma, postnasal drip (also known as upper airway cough syndrome [UACS]), or gastroesophageal reflux disease (GERD). Other common causes in immunocompetent patients include chronic bronchitis due to cigarette smoking or other irritants, bronchiectasis, and eosinophilic bronchitis. The physician should assess the likelihood of the most common causes using empiric therapy trials and trials that involve the avoidance of irritants and drugs, along with focused laboratory testing, such as chest radiography or methacholine challenge.

A normal chest radiograph in an immunocompetent patient makes postnasal drip syndrome, asthma, GERD, chronic bronchitis, and eosinophilic bronchitis more likely and makes bronchogenic carcinoma, tuberculosis, bronchiectasis, and sarcoidosis unlikely. If the chest radiograph is abnormal, the patient should be evaluated on the basis of the diseases suggested by the radiographic findings.

Postnasal drip syndrome is the most common cause of chronic cough; no diagnostic test exists, so the patient should be evaluated for this condition first. Suggestive findings on the history and physical include drainage in the posterior pharynx, throat clearing, nasal discharge, cobble stoning of the oropharyngeal mucosa, and mucus in the oropharynx. A trial of therapy with a decongestant and first-generation histamine H_1 receptor antagonist is reasonable.

Cough-variant asthma may also be considered as a cause of chronic cough. Spirometry can demonstrate airflow obstruction and reversibility of the condition. If asthma is suspected, but physical examination and spirometry are nondiagnostic, a methacholine challenge should be considered because its negative predictive value is 100%.

For GERD, an empiric trial of a proton pump inhibitor is recommended. The cough should nearly or completely resolve with treatment if it is due to GERD. If GERD is suspected but a therapeutic trial is ineffective, 24-hour monitoring of the esophagus may be considered, although it is inconvenient for patients and is not widely available.

Although most long-term smokers have a cough, it should not be assumed that the cough is due to the smoking, unless they stop smoking and the cough resolves. It is also important to recognize that multiple conditions often simultaneously contribute to cough. Chronic cough has two or more causes in 18% to 62% of patients and three causes in up to 42% of patients. The definitive diagnosis of the cause of chronic cough is established on the basis of an observation of which specific therapy eliminates the cough. Therapy that is partially successful should not be stopped but should instead be sequentially supplemented.

If the patient has a history of smoking, is exposed to environmental irritants, or is currently being treated with an ACE inhibitor, the patient should be instructed to eliminate the irritant or discontinue the medication for 4 weeks. If the cough improves or resolves, the cough is partially or entirely due to chronic bronchitis or to the ACE inhibitor.

Eosinophilic bronchitis can be distinguished from asthma by the lack of bronchial hyper-responsiveness or variable airflow obstruction. Patients with nonasthmatic eosinophilic bronchitis have normal spirometry and respond to inhaled and systemic corticosteroids. Eosinophilic bronchitis can be ruled out as a cause of chronic cough if eosinophils make up less than 3% of the nonsquamous cells in a sample of induced sputum.

Tuberculosis (TB) should be considered early in the evaluation of patients with chronic cough when the likelihood of tuberculosis is high. This includes places where the prevalence of TB is high and in populations at high risk of TB (e.g., HIV-infected persons). TB should also be considered in patients with chronic cough who have sputum production, hemoptysis, fever, or weight loss.

Causes of Chronic Cough

Aberrant innominate artery
ACE inhibitor use
Arteriovenous malformation
Aspiration
Asthma
Bronchiectasis
Bronchiolitis
Bronchogenic carcinoma
Chronic aspiration
Chronic bronchitis due to smoking or other irritants
Cystic fibrosis
Environmental exposure
Eosinophilic bronchitis
Foreign body aspiration
GERD
Immune deficiencies
Interstitial lung disease

Irritable larynx
Irritants
Irritation of external auditory meatus
Left ventricular failure
Lower respiratory tract infection
Lymphoma
Metastatic carcinoma
Persistent pneumonia
Pertussis infection
Postinfectious cough
Postnasal drip (also known as UACS, which includes chronic sinusitis,
    allergic rhinitis, vasomotor rhinitis, and nonallergic rhinitis)
Psychogenic cough
Pulmonary abscess
Sarcoidosis
Tracheitis
Upper respiratory tract infection
TB

Key Historical Features

✓ Fever
✓ Symptoms of asthma
✓ Heartburn or regurgitation
✓ Symptoms of postnasal drip (throat clearing, nasal discharge, excessive
    phlegm production)
✓ Exacerbating factors
✓ Diurnal variation
✓ Hemoptysis
✓ Purulent sputum
✓ Night sweats
✓ Weight loss
✓ Medical history
✓ Medications, especially ACE inhibitors
✓ Tobacco use
✓ Environmental exposures
✓ HIV risk factors

Key Physical Findings

✓ Vital signs
✓ Head and neck examination for lymphadenopathy, nasal discharge, sinus
    tenderness, a cobblestone appearance of the oropharynx, mucus in the
    oropharynx
✓ Cardiac examination for evidence of left ventricular failure

✓ Pulmonary examination for any abnormal breath sounds
✓ Extremity examination for cyanosis or clubbing

Suggested Work-Up

Chest x-ray	Optional in the initial evaluation of younger nonsmokers with suspected postnasal drip syndrome or sinusitis

Additional Work-Up

Pulmonary function testing	To evaluate for asthma
Methacholine challenge	If spirometry is nondiagnostic, methacholine challenge may be useful in ruling out asthma because it has a negative predictive value of 100% in the context of cough.
Bronchoscopy	Should be considered when the cause of cough remains unclear after an initial evaluation
Evaluation of induced sputum	May be helpful in diagnosing nonasthmatic eosinophilic bronchitis
High-resolution computed tomography of the chest	Helpful in evaluating chest radiograph abnormalities
24-h esophageal pH monitoring	May help link GERD and cough. Has a low specificity, so starting treatment for GERD usually is preferable to testing as an initial decision
Barium esophagography	May reveal reflux in cases when refluxate from the stomach has a pH value similar to that of the normal esophagus, thus preventing its detection during esophageal pH monitoring
Computed tomography of the sinuses	If chronic sinusitis is suspected
Cardiac studies	If a cardiac cause of the cough is suspected

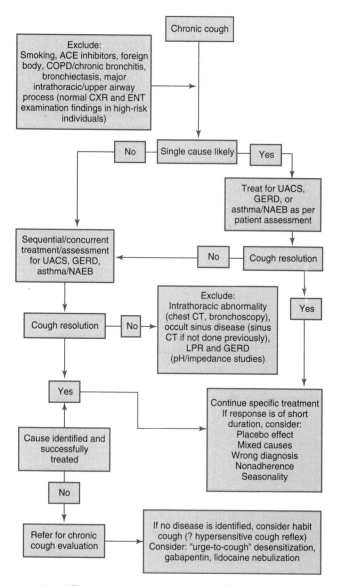

Figure 10-1. *ACE,* Angiotensin-converting enzyme; *COPD,* chronic obstructive pulmonary disease; *CT,* computed tomography; *CXR, chest x-ray; ENT, ear, nose, and throat; GERD, gastroesophageal reflux disease; LPR, laryngopharyngeal reflux; NAEB, non-asthmatic eosinophilic bronchitis; UACS,* upper airway cough syndrome. From Iyer VN, Lim KG. Evaluation of chronic cough in the immunocompetent host. Mayo Clinic Proceedings 2013;88:1115–1125.

Further Reading

Benich JJ, Carek PJ. Evaluation of the patient with chronic cough. *Am Fam Physician.* 2011;84:887–892.

Chung KF, Pavord ID. Prevalence, pathogenesis, and causes of chronic cough. *Lancet.* 2008;271:1364–1374.

Currie GP, Gray RD, McKay J. Chronic cough. *Br Med J.* 2003;326:261.

Holmes RL, Fadden CT. Evaluation of the patient with chronic cough. *Am Fam Physician.* 2004;69:2159–2166.

Irwin RS, Boulet IP, Cloutier MM, et al. Managing cough as a defense mechanism and as a symptom. A consensus panel report of the American College of Chest Physicians. *Chest.* 1998;114(2 suppl):166S.

Irwin RS, Madison JM. The diagnosis and treatment of cough. *N Engl J Med.* 2000;343:1715–1721.

Irwin RS, Madison JM. The persistently troublesome cough. *Am J Respir Crit Care Med.* 2002;165:1469–1474.

Lalloo UG, Barnes PJ, Chung KF. Pathophysiology and clinical presentations of cough. *J Allergy Clin Immunol.* 1996;98:91S–96S.

Rosen MJ. Chronic cough due to tuberculosis and other infections: ACCP evidence-based clinical practice guidelines. *Chest.* 2006;129:197S–201S.

General Discussion

The National Kidney Foundation defines chronic kidney disease (CKD) as a glomerular filtration rate (GFR) of less than 60 mL/min per 1.73 m^2 or evidence of kidney damage with or without a decreased GFR for 3 or more months. CKD can lead to progressive loss of renal function and may result in end-stage renal disease after a variable period of time following the initiating injury. Kidney damage is manifested by pathologic abnormalities or markers of kidney damage, which include abnormalities in the composition of the blood or urine (e.g., proteinuria), abnormalities in the urine sediment, and abnormalities on imaging studies.

Among individuals with CKD, the stages are classified based on the level of kidney function:

- Stage 1 Kidney damage with normal or an elevated GFR of ≥90
- Stage 2 Kidney damage with a mildly decreased GFR of 60 to 89
- Stage 3 A moderately decreased GFR of 30 to 59
- Stage 4 A severely decreased GFR of 15 to 29
- Stage 5 Kidney failure with a GFR of less than 15 or dialysis

Patients with CKD should be monitored for progression of renal failure. All individuals with a GFR of less than 60 for at least 3 months are classified as having CKD regardless of the presence or absence of kidney damage. When renal disease reaches this stage, the patient should be monitored more closely for control of hypertension, anemia, renal bone disease, and nutritional status.

Patients with CKD should be evaluated to determine the type of kidney disease, comorbid conditions, disease severity, complications, risk for loss of kidney function, and risk for development of cardiovascular disease. Patients with CKD are more likely to die of cardiovascular disease than to require dialysis. The combination of diabetes and CKD is one of the most potent predictors of adverse cardiovascular events and death. Proteinuria is a marker of kidney damage and a risk factor for accelerated progression of kidney disease. It is also increasingly recognized as an independent risk factor for all-cause and cardiovascular mortality.

Patients with CKD should be referred to a nephrologist for consultation and co-management if a clinical action plan cannot be prepared or the prescribed evaluation and recommended treatment cannot be carried out. In general, patients with a GFR less than 30 mL/min per 1.73 m^2 should be referred for nephrology consultation.

Risk Factors for Chronic Kidney Disease

Advancing age
Autoimmune diseases
Cardiovascular disease
Diabetes mellitus
Drug toxicity

Family history of kidney disease
Hyperlipidemia
Hypertension
Low birth weight
Low income and/or education
Lower urinary tract obstruction
Malignancy
Recovery from acute renal failure
Reduction in kidney mass
Smoking
Systemic infections
Urinary stones
Urinary tract infections
U.S. ethnic minority status
- African American
- Asian or Pacific Islander
- Hispanic
- Native American

Causes of Chronic Kidney Disease

Cystic diseases
- Polycystic kidney disease
Diabetic kidney disease
Glomerular diseases
- Autoimmune diseases
- Drugs
- Neoplasia
- Systemic infections
Transplant-related diseases
Tubulointerstitial diseases
- Drug toxicity
- Obstruction
- Stones
- Urinary tract infection
Vascular diseases
- Hypertension
- Large vessel disease
- Microangiopathy

Key Historical Features

✓ Symptoms during urination
✓ Recent infections
✓ Skin rash
✓ Arthritis

✓ Risk factors for HIV, hepatitis B, or hepatitis C
✓ Previous urologic evaluations
✓ Medical history (hypertension, diabetes, heart failure, cirrhosis)
✓ Medications
✓ Family history of kidney diseases

Clue	Potential Diagnosis
Review of systems	
Symptoms during urination	Usually suggest disorders of the urinary tract, such as infection, obstruction, or stones
Recent infections	May suggest postinfectious glomerulonephritis or HIV-associated nephropathy
Skin rash or arthritis	Suggests autoimmune disease, such as systemic lupus erythematosus or cryoglobulinemia
Risk factors for parenterally transmitted disease	May suggest HIV, hepatitis B, or hepatitis C infection and associated kidney diseases
Chronic diseases	
Heart failure, cirrhosis, or gastrointestinal fluid losses	Usually suggest reduced kidney perfusion ("prerenal factors")
Diabetes*	As a cause of chronic kidney disease: diabetic kidney disease usually follows a typical clinical course after onset, first with microalbuminuria, followed by clinical proteinuria, hypertension, and declining GFR.
Hypertension*	As a cause of chronic kidney disease: hypertensive nephrosclerosis is usually characterized by severely elevated blood pressure readings over a long period of time, with associated end-organ damage in addition to kidney disease. Recent worsening of hypertension, in association with findings of diffuse atherosclerosis, suggests large vessel disease due to atherosclerosis. Recent onset of severe hypertension in young women suggests large vessel disease due to fibromuscular dysplasia.
Medical history	
Findings from past "routine" examinations	May reveal a history of hypertension or proteinuria during childhood, during pregnancy, or on examinations for school, military service, or insurance.
Past urologic evaluations	Details may disclose radiologic abnormalities associated with kidney disease.
Family history of kidney diseases	
Every generation; equal susceptibility in males and females	Suggests an autosomal dominant disease, such as polycystic kidney disease.
Every generation; predominant male susceptibility	Suggests a sex-linked recessive disease, such as Alport syndrome.
Less frequent than every generation	Suggests an autosomal recessive disease, such as medullary cystic kidney disease or autosomal recessive polycystic kidney disease.

GFR, glomerular filtration rate.
*Extremely common in elderly patients and often nonspecific.
From National Kidney Foundation. K/DOQI clinical practice guidelines for chronic kidney disease: evaluation, classification, and stratification. Am J Kidney Dis. 2002;39(2 suppl 1): S1–S266.

Table 11-1. Clues to the Diagnosis of Chronic Kidney Disease from the Patient's History

Key Physical Findings

✓ Blood pressure
✓ Cardiovascular examination
✓ Skin examination for rash
✓ Joint examination for arthritis

Evaluation of Patients at Increased Risk of Chronic Kidney Disease

All patients:

Blood pressure measurement

Serum creatinine and estimate of GFR

Protein-to-creatinine ratio in a spot urine specimen

Examination of the urine sediment or dipstick for red blood cells and white blood cells

Evaluation of Patients with Chronic Kidney Disease

Serum creatinine and estimate of GFR

Protein-to-creatinine ratio in a spot urine specimen

Examination of the urine sediment or dipstick for red blood cells and white blood cells

Imaging of the kidneys, usually by ultrasound

Serum electrolytes

Additional Work-Up

The evaluation of the patient with CKD is guided by the symptoms, family history of kidney disease, medical history, physical examination findings, and findings from the urine sediment and protein-to-creatinine ratio.

Disorder	Clinical Clues	Urine Sediment	Protein-Creatinine Ratio	Additional Tests
Diabetes mellitus	Diabetes for > 15 years, retinopathy	RBCs in <25% of affected patients	>30 to >3500 mg of protein per gram of creatinine	Fasting blood sugar, A₁C
Essential hypertension	Left ventricular hypertrophy, retinopathy	Benign	>30 to 3000 mg of protein per gram of creatinine	No additional tests
Glomerulonephritis	History and physical examination: infections; rash, arthritis; patient older than 40 years	Dysmorphic >30 to > RBCs or RBC casts	3500 mg of protein per gram of creatinine	C3 and C4 for all patients. Tests for infections: anti-ASO, ASK, HIV, HBsAg, HCV, RPR, blood cultures Tests if there is rash or arthritis: ANA, ANCA, cryoglobulin, anti-GBM Tests if patient is older than 40 years: SPEP, UPEP
Interstitial nephritis	Medications, fever, rash, eosinophilia	WBCs, WBC casts, eosinophils	30 to 3000 mg of protein per gram of creatinine	ACE level; SS-A, SS-B
Low-flow states	Volume depletion, hypotension, congestive heart failure, cirrhosis, atherosclerosis	Hyaline casts, eosinophils	<200 mg of protein per gram of creatinine	FE_Na; < 1% eosinophilia
Urinary tract obstruction	Urinary symptoms	Benign or RBCs	None	KUB radiography, intravenous pyelography, spiral CT scanning, renal ultrasonography
Chronic urinary tract infection	Urinary symptoms	WBCs, RBCs	<2000 mg of protein per gram of creatinine	Pelvic examination, urine culture, voiding cystourethrography, renal ultrasonography, CT scanning
Neoplasm, paraproteinemia	Patient older than 40 years, constitutional symptoms, anemia	RBCs, RBC casts, granular casts	False-negative result or >30 to >3500 mg of protein per gram of creatinine	SPEP, UPEP, calcium level, ESR
Cystic kidney disease	Palpable kidneys with or without family history of cystic kidney disease, flank pain	RBCs	30 to 3000 mg of protein per g of creatinine	Renal ultrasonography or CT scanning if there is a complex kidney cyst or mass

Table 11-2. Diagnostic Evaluation in Chronic Kidney Disease

Disorder	Clinical Clues	Urine Sediment	Protein-Creatinine Ratio	Additional Tests
Renovascular disease	Late-onset or refractory hypertension, sudden onset of hypertension in young women, smoking history, abdominal bruit	Benign	<200 mg of protein per gram of creatinine	Renal Doppler ultrasonography, radioisotope renal scanning, MRA, renal angiography
Vasculitis	Constitutional symptoms, peripheral neuropathy, rash, respiratory symptoms	RBCs; granular casts	>30 to >3500 mg of protein per gram of creatinine	C3, C4, ANA, ANCA, HBsAg, HCV, cryoglobulins, ESR, RF, SS-A, SS-B, HIV

A1C, glycosylated hemoglobin; ACE, angiotensin-converting enzyme; ANA, antinuclear antibodies; ANCA, antineutrophil cytoplasmic antibody; anti-ASO, steptolysin O latex antibody; anti-GBM, anti-glomerular basement membrane antibody; ASK, antistreptokinase; C3, complement 3; C4, complement 4; CT, computed tomography; ESR, erythrocyte sedimentation rate; FE_{Na}, fractional excretion of sodium; HBsAg, hepatitis B surface antigen; HCV, hepatitis C virus; KUB, kidney, ureters, and bladder; MRA, magnetic resonance angiography; RBC, red blood cell; RF, rheumatoid factor; RPR, rapid plasma reagin; SPEP, serum protein electrophoresis; UPEP, urine protein electrophoresis; WBC, white blood cell; SS-A, anti-Ro antibody; SS-B, anti-La antibody. Adapted from Chronic kidney disease and pre-ESRD. Management in the primary care setting. From Snyder S, Pendergraph B. Detection and evaluation of chronic kidney disease. American Family Physician 2005;72:1723–1732.

Table 11-2. Diagnostic Evaluation in Chronic Kidney Disease

Renal biopsy is indicated when the cause of CKD cannot be determined by the history and laboratory evaluation, or when the patient's signs and symptoms suggest renal parenchymal disease. Biopsy is more commonly required in patients with CKD that is not related to diabetes. Biopsy is often indicated in adult patients with nephrotic syndrome or suspected glomerulonephritis.

Further Reading

Foley RN, Murray AM, Li S, et al. Chronic kidney disease and the risk for cardiovascular disease, renal replacement, and death in the United States Medicare population, 1998 to 1999. *J Am Soc Nephrol.* 2005;16:489–495.

Greenberg A, Cheung AK. National Kidney Foundation. *Primer on Kidney Diseases.* 3rd ed. San Diego: Academic Press; 2001.

Johnson CA, Levey AS, Coresh J, Levin A, Lau J, Eknoyan G. Clinical practice guidelines for chronic kidney disease in adults: part I: definition, disease stages, evaluation, treatment, and risk factors. *Am Fam Physician.* 2004;70:869–876.

Kidney Disease Outcomes Quality Initiative (KDOQI). KDOQI clinical practice guidelines and clinical practice recommendations for diabetes and chronic kidney disease. *Am J Kidney Dis.* 2007;49(2 suppl 2):S12–S154.

Levin A, Stevens LA. Executing change in the management of chronic kidney disease: perspectives on guidelines and practice. *Med Clin North Am.* 2005;89:701–709.

McClellan WM. Epidemiology and risk factors for chronic kidney disease. *Med Clin North Am.* 2005;89:419–445.

National Kidney Foundation. K/DOQI clinical practice guidelines for chronic kidney disease: evaluation, classification, and stratification. *Am J Kidney Dis.* 2002;39(2 suppl 1):S1–S266.

Rivera JA, O'Hare AM, Harper GM. Update on the management of chronic kidney disease. *Am Fam Physician.* 2012;86:749–754.

Snyder S, Pendergraph B. Detection and evaluation of chronic kidney disease. *Am Fam Physician.* 2005;72:1723–1732.

General Discussion

Meningitis can be defined based on time course, associated cerebrospinal fluid (CSF) profile, and underlying cause. Chronic meningitis is arbitrarily defined as meningitis that persists for 4 or more weeks. It is important to document that patients are not in a slow recovery phase because this distinguishes them from patients with resolving acute meningitis.

Chronic meningitis is uncommon and accounts for less than 10% of all meningitis cases. It has the widest spectrum of causes and occurs in both immunocompetent and immunocompromised individuals. Chronic meningitis may be caused by many different pathogens and by noninfectious causes. The major infectious causes are tuberculous meningitis and cryptococcal meningitis. The major noninfectious causes are neoplastic disease, neurosarcoidosis, and vasculitis.

The CSF examination is helpful in differentiating the patient with chronic meningitis from the patient with acute meningitis, encephalitis, or recurrent meningitis. A mildly decreased glucose in the setting of mononuclear pleocytosis should raise the possibility of chronic meningitis.

Causes of Chronic Meningitis

Bacterial
- Agents causing sinus tracts (*Actinomycetes, Arachnia, Nocardia*)
- *Brucella*
- *Francisella tularensis*
- *Listeria monocytogenes*
- Mycobacterial (*Myobacterium tuberculosis, M. avium*)
- *Neisseria meningitidis*
- Spirochetal (*Borrelia burgdorferi, Leptospira interrogans, Treponema pallidum*)
- *Tropheryma whippelii*

Fungal
- *Candida* spp.
- *Cryptococcus neoformans*
- *Coccidioides immitis*
- *Histoplasma capsulatum*
- Other mycoses (*Aspergillus, Blastomyces, Dematiaceous* spp., *Paracoccidioides, Pseudoallescheria, Sporothrix, Trichosporon beigelii, Zygomycetes*)

Parasitic
- *Acanthamoeba*
- *Angiostrongylus*
- *Coenuris cerebralis*

- *Schistosoma* spp.
- *Taenia solium* (cysticercosis)
- *Toxoplasma gondii*

Viral

- Enteroviruses
- Herpesvirus
- Retroviruses (HIV-1, Human T-Lymphotropic Virus [HTLV]-1)

Noninfectious

- Behçet disease
- Chemical meningitis
- Fabry disease
- Hypertrophic pachymeningitis
- Neoplastic
- Neurosarcoidosis
- Systemic lupus erythematosus
- Uveomeningoencephalitides
- Vasculitis

Idiopathic

- Chronic benign lymphocytic meningitis

Key Historical Features

- ✓ Fever
- ✓ Headache
- ✓ Stiff neck
- ✓ Nausea and vomiting
- ✓ Photophobia
- ✓ Drowsiness
- ✓ Malaise
- ✓ Chronicity of symptoms
- ✓ Previous systemic infections (tuberculosis, fungal infection, syphilis)
- ✓ Medical history, especially malignancy, autoimmune disease, systemic vasculitis, or immunocompromised status
- ✓ Travel history
- ✓ Geographic risk factors
- ✓ Animal exposures
- ✓ Work exposures

Key Physical Findings

- ✓ Vital signs
- ✓ Funduscopic examination for papilledema
- ✓ Opthalmologic examination for eye lesions
- ✓ Neck examination for meningismus
- ✓ Lymph node examination for lymphadenopathy

✓ Dermatologic examination for skin lesions
✓ General examination for evidence of infection or systemic disease
✓ Neurologic examination

Suggested Work-Up for Chronic Meningitis

(Not all are necessary in all cases and should be guided by clinical suspicion.)

Blood tests
- Complete blood count with differential
- Serum chemistries
- Erythrocyte sedimentation rate
- Antinuclear antibodies
- HIV serology
- Rapid plasma regain (RPR)
- Consider angiotensin-converting enzyme (ACE), antineutrophilic cytoplasmic antibodies, specific serologies, blood smears
- CSF
- Cell count with differential, protein, glucose
- Cytology
- Venereal Disease Research Laboratory (VDRL) test
- Cultures (tuberculosis, fungal, bacterial, viral)
- Stain (Gram, acid fast, India ink)
- Cryptococcal antigen
- Oligoclonal bands, immunoglobulin-G index
- Consider ACE; polymer chain reaction (viruses, mycobacteria, *T. whippelii*); histoplasma antigen, immunocytochemistry (*T. whippelii* and other selected agents); paired antibodies for *B. burgdorferi, Brucella*, histoplasma, *Coccidioides*, other fungal agents; neoplastic markers

Neuroimaging
- Brain magnetic resonance (MR) imaging with contrast
- Consider computed tomography (CT), spinal MR imaging, angiography

Cultures
- Blood (parasites, fungi, viruses, rare bacteria)
- Urine (mycobacteria, viruses, fungi)
- Sputum (mycobacteria, fungi)
- Consider gastric washings, stool, bone marrow, liver (mycobacteria, fungi)

Ancillary
- Chest radiograph
- Electrocardiogram
- Selected testing (mammogram, CT chest/abdomen)

Biopsy
- Extraneural sites (bone marrow, lymph node, peripheral nerve, liver, lung, skin, small bowel)

Useful Serologic Tests in the Chronic Meningitis Syndrome

Bacteria
- *Borrelia burgdorferi*
- *Brucella*
- *Leptospira*
- *Treponema pallidum* (RPR, VDRL)

Fungi
- *Aspergillus* spp.
- *Coccidioides immitis*
- *Histoplasma capsulatum*
- *Sporothrix schenckii*
- *Zygomycetes*

Parasites
- *Taenia solium*
- *Toxoplasma gondii*

Viruses
- HIV-1
- HTLV-1

Further Reading

Coyle PK. Overview of acute and chronic meningitis. *Neurol Clin.* 1999;17:691–710.
Goetz. *Textbook of Clinical Neurology.* 2nd ed. Philadelphia: Saunders; 2003:511–514.

General Discussion

A complaint of constipation may mean very different things to different patients. Patients tend to define constipation differently than physicians, so a complaint of constipation may mean infrequent bowel movements, straining while stooling, incomplete evacuation, abdominal pain, abdominal bloating, hard stools, small stools, or a need for digital manipulation to enable defecation.

The Rome III diagnostic criteria are widely used in research and provide a reproducible definition of functional constipation. The criteria must be fulfilled for the last 3 months, with symptom onset at least 6 months before diagnosis:

1. Must include two or more of the following:
   - Straining during at least 25% of defecations
   - Lumpy or hard stool in at least 25% of defecations
   - Sensation of incomplete evacuation for at least 25% of defecations
   - Sensation of anorectal obstruction/blockage for at least 25% of defecations
   - Manual maneuvers to facilitate at least 25% of defecations (e.g., digital evacuation, support of the pelvic floor)
   - Less than three defecations per week
2. Loose stools are rarely present without the use of laxatives
3. Insufficient criteria for irritable bowel syndrome

Chronic constipation can be divided into functional (primary) and secondary constipation. The Rome III diagnostic criteria define functional constipation, which can be further divided into normal transit (perception of constipation by patient but with normal stool movement throughout the colon), slow transit (prolonged transit time through the colon), and outlet constipation (also known as pelvic floor dysfunction, which is incoordination of the muscles of the pelvic floor during attempted evacuation). Constipation is not a normal part of aging, but may result from inadequate consumption of fluids, immobility, and secondary causes. Secondary constipation is caused by the medical conditions or medications listed in the following.

There are a wide variety of potential causes of constipation, and the majority of individuals with constipation do not have an identifiable cause to explain their symptoms. Constipation may occur due to an alteration in stool consistency, stool caliber, or colonic motility. Constipation also may result from a change in the process of rectal evacuation, usually due to an obstruction of the movement of luminal contents or poor colonic propulsive activity. It is important to distinguish functional constipation from other disorders that may be associated with altered bowel habits. The evaluation of constipation aims to exclude systemic disease or a structural disorder of the intestines.

Medications Associated with Constipation

Adrenergic agents
Antacids (aluminum or calcium)
Anticholinergic agents
Anticonvulsants
Antidiarrheal agents
Antihistamines
Antiparkinson drugs
Antipsychotics
Antispasmodics
Barium sulfate
Beta-blockers
Calcium supplements
Calcium channel blockers
Diuretics
Iron supplements
Nonsteroidal anti-inflammatory drugs
Opioids
Sucralfate
Sympathomimetics
Tricyclic antidepressants

Causes of Constipation

Adhesions
Amyloidosis
Anal fissures
Anorexia nervosa
Autonomic neuropathy
Bulimia nervosa
Cerebrovascular disease
Cognitive impairment
Colorectal cancer
Congenital megacolon (Hirschsprung disease)
Depression
Dermatomyositis
Diabetes mellitus
External compression
Heavy metal poisoning
Hirschsprung disease
Hypercalcemia
Hypokalemia

Hypomagnesemia
Hypopituitarism
Hypothyroidism
Immobility
Inflammatory stricture
- Diverticulitis
- Inflammatory bowel disease
- Postischemic injury

Irritable bowel syndrome (constipation: predominant type)
Leiomyoma
Lipoma
Medications
Multiple sclerosis
Muscular dystrophies
Myopathy
Myotonic dystrophy
Neurofibromatosis
Neuropathy
- Aganglionosis
- Hyperganglionosis
- Chagas disease
- Idiopathic
- Paraneoplastic

Parkinson disease
Pelvic floor weakness
Pelvic outlet obstruction
Pheochromocytoma
Porphyria
Pregnancy
Primary functional constipation
- Slow-transit constipation
- Pelvic floor dysfunction

Rectocele
Shy Drager syndrome
Spinal cord injury
Systemic sclerosis
Uremia

Key Historical Features

✓ Size, consistency, and frequency of the bowel movements
✓ Onset and duration of the symptoms
✓ Sense of incomplete evacuation
✓ Stool caliber
✓ Pain, bloating, or intestinal cramping between bowel movements (could be symptoms of irritable bowel syndrome)

✓ Prolonged and excessive straining with soft stools, or a need for digital manipulation to pass stools (suggests pelvic floor dysfunction)
✓ Red flag symptoms
  • Weight loss
  • Melena
  • Rectal bleeding
  • Changes in bowel habits or stool caliber
  • Fever
  • Abdominal pain or cramping
  • Nausea or vomiting
  • Rectal pain
✓ Dietary habits and fluid intake
✓ Bowel habits
✓ History of fecal incontinence
✓ Work habits
✓ Level of physical activity
✓ Medical history
✓ Surgical and obstetrical history
✓ Medications
✓ Laxative, supplement, and vitamin use

Key Physical Findings

✓ Vital signs
✓ Abdominal examination for bowel sounds, masses, distention, tenderness, organomegaly, and surgical scars
✓ Perineal examination for hemorrhoids, skin tags, fissures, warts, or rectal prolapse
✓ Assessment of the anocutaneous reflex
✓ Digital rectal examination
✓ Color and consistency of the stool
✓ Detailed neurological examination
✓ Body hair and skin examination for signs of hypothyroidism
✓ Signs of depression or anxiety

Suggested Work-Up

Diagnostic tests are not routinely recommended in the initial evaluation of a patient with chronic constipation in the absence of red flag signs or symptoms. If the history and physical examination suggest organic disease, the following studies may be appropriate:

Complete blood count	To evaluate for anemia or infection
Thyroid-stimulating hormone	To evaluate for hypothyroidism
Calcium	To evaluate for hypercalcemia
Glucose	To evaluate for diabetes mellitus
Electrolytes	To evaluate for hyopkalemia

Magnesium	To evaluate for hypomagnesemia
Blood urea nitrogen and creatinine	To evaluate for renal disease
Stool for occult blood	To evaluate for gastrointestinal malignancy or other causes of bleeding
Endoscopic evaluation	American Society for Gastrointestinal Endoscopy indications for endoscopy in patients with constipation:

- Age older than 50 years with no previous colorectal cancer screening
- Before surgery for constipation
- Change in stool caliber
- Heme-positive stools
- Iron deficiency anemia
- Obstructive symptoms
- Recent onset of constipation
- Rectal bleeding
- Rectal prolapse
- Weight loss

Additional Work-Up

Abdominal radiographs	Can detect retained stool and suggest evidence of impaction or volvulus
Serum protein electrophoresis and urine protein electrophoresis	If multiple myeloma is suspected
Anorectal manometry	To assess the anal sphincter, pelvic floor, and associated nerves. Helps to exclude Hirschsprung disease.
Balloon insertion	To evaluate for pelvic floor dysfunction
Defecography	For patients with intractable constipation or pelvic floor disorders to evaluate evacuatory disorders, such as rectal prolapse and rectocele
Colonic transit studies	To evaluate the rate of colonic transit and to rule out pelvic outlet obstruction

Further Reading

Arce DA, Ermocilla CA, Costa H. Evaluation of constipation. *Am Fam Physician*. 2002;65:2283–2290.

Borum ML. Constipation: evaluation and management. *Prim Care Clin Office Pract*. 2001;28:577–590.

Drossman DA, Dumitrascu DL. Rome III: new standard for functional gastrointestinal disorders. *J Gastrointest Liver Dis*. 2006;15:237–241.

Faigel DO. A clinical approach to constipation. *Clin Cornerstone*. 2002;4:11–21.

Jamshed N, Zone-En L, Olden KW. Diagnostic approach to chronic constipation in adults. *Am Fam Physician*. 2011;84:299–306.

Locke III GR, Pemberton JH, Phillips SF. AGA technical review on constipation. American Gastroenterological Association. *Gastroenterology*. 2000;119:1766–1778.

Longstreth GF, Thompson WG, Chey WD, et al. Functional bowel disorders. *Gastroenterology*. 2006;130:1486 [published correction appears in *Gastroenterology*. 2006;131(2):688].

Qureshi W, Adler DG, Davila RE, et al. ASGE guideline: guideline on the use of endoscopy in the management of constipation. *Gastrointest Endosc*. 2005;62:199–201.

Rao SSC. Constipation: evaluation and treatment. *Gastroenterol Clin N Am*. 2003;32:659–683.

Thompson WG, Longstreth GF, Drossman DA, et al. Functional bowel disorders and functional abdominal pain. *Gut*. 1999;45(suppl II):43–47.

General Discussion

Delirium is an acute disturbance in mental status characterized by fluctuating levels of consciousness and attention impairment. Fluctuations in cognitive skills such as memory, language, and organization are common. In general, any patient with acute onset of confusion or mental deterioration should be considered to be delirious until another diagnosis is found. The following is a list of the *Diagnostic and Statistical Manual of Mental Disorders-V* criteria for delirium:

1. A disturbance in attention (i.e., reduced ability to direct, focus, sustain, and shift attention) and awareness (reduced orientation to the environment).

2. The disturbance develops over a short period of time (usually hours to a few days), represents a change from baseline attention and awareness, and tends to fluctuate in severity during the course of a day.

3. An additional disturbance in cognition (e.g., memory deficit, disorientation, language, visuospatial ability, or perception).

4. The disturbances in criteria 1 and 3 are not explained by another preexisting, established, or evolving neurocognitive disorder and do not occur in the context of a severely reduced level of arousal, such as coma.

5. There is evidence from the history, physical examination, or laboratory findings that the disturbance is a direct physiological consequence of another medical condition, substance intoxication or withdrawal (i.e., due to drug abuse or to a medication), or exposure to a toxin or is due to multiple etiologies.

The three subtypes of delirium are hyperactive, hypoactive, and mixed. Patients with the hyperactive subtype may demonstrate restlessness, anxiety, sleep disturbances, irritability, increased psychomotor activity, emotional lability, anger, and euphoria. The presentation of the hyperactive subtype may mimic schizophrenia, psychotic disorder, or agitated dementia. Patients with the hypoactive subtype may demonstrate reduced attention, altered arousal, decreased psychomotor activity, sadness, and disorientation. The mixed subtype is characterized by fluctuations between the hyperactive and hypoactive subtypes.

Other clinical features of delirium include delusions, hallucinations, disorganized thinking, incoherent speech, memory impairment, and disorientation to time, place, or person. Neurologic abnormalities may be present, including dysgraphia, tremor, myoclonus, reflex changes, and tone changes.

Delirium is often initially misdiagnosed as depression or dementia. In distinguishing delirium from depression, an evaluation of the onset and timeline of depressive and cognitive symptoms is important. The degree of cognitive impairment in delirium is much more severe and pervasive than in depression, with a more abrupt temporal onset. In addition, delirium manifests a disturbance in arousal or consciousness, whereas this is usually not a feature of depression. When considering dementia, it is important to remember that the patient with dementia is alert and does not have the disturbance of consciousness or arousal that is characteristic of delirium. Dementia is characterized by a more gradual onset of symptoms and is chronically progressive, with less impairment of the sleep–wake cycle.

Despite advances in medical technology, the cornerstone in the evaluation of delirium remains the history and physical examination. After a thorough evaluation, laboratory testing and diagnostic imaging may be warranted, but these should be individualized on a case-by-case basis. It may be helpful to keep in mind the five leading causes of delirium: (1) fluid/electrolyte disturbances; (2) infection; (3) medication toxicity; (4) metabolic derangement; and (5) sensory and environmental disturbances.

Medications Associated with Delirium

Antiarrhythmics
- Amiodarone
- Disopyramide
- Quinidine

Antibiotics
- Antimalarials
- Isoniazid
- Linezolid
- Macrolides
- Quinolones

Anticholinergic agents

Antiemetics

Anticonvulsant agents
- Carbamazepine
- Phenytoid

Antihistamines
- Diphenhydramine
- Histamine H_2 blockers
- Gastrointestinal antispasmodics
- Urinary antispasmodics

Antihypertensives
- Beta-blockers
- Clonidine
- Methyldopa
- Reserpine

Antiparkinson drugs
- Amantadine
- Bromocriptine

- Levodopa/carbidopa
- Pergolide

Antipsychotic agents

Antivirals

- Acyclovir
- Interferon

Aspirin

Benzodiazepines

- Diazepam
- Lorazepam
- Temazepam

Benztropine

Beta-blockers

Calcium channel blockers

Chemotherapeutic agents

- Asparaginase
- Bleomycin
- Carmustine
- Cisplatin
- Fluorouracil
- Procarbazine
- Methotrexate
- Vinblastine
- Vincristine

Cold remedies

Corticosteroids

Cyclosporine

Diphenhydramine

Digoxin

Diuretics

Gastrointestinal antispasmodics

Histamine$_2$-receptor blockers

- Cimetidine
- Famotidine
- Nizatidine
- Ranitidine

Hypoglycemic agents

- Glimepiride
- Glipizide
- Glyburide

Ipratropium (inhaled)

Lithium

Meperidine

Metoclopramide

Muscle relaxants

Narcotics
- Hydromorphone
- Levorphanol
- Meperidine
- Morphine sulfate

Nonsteroidal anti-inflammatory drugs

Oxybutynin

Sleep aids and/or sedative hypnotics

Tricyclic antidepressants

Causes of Delirium

Anemia

Cardiovascular disease
- Acute myocardial infarction
- Arrhythmia
- Congestive heart failure
- Hypertensive encephalopathy
- Hypotension
- Ischemia

Fluid and electrolyte disturbances
- Dehydration
- Hypercalcemia
- Hyperkalemia
- Hypernatremia
- Hypocalcemia
- Hypokalemia
- Hypomagnesemia
- Hyponatremia
- Hypotension

Fracture

Hepatic disease
- Hepatic insufficiency

Infection
- Bacteremia
- Cholecystitis
- Diverticulitis
- Encephalitis
- Herpes zoster
- HIV infection
- Meningitis
- Pneumonia
- Sepsis
- Tetanus
- Tuberculosis
- Urinary tract infection

Malignancy and paraneoplastic syndromes
Medications
Metabolic abnormalities
- Hypoglycemia
- Hypoxia
- Parathyroid dysfunction
- Renal insufficiency
- Thyroid dysfunction
- Vitamin deficiencies

Neurologic disease
- Cerebral vasculitis
- Cerebrovascular accident
- Seizure
- Subdural hematoma (acute and chronic)
- Temporal arteritis

Physical restraints
Pulmonary disease
- Pulmonary embolism

Shock
Sleep deprivation
Surgery
Toxins
- Alcohol
- Drugs

Uncontrolled pain
Urinary or stool retention
Withdrawal syndromes
- Alcohol
- Benzodiazepines
- Other sedatives

Key Historical Features

✓ Patient age
✓ Premorbid condition and functional level
- Occupation
- Level of alertness
- Ability for self-care
- Intellectual activity
✓ History of present illness
- Onset
- Rate of symptom development
- Course over the last 24 hours
- Patient's physical complaints
- Recent falls or head trauma

- ✓ Medical history
- ✓ Surgical history, especially recent surgery
- ✓ Medications
- ✓ Over-the-counter medications, herbal remedies, and supplements
- ✓ Substance use (alcohol, tobacco, recreational drugs)

Key Physical Findings

- ✓ Vital signs
- ✓ Pulse oximetry
- ✓ Funduscopic examination
- ✓ Head, ears, eyes, nose, throat examination for dilated pupils or flushing
- ✓ Cardiovascular examination
- ✓ Pulmonary examination
- ✓ Abdominal examination for evidence of gastrointestinal pathology
- ✓ Evidence of trauma, metabolic disturbance, dehydration, or sepsis
- ✓ Neurologic examination for focal deficits, asterixis, tremor, myoclonus, or evidence of central nervous system infection
- ✓ Mini mental status examination

Suggested Work-Up

Mini mental status examination	To assess cognitive status
Complete blood count	To assess for infection or anemia
Electrolytes	To evaluate for sodium or potassium disturbances
Blood urea nitrogen and creatinine	To assess renal function
Blood glucose	To evaluate for hypo- or hyperglycemia
Calcium	To evaluate for calcium disturbances
Aspartate aminotransferase, alanine aminotransferase, and albumin	To evaluate for hepatic abnormalities
Urinalysis	To evaluate for urinary tract infection
Chest x-ray	To evaluate for pulmonary infection or cardiopulmonary disease
Electrocardiogram	For elderly patients or patients with a cardiac history or cardiac risk factors
Head computed tomography or magnetic resonance imaging	For patients with a history of falls, suspected trauma, or focal neurologic findings

Additional Work-Up

Encephalogram	May be used to differentiate delirium from other conditions and to rule out ictal and postictal seizure activity (delirium demonstrates a diffuse slowing of the background rhythm)
Troponin	If acute myocardial infarction is suspected
Erythrocyte sedimentation rate	If vasculitis or an inflammatory or rheumatologic condition is suspected
Lumbar puncture/cerebrospinal fluid examination	For febrile patients when meningitis or encephalitis is suspected
Toxicology screening	When toxin exposure is suspected
Levels of prescribed drugs	For appropriate drugs in which elevated levels may cause delirium
Arterial blood gas	To further evaluate hypoxia or acid/base disturbances

Further Reading

American Psychiatric Association. *Diagnostic and Statistical Manual of Mental Disorders.* 5th ed. Washington, DC: American Psychiatric Association; 2013.

Breitbart W, Strout D. Delirium in the terminally ill. *Clin Geriatr Med.* 2000;16:357–372.

Gleason OC. Delirium. *Am Fam Physician.* 2003;67:1027–1034.

Inouye SK. Delirium in older persons. *New Engl J Med.* 2006;354:1157–1165 [published correction appears in *New England Journal of Medicine* 2006;354:1655].

Jacobson SA. Delirium in the elderly. *Psychiatr Clin North Am.* 1997;20:91–110.

Kalish VB, Gillham JE, Unwin BK. Delirium in older persons: evaluation and management. *Am Fam Physician.* 2014;90:150–158.

Marsh CM. Psychiatric presentations of medical illness. *Psychiat Clin North Am.* 1997;20:181–204.

Murphy BA. Delirium. *Emerg Med Clin North Am.* 2000;18:243–252. Washington, DC, American Psychiatric Association, 2000.

Winawer N. Postoperative delirium. *Med Clin North Am.* 2001;85:1229–1239.

General Discussion

Diarrhea is a change in stools, usually defined clinically as the passage of three or more loose or watery stools or one or more bloody stool in 24 hours. Acute diarrhea lasts less than 14 days, persistent diarrhea lasts more than 14 days, and chronic diarrhea lasts more than 4 weeks.

Patients who present with acute diarrhea are more likely to have an infectious cause. Viral infections are the most common cause of acute diarrhea. Bacterial infections are more often associated with travel, comorbidities, and foodborne illness. Parasite infections are less common. Noninfectious causes include medication adverse effects, acute abdominal processes, gastroenterological disease, and endocrine disease. Most cases of acute diarrhea are self-limited and do not require further evaluation. Indications for stool studies in acute diarrhea include fever, bloody diarrhea, history of travel to an endemic area, recent antibiotic use, a history of inflammatory bowel disease, exposure to infants in day care centers, and a history of anal intercourse. If the patient does not meet these criteria, but the diarrhea persists for more than a few days, a more detailed evaluation is warranted.

Patients with chronic diarrhea have a much broader group of diagnoses to consider. Chronic diarrhea may be divided into categories such as watery, malabsorptive, or inflammatory; however, some categories overlap. Watery diarrhea may be subdivided into osmotic (water retention due to poorly absorbed substances), secretory (reduced water absorption), and functional (hypermotility). Secretory diarrhea can be differentiated from osmotic and functional diarrhea by higher stool volumes that continue despite fasting, and it occurs at night. The following list provides an outline of most causes for diarrhea.

The medical history is the key to the evaluation of most patients presenting with diarrhea and can help guide the diagnostic workup. Important historical features are outlined in the following.

Causes of Acute Diarrhea

Endocrine causes
- Addison disease
- Carcinoid syndrome
- Gastrinoma
- Hyperthyroidism
- Mastocytosis
- Medullary carcinoma of the thyroid
- Somatostatinoma
- Vasoactive intestinal peptide (VIP)

Gastrointestinal causes
- Bowel obstruction
- Celiac disease
- Colorectal cancer
- Constipation with overflow
- Crohn disease
- Irritable bowel syndrome
- Ischemic colitis
- Lactose intolerance
- Malabsorption
- Short bowel syndrome
- Ulcerative colitis

Infectious causes

Bacteria
- Aeromonas
- *Bacillus cereus*
- Campylobacter
- Chlamydia
- *Clostridium difficile*
- *Clostridium perfringens*
- Enterotoxigenic *Escherichia coli*
- Gonorrhea
- Listeria
- *Mycobacterium avium-intracellulare* complex
- Other *E. coli*
- Salmonella
- *Staphylococcus aureus*
- Shigella
- Syphilis
- Tuberculosis
- *Vibrio cholera*
- *Vibrio parahaemolyticus*
- Yersinia

Parasites
- *Cryptosporidium*
- *Cyclospora*
- *Entamoeba histolytica*
- *Giardia*
- *Isospora belli*
- *Microsporida*
- *Schistosoma*
- *Strongyloides*
- *Trichuris*

Viruses
- Cytomegalovirus
- Herpes simplex

- Noroviruses
- Rotavirus

Medications
- Angiotensin-converting enzyme inhibitors
- Antacids
- Antibiotics
- Chemotherapy
- Cholesterol-lowering medications
- Colchicine
- Laxatives
- Lithium
- Mannitol
- Nonsteroidal anti-inflammatory drugs (NSAIDs)
- Proton pump inhibitors

Other
- Adnexitis
- Appendicitis
- Amyloidosis
- Diverticulitis
- HIV infection
- Pelvic radiation therapy
- Postvagotomy diarrhea
- Systemic infections
- Vasculitis

Causes of Chronic Diarrhea

Watery

Secretory
- Alcoholism
- Bacterial enterotoxins (e.g., cholera)
- Bile acid malabsorption
- Brainerd diarrhea (epidemic secretory diarrhea)
- Congenital syndromes
- Crohn disease
- Endocrine disorders
- Medications
    - Antiarrhythmics (e.g., quinine)
    - Antibiotics
    - Antineoplastics
    - Biguanides
    - Calcitonin
    - Colchicine
    - Digitalis
    - NSAIDs

- - Prostaglandins
    - Ticlopidine
  - Microscopic colitis
  - Neuroendocrine tumors
  - Nonosmotic laxatives
    - Docusate
    - Senna
  - Postsurgical
    - Cholecystectomy
    - Gastrectomy
    - Intestinal resection
    - Vagotomy
  - Vasculitis

Osmotic
- Carbohydrate malabsorption syndromes
- Celiac disease
- Osmotic laxatives and antacids
  - Magnesium
  - Phosphate
  - Sulfate
- Sugar alcohols
  - Mannitol
  - Sorbitol
  - Xylitol

  Functional
  - Irritable bowel syndrome
  - Hypermotility from medications
    - Macrolides
    - Metoclopramide
    - Stimulant laxatives

Fatty

Malabsorptive
- Amyloidosis
- Carbohydrate malabsorption (e.g., lactose intolerance)
- Celiac disease
- Gastric bypass
- Giardiasis
- Lymphatic damage
  - Congestive heart failure
  - Lymphoma
- Medications
  - Acarbose
  - Aminoglycosides
  - Orlistat

- • Thyroid supplements
- • Ticlopidine
- • Mesenteric ischemia
- • Postresection diarrhea
- • Short bowel syndrome
- • Small bowel bacterial overgrowth
- • Tropical sprue
- • Whipple disease (*Tropheryma whippelii* infection)

Maldigestive
- • Hepatobiliary disorders
- • Inadequate luminal bile acid
- • Loss of regulated gastric emptying
- • Pancreatic exocrine insufficiency

Inflammatory or Exudative

Inflammatory bowel disease
- • Crohn disease
- • Diverticulitis
- • Ulcerative colitis
- • Ulcerative jejunoileitis

Invasive infectious diseases
- • *Clostridium difficile*
- • Invasive bacterial infections
  - • Tuberculosis
  - • Yersiniosis
- • Invasive parasitic infections
  - • *Entamoeba*
- • Ulcerating viral infections
  - • Cytomegalovirus
  - • Herpes simplex virus

Neoplasia
- • Colon carcinoma
- • Lymphoma
- • Villous adenocarcinoma

Radiation colitis

Key Historical Features

- ✓ Onset of illness
- ✓ Duration of symptoms
- ✓ Severity of symptoms
- ✓ Frequency of diarrhea
- ✓ Characterization of the stools
  - • Watery
  - • Bloody

- Mucus-filled
- Purulent
- Bilious

✓ Weight loss
✓ Presence of nocturnal diarrhea
✓ Presence of other gastrointestinal symptoms
- Nausea and vomiting
- Abdominal pain
- Fever
- Fecal urgency
- Grossly bloody stool

✓ Volume status
- Thirst
- Dizziness
- Urine output
- Syncope

✓ Travel to endemic areas
✓ Exposure to untreated water
✓ Dietary history
✓ Medication use (especially antibiotics or laxatives)
✓ Medical history, including history of radiation
✓ Surgical history
✓ Occupational exposures
✓ Immune status
✓ Sexual practices

Key Physical Findings

✓ Vital signs
- Fever
- Tachycardia
- Postural hypotension

✓ Findings of dehydration
- Mucous membranes
- Capillary refill
- Skin turgor

✓ Eye examination for evidence of episcleritis suggesting inflammatory bowel disease or exophthalmia suggesting hyperthyroidism
✓ Lymph node examination
✓ Skin examination or dermatitis herpetiformis suggesting celiac disease
✓ Abdominal examination
✓ Rectal examination (also consider anoscopy)
- Stool character
- Presence of blood
- Anal fistula

Suggested Work-Up for Acute or Persistent Diarrhea

Most watery diarrhea is self-limited, so testing is not usually indicated. Diagnostic investigation generally can be reserved for patients with severe dehydration, more severe illness, persistent fever, bloody stools, or immunosuppression. Cases of suspected nosocomial infection or outbreak also warrant further workup.

Complete blood count	To evaluate for an elevated white blood cell count, anemia, or hemoconcentration
Serum electrolytes	To evaluate for electrolyte disturbance
Blood urea nitrogen and creatinine	To evaluate for volume depletion or acute renal failure
Stool evaluation for white blood cells or lactoferrin	To evaluate for infectious causes of diarrhea
Stool occult blood testing	To evaluate for inflammatory causes of diarrhea.
Abdominal radiographs	In toxic patients to help confirm the diagnosis of colitis and to look for evidence of ileus or megacolon

Additional Work-Up for Acute or Persistent Diarrhea

Stool evaluation for ova and parasites	If a parasitic infection is suspected
Stool culture	If fecal white blood cells/lactoferrin are positive or if the stool is grossly bloody
Ameba serology	If amebiasis is suspected
Giardia antigen	If giardia infection is suspected
Clostridium difficile toxin testing	If the patient has recently been hospitalized or has been on antibiotics in the preceding 3 months or if the patient develops diarrhea in an institutional setting
Endoscopy	May be considered if the diagnosis is unclear after routine blood and stool tests or if symptoms persist

Suggested Work-Up for Chronic Diarrhea

The workup for acute or persistent diarrhea should be considered in addition to the workup outlined in the following.

Serum albumin	To evaluate protein levels/nutritional status
Erythrocyte sedimentation rate	To evaluate for inflammatory processes
Liver function testing	To evaluate liver function/inflammation
Fecal calprotectin	To evaluate for inflammatory bowel disease
Fecal fat concentration	To help detect pancreatic exocrine insufficiency. Steatorrhea suggests dysfunction of absorption by the small intestine.
Laxative screen	To detect laxative ingestion

Additional Work-Up for Chronic Diarrhea

Stool sodium and potassium concentrations	To calculate an osmotic gap in stool water to distinguish secretory from osmotic diarrhea
Stool pH	To help detect carbohydrate malabsorption or lactose intolerance. A pH of less than 5.5 suggests lactose intolerance.
Stool laxative screen	If laxative abuse is suspected
Stool magnesium level	If magnesium ingestion is suspected
Thyroid-stimulating hormone	To evaluate for hyperthyroidism if it is suspected clinically
Celiac panel	If celiac disease is suspected
Blood glucose	To evaluate for diabetes mellitus if it is suspected
Blood tests for hormone-secreting tumors	If hormone-secreting tumor is suspected
Adrenocorticotrophic hormone level	If adrenal insufficiency is suspected
Secretin test	If pancreatic insufficiency is suspected
Urine test for metanephrines	If pheochromocytoma is suspected
Computed tomography scan of the abdomen	To help detect small bowel disease, colonic disease, and pancreatic tumors
Sigmoidoscopy or colonoscopy	To evaluate for inflammatory bowel disease and tumors. Also allows biopsy to be performed.

Further Reading

Feldman M, Friedman LS, Sleisenger MH, eds. *Sleisenger & Fordtran's Gastrointestinal and Liver Disease: Pathophysiology, Diagnosis, and Management.* 7th ed. Philadelphia: Saunders; 2002:137.

Fine KD, Schiller LR. AGA technical review on the evaluation and management of chronic diarrhea. *Gastroenterology.* 1999;116:1464–1486.

Gore JI, Surawicz C. Severe acute diarrhea. *Gastroenterol Clin North Am.* 2003;32:1249–1267.

Lee SD, Surawicz CM. Infectious causes of chronic diarrhea. *Gastroenterol Clin.* 2001;30:679–692.

Schiller L, Sellin J. Diarrhea. In: Feldman LF, Sleisenger M, eds. *Gastrointestinal and Liver Disease,* vol. 1. 7th ed. Philadelphia: WB Saunders; 2002.

Schiller LR. Diarrhea. *Adv Gastroenterol.* 2000;84:1259–1274.

Yates J. Traveler's diarrhea. *Am Fam Physician.* 2005;71:2095–2100.

16 DYSPNEA

General Discussion

In its consensus statement, the American Thoracic Society has defined dyspnea as "a subjective experience of breathing discomfort that consists of qualitatively distinct sensations that vary in intensity." The experience of dyspnea derives from interactions among multiple physiological, psychological, social, and environmental factors. One of the more popular theories of dyspnea states that dyspnea results from a disassociation or a mismatch between central respiratory motor activity and incoming afferent information from receptors in the airways, lungs, and chest wall structures.

The development of shortness of breath is an expected outcome of over-exertion, such as occurs after running or heavy lifting. However, when dyspnea occurs at rest or during exertion that is less than expected, it is considered pathologic and a symptom of a disease state.

Many patients have a likely cause of dyspnea, such as exacerbation of known congestive heart failure, chronic obstructive pulmonary disease (COPD), or asthma. However, in other patients, the diagnosis may not be readily apparent even after a thorough history and physical examination. The first step in the evaluation of the patient with dyspnea is to determine the status of the patient: (1) distress with unstable vital signs; (2) distress with stable vital signs; or (3) no distress and stable vital signs. The next step in the evaluation of patients with dyspnea is to establish the primary organ system involved: pulmonary, cardiac, both, or neither.

Asthma, congestive heart failure, myocardial ischemia, COPD, interstitial lung disease, pneumonia, and psychogenic disorders account for approximately 85% of all cases of dyspnea. In the elderly patient, dyspnea is generally due to one of five major etiologies: (1) cardiac disease; (2) respiratory disease; (3) deconditioning/obesity; (4) respiratory muscle dysfunction; or (5) psychological disorders. The patient's age, comparison with peers, daily or usual activities, overall fitness level, and any other medical problems must be considered.

In most patients, the cause or causes of dyspnea can be determined by using the history and physical examination to identify common etiologies, particularly cardiac and pulmonary causes. In some cases, specific diagnostic testing or consultation may be required to establish or confirm the diagnosis.

Medications Associated with Dyspnea

Amiodarone (pneumonitis)
Aspirin overdose
Beta-blockers (may aggravate obstructive airway disease)
Methotrexate
Nitrofurantoin (pneumonitis)

Causes of Dyspnea

Cardiac causes
- Arrhythmia
  - Atrial fibrillation
  - Inappropriate sinus tachycardia
  - Sick sinus syndrome/bradycardia
- Asymmetric septal hypertrophy
- Cardiomyopathies
- Congestive heart failure
- Coronary artery disease/ischemia
- Myocardial infarction
- Pericardial effusion/tamponade
- Pericarditis
- Valvular disease
  - Aortic insufficiency/stenosis
  - Congenital heart disease
  - Mitral valve insufficiency/stenosis

Gastrointestinal
- Aspiration
- Gastroesophageal reflux disease

Metabolic and endocrine causes
- Carbon monoxide poisoning
- Metabolic acidosis
- Salicylate poisoning
- Thyroid disease
- Uremia

Medications

Neuromuscular causes
- Acidosis
- Amyotrophic lateral sclerosis
- Guillain-Barré syndrome
- Muscular dystrophies
- Myasthenia gravis
- Phrenic nerve palsy
- Poliomyelitis

Psychogenic causes
- Anxiety
- Depression
- Hyperventilation
- Pain
- Panic attacks
- Post-traumatic stress disorder
- Secondary gain/malingering
- Somatization disorder

Pulmonary causes
- Asbestosis
- Aspiration (may be due to gastroesophageal reflux disease)
- Asthma
- Berylliosis
- Bronchiectasis
- Bronchiolitis obliterans
- Bronchitis
- COPD
- Coal workers' lung
- Hypersensitivity pneumonitis
- Malignancy (primary or metastatic)
- Pleural effusion
- Pleural thickening
- Pneumoconiosis
- Pneumonia
- Pneumothorax
- Pulmonary edema
- Pulmonary embolism
- Pulmonary hypertension
- Radiation pneumonitis
- Restrictive lung disease
- Silicosis

Upper airway obstruction
- Croup
- Epiglottitis
- Foreign body aspiration
- Laryngeal disease
- Tracheal stenosis
- Tracheomalacia
- Vocal cord paralysis

Other causes
- Abdominal mass
- Anemia
- Aspirin overdose
- Chest wall deformities
- Deconditioning
- Food allergy
- Kyphoscoliosis
- Liver cirrhosis
- Obesity
- Opportunistic infection in an immunosuppressed patient
- Pain/splinting
- Thoracic burn with eschar formation
- Trauma

Key Historical Features

✓   Onset
✓   Duration
✓   Frequency
✓   Descriptive qualities
✓   Intensity
✓   Triggers
✓   Relieving factors
✓   Occurrence at rest or with exertion
✓   Orthopnea
✓   Paroxysmal nocturnal dyspnea
✓   Wheezing
✓   Edema
✓   Presence of cough or sputum production
✓   Fever
✓   Chest pain, radiation of pain, nausea, or diaphoresis
✓   Leg swelling, redness, warmth, or pain
✓   Sore throat
✓   Indigestion
✓   Dysphagia
✓   Hemoptysis
✓   Anxiety symptoms
✓   History of trauma
✓   History of scuba diving
✓   Medical history, especially heart disease
✓   Surgical history, especially recent surgery
✓   Medications
✓   Family history
✓   Smoking history and exposure to secondhand smoke
✓   Occupational exposures to asbestos, dust, or volatile chemicals

Key Physical Findings

✓   Vital signs
✓   Body weight to compare with previous values
✓   General appearance, mental status, ability to speak
✓   Observation of breathing pattern and use of accessory muscles
✓   Neck examination for distended neck veins, thyroid enlargement, tracheal position, and stridor
✓   Chest examination for dullness to percussion, subcutaneous emphysema, or kyphoscoliosis
✓   Cardiac examination for heart rate, murmurs, or extra heart sounds
✓   Pulmonary examination for breath sounds, wheezing, or rales

✓ Abdominal examination for hepatomegaly, masses, ascites, or hepatojugular reflux

✓ Extremity examination for edema or evidence of deep venous thrombosis. Digit examination for cyanosis or clubbing.

Suggested Work-Up

Pulse oximetry	To determine oxygenation level. Useful to measure at rest and after exercise.
Chest radiograph	To evaluate for conditions such as congestive heart failure, pulmonary edema, pneumonia, pneumothorax, or COPD
Electrocardiogram	To evaluate for ischemia, arrhythmia, or left ventricular hypertrophy
Spirometry	To distinguish obstructive lung disorders from restrictive lung disorders
Complete blood count	To evaluate for anemia, infection, or erythrocytosis
Electrolytes, blood urea nitrogen, creatinine, magnesium, and calcium	To evaluate for acid-base disturbances, intravascular volume disturbances, electrolyte abnormalities, or uremia

Additional Work-Up

Echocardiogram	To evaluate for heart failure, ventricular hypertrophy, valvular dysfunction, or elevated pulmonary artery pressures
Pulmonary function testing	To measure lung volumes and carbon monoxide diffusion in the lung
Brain natriuretic peptide	To distinguish between heart failure and pulmonary causes of dyspnea
Arterial blood gas	To provide information about altered pH, hypercapnia, hypocapnia, or hypoxemia
Troponin	If ischemia or infarction is suspected
Thyroid-stimulating hormone	If thyroid abnormality is suspected as a cause of dyspnea
Digoxin level	For patients taking digoxin
Treadmill stress test, stress thallium, or stress echocardiogram	For patients with known or suspected coronary artery disease in whom dyspnea may represent an anginal equivalent

Neck radiographs	If stridor is present or upper airway obstruction is suspected
D-Dimer	If deep venous thrombosis or pulmonary embolism is suspected
Bilateral venous compression ultrasonography plus either ventilation-perfusion scan or pulmonary computed tomography (CT) angiography, or pulmonary angiography	If pulmonary embolism is suspected
High-resolution computed tomography	May be helpful in diagnosing interstitial lung disease, pulmonary fibrosis, bronchiectasis, and pulmonary embolism
Holter monitor	To help diagnose intermittent arrhythmias that may result in dyspnea
Cardiac catheterization	May be required to confirm or diagnose less common causes of pulmonary hypertension
Esophageal pH monitoring	To help establish gastroesophageal reflux as the cause of dyspnea
Cardiopulmonary exercise testing	Helps quantify cardiac function, pulmonary gas exchange, ventilation, and physical fitness. May be useful in cases in which no apparent cause for dyspnea is found after a thorough evaluation.
Lung biopsy	May be indicated if interstitial lung disease or malignancy is suspected

Further Reading

American Thoracic Society. Dyspnea: mechanisms, assessment, and management: a consensus statement. *Am J Respir Crit Care Med.* 1999;159:321–340.

Karnani NG, Reisfield GM, Wilson GR. Evaluation of chronic dyspnea. *Am Fam Physician.* 2005;71:1529–1537.

Mahler DA, Fierro-Carrion G, Baird JC. Evaluation of dyspnea in the elderly. *Clin Geriatr Med.* 2003;19:19–33.

Morgan WC, Hodge HL. Diagnostic evaluation of dyspnea. *Am Fam Physician.* 1998;57:711–716.

Sarkar S, Amelung PJ. Evaluation of the dyspneic patient in the office. *Prim Care.* 2006;33:643–657.

Shiber JR, Santana J. Dyspnea. *Med Clin North Am.* 2006;90:453–479.

Wahls SA. Causes and evaluation of chronic dyspnea. *Am Fam Physician.* 2012;86:173–180.

Zoorob RJ, Campbell JS. Acute dyspnea in the office. *Am Fam Physician.* 2003;68:1803–1810.

General Discussion

Dysuria is the sensation of burning, pain, or discomfort on urination that is most often the result of infection or inflammation of the bladder and/or urethra. Infection may present as urethritis, cystitis, prostatitis, or pyelonephritis. Although dysuria is often equated with urinary tract infection, dysuria also may result from vaginitis, malformations of the urinary tract, malignancy, hormonal conditions, trauma, interstitial cystitis, neurogenic conditions, and psychogenic disorders.

The timing of the dysuria may help predict the location of the problem in the urinary tract. Discomfort at the start of urination suggests a urethral source of inflammation, whereas pain occurring over the suprapubic area upon completion of urination often indicates inflammation of the bladder.

Dysuria is much more common in women than in men, and it affects older men more than younger men, reflecting the impact of benign prostatic hyperplasia (BPH).

Urinary symptoms suggestive of cystitis may occur in the absence of an identifiable infection, a condition known as painful bladder syndrome and/or interstitial cystitis. The current understanding of this syndrome involves a disruption of bladder mucous produced by the urothelium to provide a protective coating for the bladder. Toxins in the urine are then able to penetrate the bladder wall, causing pelvic pain, bladder pain, urinary urgency, and/or urinary frequency. In the diagnostic evaluation, cystoscopy is indicated principally to rule out other pathologies in the bladder, including bladder cancer.

Medications and Supplements Associated with Dysuria

Anticholinergics
Cantharidin
Cyclophosphamide
Dopamine
Nonsteroidal anti-inflammatory drugs
Penicillin G
Pumpkin seeds
Saw palmetto
Ticarcillin

Causes of Dysuria

Anatomic issues
- BPH
- Bladder diverticula
- Urethral stricture

Infection
- Cervicitis
- Cystitis
- Epididymo-orchitis
- Prostatitis
- Schistosomiasis
- Urethritis (herpes simplex, chlamydia, gonorrhea)
- Vulvovaginitis

Hormonal causes
- Atrophy and dryness in postmenopausal women

Inflammatory disorders
- Autoimmune disorders
- Behcet syndrome
- Reactive arthritis

Medication and supplement side effects

Neoplasm
- Bladder cancer
- Penile cancer
- Prostate cancer
- Renal cell tumor
- Vaginal cancer
- Vulvar malignancy

Psychogenic disorders
- Anxiety
- Chemical dependency
- Chronic pain syndromes
- Depression
- Somatization
- Stress

Trauma
- Urethral instrumentation or catheter placement
- Urethral trauma during intercourse

Other causes
- Bicycle riding
- Horseback riding
- Interstitial cystitis
- Sensitivity to creams, sprays, soaps, or toilet paper
- Stones (renal, ureteral, and bladder)
- Urethral syndrome

Key Historical Features

✓ Onset and duration of dysuria
✓ Fever, chills, nausea, or vomiting
✓ Timing of dysuria, particularly if related to menstrual cycle

- ✓ Frequency of dysuria
- ✓ Severity
- ✓ Location of discomfort
- ✓ External versus internal dysuria
- ✓ Pain at onset of urination versus suprapubic pain after voiding
- ✓ Presence of hematuria
- ✓ Urinary frequency, urgency, or hesitation
- ✓ Nocturia
- ✓ Sexual habits
- ✓ Penile discharge
- ✓ Scrotal pain
- ✓ Perineal pain
- ✓ Vaginal discharge
- ✓ Dyspareunia
- ✓ Use of topical irritants, such as lubricants, douches, or soaps
- ✓ Back pain
- ✓ Joint pain
- ✓ Ocular symptoms
- ✓ Oral mucosal symptoms
- ✓ Medical history
- ✓ Surgical history
- ✓ Sexual history, including history of sexually transmitted diseases
- ✓ Tobacco use
- ✓ Medications
- ✓ Family history

Key Physical Findings

- ✓ Fever
- ✓ Head and neck examination for conjunctivitis or oral ulcers
- ✓ Abdominal examination to assess the kidneys and bladder
- ✓ Back examination for costovertebral angle tenderness
- ✓ Pelvic examination in women
- ✓ Perineal, penile, and testicular examination in men
- ✓ Digital rectal examination
- ✓ Inguinal lymphadenopathy
- ✓ Extremity examination for joint swelling or tenderness
- ✓ Skin examination for rash

Suggested Work-Up

Urinalysis	To evaluate for pyuria or hematuria
Urine culture	To accurately diagnose infection and determine antimicrobial susceptibility of infecting bacteria

Vaginal wet-mount preparation	To detect *Trichomonas vaginalis* and Candida species
Urethral smear or urine ligase chain reaction and polymerase chain reaction tests for *Neisseria gonorrhoeae* and *Chlamydia trachomatis*	To detect *N. gonorrhoeae* and *C. trachomatis* infections

Additional Work-Up

Urine cytology	If urinary tract malignancy is suspected
Cystoscopy	To detect bladder or urethral pathology and confirm the diagnosis of interstitial cystitis. Used in the evaluation of noninfectious hematuria.
Renal ultrasonography	If kidney or ureter pathology, such as abscess or hydronephrosis, is suspected
Bladder ultrasonography	If bladder or urethral stones are suspected or if bladder diverticula are suspected
Plain films of kidneys, ureters, and bladder	For rapid evaluation of suspected renal stones
Contrast computed tomography (CT) scan (preferred)	To visualize avascular structures such as infarcts, cysts, abscesses, and necrotic tumors
Noncontrast CT scan	To evaluate for renal stones/calcifications and to evaluate solid tissue in the urinary tract
Voiding cystourethrogram	To assess for abnormalities such as vesicoureteral reflux, neurogenic bladder, urethral strictures, diverticula, and benign prostatic hyperplasia
Intravenous pyelography	To evaluate recurrent urinary tract infection or localize ureteral calculi
Magnetic resonance imaging with gadolinium enhancement	To identify urinary obstruction or mass in patients with renal insufficiency or allergy to iodinated contrast media

Further Reading

Bremnor JD, Sadovsky R. Evaluation of dysuria in adults. *Am Fam Physician*. 2002;65:1589–1596.

French L, Phelps K, Pothula NR, Mushkbar S. Urinary problems in women. *Prim Care Clin Office Pract.* 2009;36:53–71.

Roberts RG, Hartlaub PP. Evaluation of dysuria in men. *Am Fam Physician.* 1999;60:865–872.

Thomas A, Woodard C, Rovner ES, Wein AJ. Urologic complications of nonurologic medications. *Urol Clin North Am.* 2003;30:123–131.

General Discussion

Edema is an accumulation of fluid in the intercellular tissue that occurs when local or systemic conditions disrupt the equilibrium between the interstitial and intravascular fluid spaces. This equilibrium is regulated by the capillary hydrostatic pressure gradient and the oncotic pressure gradient across the capillary. Increased capillary hydrostatic pressure, increased plasma volume, decreased plasma oncotic pressure (hypoalbuminemia), increased capillary permeability, or lymphatic obstruction can lead to the development of edema. The major causes of each of these events is reviewed in the following.

Edema may be benign or may indicate a systemic disease. As such, the etiology of edema should always be determined. Acute swelling of a limb (72 hours or less) suggests deep venous thrombosis (DVT), cellulitis, ruptured popliteal cyst, acute compartment syndrome, or a side effect of a calcium channel blocker. Generalized edema is more suggestive of chronic systemic conditions, such as congestive heart failure, renal disease, or hepatic disease. Dependent edema from venous insufficiency typically improves with elevation of the extremities and worsens with dependency.

Causes of Peripheral Edema

Increased capillary hydraulic pressure
- Acute pulmonary edema
- Cirrhosis
- Compartment syndrome
- Compression of the inferior vena cava or iliac veins
- Constrictive pericarditis
- DVT
- Heart failure (right ventricular failure)
- Hepatic venous obstruction
- Medications (see the following)
- Pregnancy
- Premenstrual edema
- Primary renal sodium retention
- Re-feeding edema
- Renal disease and nephritic syndrome
- Restrictive cardiomyopathy
- Tricuspid valvular disease
- Venous obstruction in an extremity

Decreased plasma oncotic pressure
- Cirrhosis
- Malabsorption
- Malnutrition

- Nephrotic syndrome
- Preeclampsia

Increased capillary permeability
- Adult respiratory distress syndrome
- Allergic reactions
- Angioedema
- Burns
- Cellulitis
- Chronic venous insufficiency
- Compartment syndrome
- Inflammation or local infection
- Interleukin-2 therapy
- Malignant ascites
- May-Thurner syndrome
- Reflex sympathetic dystrophy
- Trauma
- Urticaria

Lymphatic obstruction or increased interstitial oncotic pressure
- Congenital lymphedema
- Filariasis
- Hypothyroidism
- Lymphatic compression from tumor
- Lymphedema praecox
- Lymphedema tarda
- Malignant ascites
- Nodal enlargement from malignancy
- Postradiation
- Postsurgical (after axillary lymph node dissection, inguinal lymphadenectomy, or coronary artery bypass graft)
- Trauma

Other
- Idiopathic
- Medications
- Myxedema

Medications Associated with Peripheral Edema

Acyclovir
Beta-blockers
Calcium channel blockers (particularly dihydropyridines)
Celecoxib
Clonidine
Corticosteroids
Cyclophosphamide
Cyclosporine
Cytosine arabinoside

Docetaxel
Estrogens
Fludrocortisone
Granulocyte colony-stimulating factor
Granulocyte-macrophage colony-stimulating factor
Guanethidine
Hydralazine
Interferon-alfa
Interleukin-2
Interleukin-4
Methyldopa
Minoxidil
Mithramycin
Monoamine oxidase inhibitors
Nonsteroidal anti-inflammatory drugs
Phenylbutazone
Pramipexole
Progesterones
Reserpine
Testosterone
Thiazolidinediones (pioglitazone, rosiglitazone)
Trazodone
Vasodilators (diazoxide, hydralazine, minoxidil)

Key Historical Features

- ✓ Unilateral or bilateral edema
- ✓ Timing of the edema
- ✓ Improvement with changes in position
- ✓ Cardiopulmonary symptoms
- ✓ Abdominal symptoms
- ✓ Symptoms or history of sleep apnea
- ✓ Medical history (especially cardiac, renal, hepatic, and thyroid disease)
- ✓ Surgical history
- ✓ History of irradiation
- ✓ Medications

Key Physical Findings

- ✓ Eye examination for exophthalmos
- ✓ Thyroid examination
- ✓ Cardiovascular examination for evidence of jugular venous distension
- ✓ Pulmonary examination for crackles
- ✓ Abdominal examination for hepatomegaly or ascites
- ✓ Extremity examination for pitting, tenderness, or changes in skin temperature

✓ Skin examination for jaundice, erythema, hyperpigmentation, or ulceration

✓ Neurologic examination for tremor or asterixis

Suggested Work-Up

Blood urea nitrogen, creatinine, and urinalysis	To evaluate renal function
Liver enzymes	To evaluate for hepatic disease
Albumin level	To assess nutritional status and detect hepatic synthetic dysfunction
Thyroid-stimulating hormone	To evaluate for hypothyroidism
Brain natriuretic peptide (BNP)	To evaluate for congestive heart failure
D-dimer, electrocardiogram, and chest x-ray	To evaluate for cardiopulmonary disease

Additional Work-Up

The following studies may be indicated when preliminary findings warrant them.

D-dimer	If DVT is a consideration in a low-risk patient
Venous compression ultrasonography	If DVT is suspected
Duplex ultrasonography	If suspected chronic venous insufficiency requires confirmation
Serum and protein electrophoresis	To evaluate for multiple myeloma
24-hour urine collection or spot urine protein to creatinine ratio	To quantify the amount of proteinuria if proteinuria is found on the urinalysis
Echocardiography	If heart failure is suspected or suggested by an elevated BNP or for patients with sleep apnea
Sleep study	If sleep apnea is suspected
Magnetic resonance angiography with venography of the lower extremity and pelvis	For suspected proximal DVT if ultrasonography is negative
Invasive studies such as cardiac catheterization or biopsy	If warranted based upon clinical findings

Further Reading

Cho S, Atwood JE. Peripheral edema. *Am J Med.* 2002;113:580–586.

Davison JM. Edema in pregnancy. *Kidney Int.* 1997;51(suppl):S90–S96.

Ely JW, Osheroff JA, Chambliss ML, Ebell MH. Approach to leg edema of unclear etiology. *J Am Board Fam Med.* 2006;19:148–160.

Halperin AK, Cubeddu LX. The role of calcium channel blockers in the treatment of hypertension. *Am Heart J.* 1986;111:363–382.

Markham Jr RV, Gilmore A, Pettinger WA, et al. Central and regional hemodynamic effects and neurohumoral consequences of minoxidil in severe congestive heart failure and comparison to hydralazine and nitroprusside. *Am J Cardiol.* 1983;52:774–781.

O'Brien JG, Chennubhotla RV. Treatment of edema. *Am Fam Physician.* 2005;71:2111–2117.

Rose BD. Pathophysiology and etiology of edema. In: Rose BD, ed. *UpToDate.* Wellesley, MA: UpToDate; 2004.

Rose BD. *Renal Pathophysiology: The Essentials.* Baltimore: Williams & Wilkins; 1994.

Thomas ML, Lloyd SJ. Pulmonary edema associated with rosiglitazone and troglitazone. *Ann Pharmacother.* 2001;35:123–124.

Trayes KP, Studdiford JS, et al. Edema: diagnosis and management. *Am Fam Physician.* 2013;88:102–110.

Valentin JP, Ribstein J, Halimi JM, Mimran A. Effect of different calcium antagonists on transcapillary fluid shift. *Am J Hypertens.* 1990;3:491–495.

General Discussion

Cholestasis refers to the pathologic condition in which the liver's ability to secrete bile is impaired. Cholestasis is characterized by elevated serum alkaline phosphatase (AP) and γ-glutamyltransferase (GGT) out of proportion to elevation of aminotransferase enzymes. Cholestasis develops either from a defect in bile synthesis, impairment in bile secretion, or obstruction to bile flow. It may occur as a result of an acute or chronic process involving either the extrahepatic or intrahepatic biliary tree.

The highest concentration of AP is present in the liver and bone, so an elevation usually is attributed to either liver or bone disease. However, AP also is present in the intestines, kidneys, placenta, and leukocytes.

The first step in evaluating a patient with an elevated AP level is to try and identify the source of the AP. This can be performed either through fractionation of the isoenzymes by electrophoresis or by obtaining 5′-nucleotidase and GGT levels, both of which are elevated in hepatobiliary disease. The next step is to determine whether cholestasis is due to an intrahepatic or extrahepatic disease process. Cholestasis is considered intrahepatic when impairment in bile excretion occurs at the hepatocellular level, and it is extrahepatic when the bile duct is obstructed.

Drug-induced liver injury should be considered in the differential diagnosis in a patient with cholestasis and normal hepatobiliary imaging. An asymptomatic increase in liver enzymes can be observed, particularly increased AP, but jaundice with or without pruritis is a common presentation. When a drug-induced liver injury is suspected, cholestasis is defined as an increase in AP greater than two times normal and/or an alanine aminotransferase (ALT) to AP ratio of less than two.

Individuals with blood type O or B have been shown to have an elevation in serum AP after consumption of a fatty meal. The level of serum AP also varies by age. Women in the third trimester of pregnancy can have elevated serum AP levels because of influx from the placenta.

Medications Commonly Associated with Cholestatic Liver Injury

Anabolic steroids
Antibiotics

- Amoxicillin/clavulanate
- Cephalosporins
- Ciprofloxacin
- Clindamycin
- Macrolides
- Nitrofurantoin
- Penicillins
- Sulfonamides

- Tetracyclines
- Trimethoprim/sulfamethoxazole

Anticonvulsants
- Carbamazepine
- Phenytoin

Antifungals
- Terbinafine

Antihypertensives
- Enalapril
- Irbesartan
- Verapamil

Anti-inflammatory drugs
- Azathioprine
- Diclofenac
- Ibuprofen

Clopidogrel

Dietary supplements containing anabolic steroids

HIV medications
- Didanosine
- Nevirapine
- Stavudine

Oral contraceptives

Psychotropic medications
- Chlorpromazine
- Duloxetine
- Tricyclic antidepressants

Trazodone

Causes of Elevated Alkaline Phosphatase

Extrahepatic cholestasis
   Extrinsic obstruction
- Stones (choledocholithiasis)
   Malignancy
- Ampullary cancer
- Cholangiocarcinoma
- Gallbladder
- Metastatic
- Pancreas
    - Pancreatitis
    - Pancreatic pseudocyst
    - Parasitic infection
    - Secondary sclerosis

Intrahepatic cholestasis
- Autoimmune cholangitis (primary sclerosing cholangitis (PSC)-like)
- Autoimmune cholangiopathy

Genetic
- Benign recurrent intrahepatic cholestasis
- Drugs and herbal remedies
- Dubin-Johnson or Rotor syndrome
- Progressive familial intrahepatic cholestasis

Granulomatous liver disease
- Infections
- Sarcoidosis

Hepatitis
- Alcoholic
- Hepatitis B
- Hepatitis C

Idiopathic adult ductopenia

Malignancy
- Hepatocellular
- Metastatic

Postoperative state

Pregnancy

Primary biliary cirrhosis (PBC)

PSC

Prolonged total parenteral nutrition

Sepsis

Nonhepatic

Bone disease
- Healing fracture
- Malignancy (osteogenic sarcoma, metastatic)
- Osteomalacia
- Paget disease
- Rickets
- Vitamin D deficiency

Endocrine
- Hyperparathyroidism
- Hyperthyroidism

Heart
- Heart failure

Malignancy
- Leukemia
- Lymphoma
- Multiple endocrine neoplasia type II
- Renal cell carcinoma

Physiologic
- Adolescence
- After a fatty meal in patients with blood group O or B
- Pregnancy

Renal
- Renal failure

Physiologic	Pregnancy
	Adolescence
	Following a fatty meal in subjects with blood group O or B
Bone disease	Healing fracture
	Paget disease
	Osteomalacia
	Vitamin D insufficiency
	Rickets
	Malignancy: osteogenic sarcoma, metastatic
Renal	Renal failure
Heart	Heart failure
Endocrine	Hyperthyroid
	Hyperparathyroid
Malignancy	Lymphoma
	Leukemia
	Renal cell carcinoma
	Multiple endocrine neoplasia II

Table 19-1. Nonhepatic Causes of Elevated Alkaline Phosphatase

Intrahepatic Cholestasis	Extrahepatic Cholestasis
Hepatitis: viral (B, C), alcoholic	Extrinsic obstruction
Genetic	• Stones
• Benign recurrent intrahepatic cholestasis	Malignancy
• Progressive familial intrahepatic cholestasis	• Pancreas
• Dubin-Johnson, Rotor syndrome	• Gallbladder
• Drugs and herbal remedies	• Metastatic
Pregnancy	• Cholangiocarcinoma
PBC	• Ampullary cancer
PSC	Pancreatitis
Granulomatous liver disease	Pancreatic pseudocyst
• Infections	Parasitic infection
• Sarcoidosis	Secondary sclerosis (surgery, chemotherapy)
Infiltrative	
• Amyloidosis	
• Lymphoma	
Idiopathic adult ductopenia	
Autoimmune cholangitis (PSC-like)	
Autoimmune cholangiopathy (PBC-like)	
Prolonged TPN	
Postoperative state	
Sepsis	
Malignancy	
• Hepatocellular	
• Metastatic	

PBC, Primary biliary cirrhosis; *PSC,* primary sclerosing cholangitis; *TPN,* total parenteral nutrition.

From Siddique A, Kowdley KV. Approach to a patient with elevated serum alkaline phosphatase. *Clin Liver Dis* 2012;16:199–229.

Table 19-2. Causes of Cholestatic Liver Disease

Key Historical Features

✓ Fever
✓ Chills
✓ Right upper quadrant pain
✓ Jaundice
✓ Pruritis
✓ Fatigue
✓ Medical history
✓ Surgical history
✓ Family history of cholestatic liver disease
✓ Medications, herbal remedies, and over-the-counter medications
✓ Social history, especially alcohol consumption and recreational drug use

Key Physical Findings

✓ Cardiopulmonary examination for evidence of pleural effusion, suggesting ascites
✓ Abdominal examination for pain, hepatomegaly, or ascites
✓ Stigmata of liver disease, such as gynecomastia, palmar erythema, spider nevi, and caput medusa
✓ Lymph node examination for enlarged left supraclavicular node or periumbilical nodule, suggesting abdominal malignancy
✓ Genitourinary examination for testicular atrophy, suggesting advanced cirrhosis

Suggested Work-Up

Fractionation of the AP isoenzymes by electrophoresis or 5′-nucleotidase and GGT levels	To determine the source of the AP

If the liver is the source of the elevated AP:

Abdominal ultrasound	To evaluate for intrahepatic and extrahepatic biliary dilatation

If ultrasound shows no biliary dilatation, proceed to evaluation for intrahepatic cholestasis:

Complete blood count with differential	To evaluate for infection or hematologic malignancy
Aspartate aminotransferase, ALT, GGT	To evaluate for hepatocellular disease
Albumin, bilirubin, prothrombin time	To evaluate liver synthetic function
Antinuclear antibody	May suggest autoimmune hepatitis

Smooth muscle antibody	To evaluate for autoimmune hepatitis
Antimitochondrial antibody (AMA)	Positive AMA is highly suggestive of PBC
Pronuclear antineutrophil cytoplasmic antibody	To evaluate for primary sclerosing cholangitis
Immunoglobulin levels	Elevated immunoglobulin-M (IgM) suggests PBC, elevated IgA suggests alcoholic liver disease, and elevated IgG suggests autoimmune hepatitis

Additional Work-Up

Magnetic resonance cholangiopancreatography	To evaluate for lesions causing extrahepatic obstruction. Indicated if patient presents with jaundice and weight loss to evaluate for pancreatic cancer or cholangiocarcinoma.
Endoscopic ultrasound	To evaluate (and help biopsy) the pancreas, pancreatic ducts, and bile ducts
Endoscopic cholangiopancreatography	The gold standard for visualizing the biliary tract to identify the cause and level of obstruction. Brushings and biopsy can be obtained, and therapeutic intervention (e.g., stone extraction or dilation, and stenting of biliary strictures) can be performed.
Liver biopsy	May be required when the diagnosis is unclear or for staging purposes

Further Reading

Bjornsson ES, Jonasson JG. Drug-induced cholestasis. *Clin Liver Dis*. 2013;17:191–209.

Leise MD, Poterucha JJ, Talwalkar JA. Drug-induced liver injury. *Mayo Clin Proc*. 2014;89:95–106.

Siddique A, Kowdley KV. Approach to a patient with elevated serum alkaline phosphatase. *Clin Liver Dis*. 2012;16:199–229.

Woreta TA, Alqahtani SA. Evaluation of abnormal liver tests. *Med Clin North Am*. 2014;98:1–16.

General Discussion

Amylase traditionally has been used to diagnose pancreatitis, although with the increased availability of serum lipase, it is relied upon less frequently. The two main sources of amylase are the pancreas and salivary glands, although lower levels can be found in other tissues, including the small intestine, ovaries, fallopian tubes, testes, lungs, thyroid, mammary glands, and tonsils. Serum amylase can be broken down into its two amylase isoenzymes, p-type and s-type, which predominantly reflect pancreatic and/or intestinal and salivary gland activity, respectively.

Amylase was first used in clinical medicine in the early 20th century when its link to pancreatic inflammation was discovered, and for many years, it served as the laboratory gold standard for diagnosing pancreatitis. It has since been found that hyperamylasemia is found in many other diseases. In addition, amylase is rapidly cleared through a combination of renal and extra-renal pathways, with a half-life of approximately 2 hours, making its application in clinical care somewhat limited. Serum amylase levels peak within 24 to 48 hours after the onset of abdominal pain in acute pancreatitis, but because of its rapid clearance, it remains elevated for a shorter time than other markers, such as serum lipase, which carries a greater sensitivity and specificity.

Although pancreatic inflammation is the most often cited clinical association of amylase, many pancreatic, gastrointestinal, salivary, and other conditions can be associated with elevated levels. Specifically, trauma or inflammation of the gastrointestinal tract, including infection, perforation, and surgery, can result in a transient elevation in amylase. Salivary gland irritation from alcoholism, infections such as mumps, eating disorders such as anorexia and bulimia, and radiation can also cause elevated amylase levels. Even pregnancy can be associated with high amylase levels. Thus, the clinical context, with an accurate history and physical examination, is paramount when approaching hyperamylasemia.

Medications Associated with Amylase Elevation

Acetaminophen
Amphetamines
Aspariginase
Azathioprine
Carbon tetrachloride
Chlorthalidone
Cimetidine
Clofibrate
Coumadin

Corticosteroids
Cyproheptadine
Estrogen-containing contraceptives
Ethacrynic acid
Ethanol
Furosemide
Histamine
Indomethacin
Methacholine
Methanol
Narcotics
Oxyphenylbutazone
Phenylbutazone
Phenformin
Propoxyphene
Rifampin
Salicylates
Sulfonamides
Tetracycline
Thiazide diuretics
Valproic acid
Vitamin D

Causes of Elevated Amylase

Pancreatic disease
- Carcinoma
- Cystic fibrosis
- Pancreatitis
- Pancreatic abscess or pseudocyst
- Trauma or annulation (surgery, endoscopic retrograde cholangiopancreatography)
- Cystic fibrosis

Gastrointestinal disease
- Appendicitis
- Cholecystitis
- Gallbladder disease
- Hepatitis
- Liver disease/cirrhosis
- Mesenteric ischemia
- Obstructed or perforated bowel
- Peptic ulcer (perforated or penetrating)
- Peritonitis

Salivary gland disease
- Alcoholism
- Ductal obstruction (sialolith)

- Mumps/parotitis
- Radiation
- Trauma (maxillofacial)

Gynecologic disease
- Ovarian or fallopian cyst
- Pelvic inflammatory disease
- Ruptured ectopic pregnancy

Miscellaneous
- Abdominal aortic aneurysm
- Acidosis (ketotic and nonketotic)
- Burns
- Cerebral trauma
- Eating disorders (anorexia, bulimia nervosa)
- Macroamylasemia
- Medications
- Pneumonia
- Postoperative
- Pregnancy
- Prostatic disease
- Renal failure
- Renal transplant
- Solid tumors of ovary, lung, breast

Key Historical Features

✓ Fever
✓ Weight loss
✓ Alcohol use
✓ Known or suspected gallstones
✓ Abdominal pain (location, onset)
✓ Medical history
✓ Surgical history (especially abdominal)
✓ Medications
✓ Renal health
✓ Sexual history
✓ Contraception use/pregnancy status

Key Physical Findings

✓ Vital signs
✓ Dental examination for enamel loss, suggesting eating disorder
✓ Salivary gland and duct evaluation for stones, tenderness
✓ Pulmonary examination for focal findings, including rales or rhonchi
✓ Abdominal examination for location of pain, rebound, guarding, or hepatomegaly

✓ Pelvic examination for discharge, cervical motion tenderness, adnexal mass
✓ Prostate examination for hypertrophy, nodules

Suggested Work-Up

The workup should be directed by the clinical picture:

Lipase	To evaluate for pancreatitis
Liver function tests	To evaluate for cholecystitis, choledocholithiasis, hepatitis
Pregnancy test	To evaluate for possible pregnancy
Complete blood count	To evaluate for infection or severe inflammation (e.g., pneumonia, mesenteric ischemic, and so on)
Creatinine	To evaluate renal function

Additional Work-Up

Computed tomography of the abdomen/pelvis	To evaluate for pancreatitis complications (abscess, pseudocyst), carcinoma, obstruction, or mesenteric ischemia
Right upper quadrant ultrasound	If gallstones or liver cirrhosis are suspected
Chest x-ray	If pneumonia is suspected
Hepatitis serologies	If viral hepatitis is suspected
Gonorrhea and chlamydia swabs or urinary evaluation	If pelvic inflammatory disease is suspected

Further Reading

Agarwal N, Pitchumoni CS, Sivaprasad AV. Evaluating tests for acute pancreatitis. *Am J Gastroenterol.* 1990;85:356–366.

Garrison R. Amylase. *Emerg Med Clin North Am.* 1986;4:315–327.

Salt WB, Schenker S. Amylase–its clinical significance: a review of the literature. *Medicine.* 1976;55:269–289.

Visser RJ, Abu-Laban RB, McHugh DF. Amylase and lipase in the emergency department evaluation of acute pancreatitis. *J Emerg Med.* 1999;17:1027–1037.

21 ERECTILE DYSFUNCTION

General Discussion

Erectile dysfunction is the inability to achieve or maintain a penile erection sufficient for satisfactory sexual performance. Erectile dysfunction may be divided into either psychogenic or organic origin. Of the organic causes, vascular etiologies represent the largest group, although neurogenic, hormonal, anatomic, or drug-induced etiologies may be implicated. Up to 80% of cases have an organic cause, and erectile dysfunction may result from a combination of organic and psychological causes.

The evaluation of the patient with erectile dysfunction begins with a thorough history to assess the patient's sexual function and to differentiate erectile dysfunction from other sexual problems, such as a decreased libido or ejaculatory problems. History and physical examination are sufficient in making an accurate diagnosis of erectile dysfunction in most cases.

Medications and Substances Associated with Erectile Dysfunction

5-α reductase inhibitors
Alpha-blockers
Amphetamines
Antipsychotics
Barbiturates
Benzodiazepines
Beta-blockers
Bromocriptine
Butyrophenones
Calcium channel blockers
Carbamazepine
Clonidine
Cocaine
Corticosteroids
Digoxin
Dimenhydrinate
Diphenhydramine
Disopyramide
Estrogens
Fibrates
Gemfibrozil
Heroin
Histamine H_2 receptor blockers
Hydroxyzine
Interferon-alfa
Levodopa

Lithium
Luteinizing hormone–releasing hormone agonists
Ketoconazole
Marijuana
Meclizine
Methyldopa
Methotrexate
Metoclopramide
Monoamine oxidase inhibitors
Omeprazole
Opioids
Phenobarbital
Phenothiazines
Phenytoin
Progesterone
Promethazine
Reserpine
Selective serotonin reuptake inhibitors
Spironolactone
Statin medications
Thiazide diuretics
Tricyclic antidepressants
Trihexyphenidyl

Causes of Erectile Dysfunction

Addison disease
Aging
Alcohol abuse
Anatomic abnormalities
Anxiety
Atherosclerosis
Cavernosal disorders
Chronic obstructive pulmonary disease
Chronic renal failure
Cigarette smoking
Cushing syndrome
Depression
Diabetes mellitus
Heart disease
Herniated disc
Hyperlipidemia
Hyperprolactinemia
Hypertension
Hyperthyroidism

Hypogonadism
Hypothyroidism
Ischemic heart disease
Lipid disorders
Liver disease
Marijuana use
Medications
Multiple sclerosis
Narcotic use
Pelvic radiation
Pelvic surgery
Pelvic trauma
Peripheral neuropathy
Peripheral vascular disease
Peyronie disease
Renal failure
Social stressors
Spinal cord injury
Spinal disc herniation
Trauma
Vascular disease
Venous incompetence

Key Historical Features

✓ Onset, duration, and progression of the erectile dysfunction
✓ Quality of erections
✓ Presence or absence of nocturnal erections
✓ Presence or absence of dysfunction with masturbation
✓ Libido
✓ Quality and timing of orgasm
✓ Volume and appearance of ejaculate
✓ Sexually-induced genital pain
✓ Penile curvature with erection
✓ Partner sexual function
✓ Medical history
  • Cardiovascular disease
  • Diabetes mellitus
  • Hypertension
  • Hyperlipidemia
  • Obesity
  • Neurologic disorders (e.g., cerebrovascular accident, Parkinson disease, multiple sclerosis, dementia)
  • Hormonal disorders (e.g., hypothyroidism, hypogonadism, hyperprolactinemia)
  • Peyronie disease

✓   Surgical history, especially pelvic surgery such as prostatectomy
✓   History of pelvic irradiation
✓   Medication use
✓   Cigarette use
✓   Alcohol abuse
✓   Illicit drug use
✓   Psychosocial history (e.g., depression, anxiety, relationship problems, life stressors, history of sexual abuse)
✓   Physical activity level

Key Physical Findings

✓   Body habitus
✓   Cardiovascular examination
   •   Blood pressure and pulse
   •   Signs of hypertensive or ischemic heart disease
   •   Abdominal or femoral artery bruits
   •   Peripheral pulses
   •   Skin and hair patterns suggestive of peripheral vascular disease
✓   Neurologic examination
   •   Signs of anxiety or depression
   •   Anal sphincter tone and anal reflex
✓   Genitourinary systems
   •   Phimosis or hypospadias
   •   Testicular size and other evidence of hypogonadism
   •   Evidence of Peyronie disease
   •   Prostate gland for size, symmetry, and nodules

Suggested Work-Up

The American Urologic Association and World Health Organization recommend limited diagnostic testing in men with erectile dysfunction.

Fasting blood sugar	To evaluate for diabetes mellitus
Lipid panel	To evaluate for lipid disorders
Thyroid-stimulating hormone	To evaluate for thyroid disorders
Morning serum testosterone	To evaluate for low testosterone

Additional Work-Up

Complete blood count	If infection or polycythemia is suspected
Urinalysis	If renal disease or urinary tract infection is suspected

Blood urea nitrogen and creatinine	If renal disease is suspected
Serum prolactin	If hyperprolactinemia is suspected
Luteinizing hormone and follicle-stimulating hormone	In men with low testosterone, to differentiate testicular from hypothalamic–pituitary dysfunction
Magnetic resonance imaging of the brain (pituitary)	In men with elevated prolactin level, to evaluate for pituitary tumor

Further Reading

Fazio L, Brock G. Erectile dysfunction: management update. *Can Med Assoc J.* 2004;170:1429–1437.

Heidelbaugh JJ. Management of erectile dysfunction. *Am Fam Physician.* 2010;81:305–312.

Jardin A, Wagner G, Khoury S, et al. Recommendations of the 1st International Consultation on Erectile Dysfunction. In: Jardin A, Wagner G, Khoury S, et al. *Erectile Dysfunction.* Plymouth, UK: Health Publication Ltd; 2000:711–726.

McVary KT. Erectile dysfunction. *N Engl J Med.* 2007;357:2472–2481.

Miller TA. Diagnostic evaluation of erectile dysfunction. *Am Fam Physician.* 2000;61:95–104.

Montague DK, Jarow JP, Broderick GA, et al. for the Erectile Dysfunction Guideline Update Panel. Chapter 1: The management of erectile dysfunction: an AUA update. *J Urol.* 2005;174:230–239.

NIH consensus conference on impotence. *JAMA.* 1993;270:83–90.

Seftel AD, Mohammed MA, Althof SE. Erectile dysfunction: etiology, evaluation, and treatment options. *Med Clin N Am.* 2004;88:387–416.

Thomas DR. Medications and sexual function. *Clin Geriatr Med.* 2003;19:553–562.

22 FATIGUE

General Discussion

Fatigue is defined as a subjective state of sustained lack of energy or exhaustion with a decreased capacity for physical and mental work that persists despite sufficient rest. Fatigue is one of the most common complaints in adults presenting for primary care in the United States, and it must be differentiated from weakness or exertional difficulties.

Acute viral syndromes are a common cause of fatigue and usually are self-limited. Depression is the most common cause of clinically important fatigue in patients presenting for primary care. Overexertion, deconditioning, anemia, lung disease, medications, and cancer are common causes of fatigue as well. Fatigue that persists longer than 1 month generally warrants investigation. Fatigue is common in the older population and may represent part of the normal aging process. However, fatigue should not be attributed to advanced age alone. Fatigue as a consequence of advanced age should be a diagnosis of exclusion. Although fatigue usually is the symptom of which the patient complains, a careful history often will reveal associated symptoms.

A targeted physical examination may lead to additional diagnostic clues. A laboratory examination may not be required in all cases of fatigue, but targeted testing may help the clinician reveal the cause of the patient's symptoms. However, no etiology can be identified in one third of cases of fatigue.

Chronic fatigue syndrome (CFS) is a clinical diagnosis that can be made only after other etiologies of fatigue have been excluded. The etiology of CFS is unclear and is likely complex. It remains controversial whether there is a single etiology for CFS or whether there may be multiple factors involved. The Centers for Disease Control and Prevention developed specific diagnostic criteria for CFS and updated the criteria in 1994. The criteria require severe fatigue for more than 6 months, and at least four of the following symptoms:

- Headache of new type, pattern, or severity
- Multijoint pain without swelling or erythema
- Muscle pain
- Postexertional malaise for more than 24 hours
- Significant impairment in short-term memory or concentration
- Sore throat
- Tender lymph nodes
- Unrefreshing sleep

Medications Associated with Fatigue

Almost every medication may cause fatigue and should be considered in the evaluation of the patient with fatigue. The following categories of medications are the more common causes of fatigue:

Antibiotics
Antidepressants
Antihistamines
Antihypertensives
Benzodiazepines
Beta-blockers
Diuretics
Glucocorticoids
Muscle relaxants
Narcotic pain medications
Nonsteroidal anti-inflammatory drugs
Selective serotonin reuptake inhibitors
Sleeping medications
Tricyclic antidepressants

Causes of Fatigue

Addison disease
Adrenal insufficiency
Advancing age
Alcohol abuse
Allergic rhinitis
Amebiasis
Anemia
Anorexia nervosa
Bipolar disorder
Blastomycosis
Bulimia nervosa
Cancer
Carbon monoxide poisoning
Celiac disease
Chemotherapy
Chronic pulmonary disease
Chronic sinusitis
Coccidiomycosis
Cushing disease
Cytomegalovirus infection
Dementia
Depression
Dermatomyositis
Diabetes mellitus

Domestic abuse
Drug abuse
Endocarditis
Epstein-Barr virus syndrome
Fibromyalgia
Giardiasis
Heart failure
Heavy metal exposure
Helminth infestation
Hepatitis B or C
Histoplasmosis
HIV
Hypercalcemia
Hyperthyroidism
Hypothyroidism
Liver disease
Lyme disease
Lymphoma
Malignancy
Malnutrition
Medications
Mixed connective tissue disease
Multiple sclerosis
Myasthenia gravis
Narcolepsy
Obesity
Parkinson disease
Parvovirus B19 infection
Polymyalgia rheumatica
Polymyositis
Radiation therapy
Rheumatoid arthritis
Sarcoidosis
Schizophrenia
Significant weight loss
Situational stress
Sjögren syndrome
Sleep apnea
Somatoform disorder
Systemic lupus erythematosus
Temporal arteritis
Toxin exposure
Tuberculosis
Uremia
Viral infections
Vitamin deficiency

Key Historical Features

✓ Onset
✓ Nature of the fatigue
✓ Medical history, including psychiatric history
✓ Medications
✓ Family history
✓ Social history
  - Travel
  - Alcohol use
  - Drug use
  - Dietary habits
  - Caffeine consumption
  - Life events and/or stressors, relationships with family members
✓ Review of systems
  - Fever, chills
  - Night sweats
  - Weight loss or weight gain
  - Appetite
  - Arthralgias
  - Myalgias
  - Headache
  - Adenopathy
  - Paresthesias
  - Sore throat
  - Rash
  - Sleep disturbance
  - Anhedonia
  - Weakness
  - Problems with memory or concentration

Key Physical Findings

✓ Age
✓ Gender
✓ Weight
✓ Vital signs
✓ Head and neck examination for signs of anemia, sinusitis, oral ulcerations, postnasal drip, thyromegaly, or lymphadenopathy
✓ Ophthalmologic examination for signs of increased intracranial pressure, retinopathy, or anemia
✓ Cardiovascular examination, including jugular venous distension
✓ Pulmonary examination
✓ Abdominal examination for abdominal masses, hepatomegaly, splenomegaly, or ascites

- ✓ Examination of the musculature for signs of weakness or muscle atrophy
- ✓ Skin examination for color changes, rash, skin texture changes, or hair changes
- ✓ Genital examination
- ✓ Rectal examination, including stool guaiac
- ✓ Neurologic examination

Suggested Work-Up

Serial weight measurement	To help evaluate for depression or systemic illness
Monitoring of temperature	To help evaluate for infection or malignancy
Complete blood count	To evaluate for infection or malignancy
Electrolytes	To evaluate for adrenal insufficiency
Blood urea nitrogen and creatinine	To evaluate for renal failure
Glucose	To evaluate for diabetes mellitus
Alanine aminotransferase and aspartate aminotransferase	To evaluate for hepatocellular disease
Total bilirubin	To evaluate for hepatitis or hemolysis
Albumin	To evaluate for malnutrition and hepatic synthetic dysfunction
Alkaline phosphatase	To evaluate for obstructive liver disease
Creatine kinase	To evaluate for muscle disease
Calcium	To help detect hyperparathyroidism, cancer, and sarcoidosis
Phosphorus	To evaluate for hypo- or hyperphosphatemia
Erythrocyte sedimentation rate	To help detect collagen–vascular disease, malignancy, endocarditis, abscess, osteomyelitis, tuberculosis, etc.
Thyroid-stimulating hormone	To evaluate for hyper- and hypothyroidism

| Urinalysis | To evaluate for proteinuria and renal disease |
| Pregnancy test | To diagnose pregnancy, if indicated |

Additional Work-Up

Lyme serologies	If Lyme disease is suspected
HIV	If the patient is at risk for HIV infection
Antinuclear antibody (ANA)	If lupus or other collagen vascular diseases are suspected
Hepatitis B and C screening	If the patient is at risk of hepatitis B or C or if the patient has abnormal liver function tests
Purified protein derivative (PPD) skin test	If the patient is at risk for tuberculosis or if tuberculosis is suspected clinically
Chest x-ray	If cardiopulmonary disease is suspected
Brucella titers	If brucellosis is suspected clinically
Monospot or Epstein-Barr titers	If mononucleosis/Epstein-Barr infection is suspected
Cytomegalovirus (CMV) titers	If CMV infection is suspected
Blood cultures	If endocarditis or bacteremia is suspected
Histoplasma antigen	If histoplasmosis is suspected
Adrenocorticotrophic hormone test	If Cushing disease is clinically suspected
Tensilon test	If myasthenia gravis is clinically suspected
Electrocardiogram	If heart failure or arrhythmia is suspected
Echocardiogram	If heart failure is suspected
Parvovirus immunoglobulin-M	If parvovirus infection is suspected
24-hour urine for heavy metals	If heavy metal exposure is suspected
Serum angiotensin-converting enzyme level	If sarcoidosis is suspected
Pulmonary function tests	If chronic obstructive or other lung disease is suspected

Further Reading

Cho WK, Stollerman GH. Chronic fatigue syndrome. *Hosp Pract (Off Ed)*. 1992;27:221–224.

Craig T, Kakumanu S. Chronic fatigue syndrome: evaluation and treatment. *Am Fam Physician*. 2002;65:1083–1090.

Fukuda K, Straus SE, Hickie I, Sharpe MC, Dobbins JG, Komaroff A. International Chronic Fatigue Syndrome Study Group. The chronic fatigue syndrome: a comprehensive approach to its definition and study. *Ann Intern Med*. 1994;121:953–959.

Manzullo EF, Escalante CP. Research into fatigue. *Hematol Oncol Clin North Am*. 2002;619–628.

Morrison RE, Keating HJ. Fatigue in primary care. *Obstetrics and Gynecology Clinics*. 2001;28:225–240.

Rosenthal TC, Majeroni BA, Pretorius R, Malik K. Fatigue: an overview. *Am Fam Physician*. 2008;78:1173–1179.

Yancey JR, Thomas SM. Chronic fatigue syndrome: diagnosis and treatment. *Am Fam Physician*. 2012;86:741–746.

23 FEVER OF UNKNOWN ORIGIN

General Discussion

Fever of unknown origin (FUO) initially was defined as a temperature elevation of 101 °F (38.3 °C) or higher for 3 weeks or longer, the cause of which was not diagnosed after 1 week of intensive in-hospital investigation. Subsequently, it was suggested that the minimum evaluation be changed to at least three outpatient visits or 3 days of inpatient care. Today, FUO may be assumed when no reasonable diagnosis is reached after an appropriate inpatient or outpatient investigation.

Some attempts have been made to change the definition of FUO in special populations, such as classic FUO, nosocomial FUO, FUO in neutropenic patients, and FUO in HIV patients. Although such categorization has its merits, the pathogens in each of these categories merely reflect the frequency distribution of diseases that cause prolonged fevers in these categories. Such categorization does not significantly alter or improve the diagnostic approach.

Recent series show that the diseases responsible for FUO involve more than 100 disorders. The differential diagnosis of FUO can be divided into four subgroups: infection (20%–40%); malignancy (20%–30%); noninfectious inflammatory disease (10%–30%); and miscellaneous (10%–20%). Traditionally, infectious diseases represent the largest group of illnesses that cause FUOs. However, the incidence of malignancy responsible for FUO has increased, and in some published series, malignancy is the most common cause of FUOs. As the duration of the fever increases, the likelihood of an infectious etiology decreases.

Abdominal abscesses, tuberculosis, and endocarditis are the most common infectious causes of FUO. Hodgkin and non-Hodgkin lymphoma are the most common neoplastic diseases responsible for FUO. Adult Still disease and temporal arteritis are the most common noninfectious inflammatory causes of FUO.

Atypical presentation of infection is common in older adults, particularly the very old (80+ years). Normal body temperature and the amplitude of circadian rhythm is reduced in frail, older individuals, but not necessarily in healthy older persons. Twenty percent to 30% of older individuals with serious infections present with an absent or blunted fever response. Connective tissue diseases are identified as the cause of the illness, with a relatively high frequency in patients older than 65 years. This is primarily because temporal arteritis and polymyalgia rheumatica are common in this age group.

Fever may be the sole or the most prominent feature of an adverse drug reaction, which is implicated in 1% to 3% of FUO cases. Rash or eosinophilia may occur, although neither is common. Drug fever is a diagnosis of exclusion and may be confirmed by withdrawal of the offending medication.

Historical clues and physical findings, if present, provide the most useful diagnostic information in the evaluation of FUO. Repeated re-questioning and re-examination over time is extremely important because findings that were not initially apparent may become so and provide important clues to the diagnosis. Hospitalization may be considered at any time during the evaluation of FUO, especially if the patient exhibits signs of a serious illness.

Testing should be guided by the history and physical examination. It is not cost effective to order batteries of screening tests without some clinical suspicion for a diagnosis. The diagnostic objective is to use the history, physical examination, and laboratory data to establish a pattern of organ involvement.

Between 7% and 30% of FUO cases remain undiagnosed after a thorough evaluation. However, fever resolves in most of these patients within a short time, and the mortality rate is 3% 5 years later. Only rarely does a serious disorder emerge later.

Medications Associated with Fever of Unknown Origin

Allopurinol
Aminoglycosides
Amphotericin
Atropine
Barbiturates
Captopril
Carbamazepine
Carbapenems
Cephalosporins
Cimetidine
Clindamycin
Clofibrate
Erythromycin
Heparin
Hydralazine
Hydrochlorothiazide
Ibuprofen
Interferon
Interleukin-2
Isoniazid
Macrolides
Meperidine
Methyldopa
Minocycline
Nifedipine
Nitrofurantoin
Penicillins
Phenothiazines
Phenytoin

Procainamide
Quinidine
Ranitidine
Rifampin
Salicylates
Sulfonamides
Sulindac
Vancomycin

Causes of Fever of Unknown Origin

Infections
  Abdominal abscesses
  Amebiasis
  Blastomycosis
  Brucellosis
  Cat-scratch disease
  Coccidioidomycosis
  Colorado tick fever
  Complicated urinary tract infection
  Cytomegalovirus
  Dengue
Dental abscesses
Encephalitis
Endocarditis
Epstein-Barr virus
Filariasis
Histoplasmosis
HIV
Leptospirosis
Lyme disease
Lymphocytic choriomeningitis
Malaria
Meningitis (chronic)
Mycobacterium avium-intracellulare complex
Osteomyelitis
  Pelvic abscesses
  Pneumocystis carinii pneumonia
  Prostatitis
  Relapsing fever
  Salmonella
  Septic arthritis
  Sinusitis
  Syphilis
  Tuberculosis (especially extrapulmonary)

Tularemia
Typhoid fever
Urinary tract infection
Visceral leishmaniasis
Malignancies
Angio-immunoblastic lymphadenopathy with dysproteinemia
Atrial myxoma
Central nervous system malignancies
Chronic leukemia
Colorectal carcinoma
Hepatoma
Leukemia
Lymphoma (Hodgkin and non-Hodgkin)
Malignant histiocytosis
Metastatic disease
Multiple myeloma and other myelodysplastic syndromes
Pancreatic carcinoma
Pheochromocytoma
Renal cell carcinoma
Sarcomas
Noninfectious inflammatory disease
Adult Still disease
Behçet syndrome
Crohn disease
Cryoglobulinemia
Familial Mediterranean fever
Inflammatory bowel disease
POEMS syndrome
Polyarteritis nodosa
Polymyalgia rheumatica
Reiter syndrome
Rheumatoid arthritis
Rheumatoid fever
Sarcoidosis
Sjögren syndrome
Syphilis
Systemic lupus erythematosus
Temporal arteritis
Vasculitides
Wegener granulomatosis
Miscellaneous
Allergic alveolitis
Aortic dissection
Cirrhosis (especially alcoholic)
Deep venous thrombosis

Drug-induced fever
Erythema multiforme
Factitious fever
Hematoma
Hepatitis
Hypergammaglobulinemia immunoglobulin-D syndrome
Kikuchi disease (histocytic necrotizing adenitis)
Pancreatitis
Pulmonary embolism
Retroperitoneal fibrosis
Sarcoidosis
Schnitzler syndrome
Serum sickness
Subacute thyroiditis
Sweet syndrome
Thrombophlebitis
Thrombotic thrombocytopenia purpura
Thyroiditis
Tumor necrosis factor receptor–associated periodic syndrome
Vitamin B_{12} deficiency

Key Historical Features

- ✓ Fever pattern
- ✓ Recent contact with persons exhibiting similar symptoms
- ✓ Arthralgias
- ✓ Rash
- ✓ Sore throat
- ✓ Medical history
- ✓ Surgical history
- ✓ Family history
- ✓ Medications
- ✓ Exposures and living conditions
- ✓ Recent travel
- ✓ Work environment
- ✓ Exposure to pets and other animals
- ✓ Alcohol use
- ✓ Smoking history
- ✓ Intravenous drug use

Key Physical Findings

- ✓ Vital signs
- ✓ General physical appearance
- ✓ Eye examination for evidence of conjunctivitis or uveitis

✓ Head and neck examination for evidence of sinusitis, evidence of temporal arteritis, oropharyngeal lesions or ulcerations, tender teeth, lymphadenopathy, or eye findings
✓ Thyroid examination for enlargement or tenderness
✓ Cardiac examination for murmurs
✓ Pulmonary examination
✓ Abdominal examination for hepatic abnormalities, splenomegaly, masses, or adenopathy
✓ Skin and nail examination for rash, skin lesions, petechiae, splinter hemorrhages, subcutaneous nodules, or clubbing
✓ Lower extremity examination for evidence of deep venous tenderness
✓ Genital examination for testicular or epididymal nodules
✓ Rectal examination for perirectal fluctuance or tenderness. Prostate examination for prostatic tenderness or fluctuance.

Suggested Work-Up

Complete blood count with differential	To evaluate for infection or hematologic abnormalities
Erythrocyte sedimentation rate	To evaluate for infection or inflammation (level more than 100 mm/hour suggests etiologies such as abdominal/pelvic abscess, osteomyelitis, and endocarditis)
C-reactive protein	To evaluate for infection or inflammation
Electrolytes	To evaluate for metabolic abnormalities
Serum transaminases and alkaline phosphatase	To evaluate for liver disease
Urinalysis	To evaluate for urinary tract infection or other urinary abnormalities
Urine culture	To evaluate for urinary tract infection
Blood cultures	To evaluate for endocarditis and to identify blood-borne infections
Chest radiograph	To screen for infection, collagen vascular disease, or malignancy

Additional Work-Up

Ultrasound of the abdomen and pelvis	To evaluate for abscess or malignancy
Computed tomography (CT) of abdomen and pelvis	To evaluate for abscess or malignancy. Should be considered early in the diagnostic process.
Procalcitonin	Newer specific marker for bacterial infection
Serum protein electrophoresis (or interferon-γ release assay)	To evaluate for multiple myeloma
Purified protein derivative (PPD) skin test	To evaluate for tuberculosis
Lactate dehydrogenase	To evaluate for infectious and malignant causes
Ferritin	To evaluate for malignancy (myeloproliferative disorders) and noninfectious inflammatory diseases (lupus or temporal arteritis)
Lower extremity venous compression ultrasound	To evaluate for deep venous thrombosis
Urine and sputum cultures for acid fast bacillus	If pulmonary or extrapulmonary tuberculosis is suspected
Venereal disease reaction level	To evaluate for syphilis
HIV test	To evaluate for HIV infection
Antinuclear antibodies	To evaluate for noninfectious inflammatory diseases
Antineutrophil cytoplasmic	To evaluate for noninfectious inflammatory antibodies and rheumatoid factor diseases
Cryoglobulins	To evaluate for endocarditis, lupus, leukemias, and lymphomas
Complement studies	To evaluate for noninfectious inflammatory diseases
Thyroid function studies	To evaluate for thyroiditis
Serology for cytomegalovirus (CMV), Epstein-Barr virus (EBV), Antistreptolysin O (ASO) titer	If CMV, EBV, or streptococcal disease is suspected
Sinus radiographs or CT	If sinusitis is suspected

Echocardiogram (transthoracic or transesophageal)	To evaluate for bacterial endocarditis
Lumbar puncture	If central nervous system infection, malignancy, or autoimmune disease is suspected
Liver biopsy	Can reveal granulomatous hepatitis and determine its cause
Temporal artery biopsy	If temporal arteritis is suspected
Chest CT with contrast	If nonhematologic malignancy is suspected
Mammography	To evaluate for breast cancer
Stool guaiac	To evaluate for gastrointestinal blood loss
Upper/lower endoscopy	If gastrointestinal malignancy is suspected
Magnetic resonance imaging of the aortic arch and great vessels	If vasculitis is suspected
Bone scan	If nonhematologic malignancy, metastatic disease, or osteomyelitis is suspected
Nuclear imaging studies (18 F fluorodeoxyglucose positron emission tomography, gallium-67, technetium-99 m, -indium-labeled leukocytes)	To detect inflammatory conditions and neoplastic lesions that may be underdiagnosed by CT scans. 18 F fluorodeoxyglucose scans have high positive and negative values for inflammatory and malignant processes. Gallium-67 scan is best for infection and malignancy. Indium-labeled leukocytes may help diagnose occult septicemia. Technetium-99 m may help diagnose acute infection and inflammation of bones and soft tissue.
Bone marrow biopsy	If hematologic malignancy is suspected
Biopsy of suspicious lymph nodes	To help evaluate for malignancy or infectious cause
Biopsy of suspicious skin lesions	To obtain histologic clues to the diagnosis

Further Reading

Armstrong W, Kazanjian P. Fever of unknown origin in the general population and in HIV-infected persons. In: *Cohen & Powderly: Infectious Diseases.* 2nd ed. St. Louis, MO: Mosby; 2004.

Carsons SE. Fever in rheumatic and autoimmune disease. *Infect Dis Clin North Am.* 1996;10:67–84.

Cunha BA. Fever of unknown origin. *Infect Dis Clin North Am.* 1996;10:111–127.

Cunha BA. Fever of unknown origin (FUO). In: Gorbach SL, Bartlett JB, Blacklow NR, eds. *Infectious Diseases.* 2nd ed. Philadelphia: WB Saunders; 1996.

Durack DT, Street AC. Fever of unknown origin—reexamined and redefined. *Curr Clin Top Infect Dis.* 1991;11:35–51.

Hersch EC, Oh RC. Prolonged febrile illness and fever of unknown origin in adults. *Am Fam Physician.* 2014;90:91–96.

Mackowiak PA, Durack DT. Fever of unknown origin. In: *Mandell, Bennett, & Dolin: Principles and Practice of Infectious Diseases.* 6th ed. Philadelphia: Churchill Livingstone; 2005.

Norman DC, Yoshikawa TT. Fever in the elderly. *Infect Dis Clin North Am.* 1996;10:93–99.

Roth AR, Basello GM. Approach to the adult patient with fever of unknown origin. *Am Fam Physician.* 2003;68:2223–2228.

General Discussion

Fibromyalgia is a chronic, idiopathic nonarticular pain syndrome defined by widespread musculoskeletal pain and generalized tender points. Other common symptoms include fatigue, headache, sleep disturbances, morning stiffness, anxiety, and paresthesias. Fibromyalgia is not a diagnosis of exclusion and should be identified by its own characteristics. The 1990 American College of Rheumatology (ACR) classification criteria for fibromyalgia has two components: (1) the presence of widespread pain involving both sides of the body, above and below the waist, as well as the axial skeletal system, for more than 3 months; and (2) the presence of 11 tender points among 18 specified sites as outlined in the following.

Less common features that generally occur in 25% to 50% of cases of fibromyalgia include headache, light-headedness, dizziness, irritable bowel syndrome, psychological distress, depression, Raynaud phenomenon, subjective joint swelling (without objective swelling), nondermatomal parasthesias (without objective neurologic findings), and marked functional disability. Other somatic complaints include palpitations, dyspareunia and/or pelvic pain, temporomandibular pain, chronic rhinitis or "allergies," and cognitive difficulties, such as memory impairment, concentration issues, grasping for words, and poor vocabulary.

The somatic complaints distinguish fibromyalgia from rheumatoid arthritis (RA). However, fibromyalgia may coexist with other rheumatic diseases, especially systemic lupus erythematosus and RA. The differential diagnosis of fibromyalgia includes hypothyroidism, arthritis, polymyalgia rheumatica, osteomalacia, myofascial pain syndrome, metabolic and inflammatory myopathies, spondyloarthropathy, radiculopathy, and cardiac or pleuritic pain. The major challenge for the clinician is to distinguish fibromyalgia from an inflammatory or metabolic myopathy.

Muscular aching and stiffness in fibromyalgia are more proximal than distal, although the patient may complain of hurting all over. Palpation of a fibromyalgia trigger point (FTP) causes pain localized to the area of palpation, the pain does not radiate to adjacent areas, and no pain is experienced at sites proximal or distal to the examining finger.

The 2010 ACR preliminary diagnostic criteria for fibromyalgia have been provisionally approved by the ACR and have been quantitatively validated using patient data, but these criteria have not undergone validation based on an external dataset. The 2010 criteria provide an alternative approach to diagnosis and classification that does not require a tender point examination, but they do provide a scale for measurement of the severity of symptoms that are characteristic of fibromyalgia. These criteria also recognize the importance of cognitive problems and somatic symptoms that were not included in the 1990 ACR classification criteria. However, questionnaire-based criteria alone cannot be used for establishing the diagnosis of fibromyalgia and require additional validation in different patient populations.

Key Historical Features

✓   Chronicity of pain
✓   Intensity of pain
✓   Nature of pain
✓   Location(s) of pain
✓   Triggering factors
✓   Aggravating factors
✓   Presence of fatigue
✓   Presence of stiffness
✓   Sensation of joint swelling
✓   Presence of poor sleep or nonrestorative sleep
✓   Headache
✓   Cognitive difficulties
✓   Auditory/vestibular/ocular complaints
✓   Symptoms of irritable bowel syndrome
✓   Palpitations
✓   Dyspareunia
✓   Temporomandibular pain
✓   Other constitutional symptoms
✓   Mental stress, coping skills
✓   Quality of life
✓   Physical functioning and activities
✓   Perceived disability
✓   Medical history, especially conditions that may be associated with fibromyalgia:
  •   Bladder irritability
  •   Chronic fatigue syndrome
  •   Headaches
  •   Obstructive sleep apnea
  •   Raynaud phenomenon
  •   Restless legs syndrome
  •   Temporomandibular syndrome
  •   Vulvodynia
✓   Medical history of conditions that may cause musculoskeletal pain:
  •   Localized pain syndromes
  •   Myofascial pain syndrome
  •   Osteoarthritis
  •   Polymyalgia rheumatica
  •   RA
  •   Spondyloarthritis
  •   Systemic lupus erythematosus
  •   Thyroid disease

✓ Psychiatric history, especially conditions that may be associated with fibromyalgia:
- Anxiety
- Depressive disorders
- Posttraumatic stress disorder

✓ Surgical history
✓ Medications
✓ Family medical history
✓ Use of alcohol, tobacco, or drugs
✓ Current employment status
✓ Review of systems
✓ History of trauma or abuse

Key Physical Findings

American College of Rheumatology 1990 Criteria
Recommended Tender Point Locations

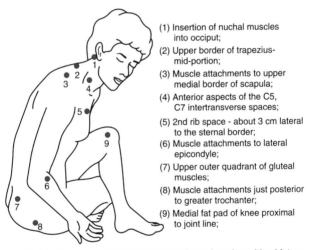

(1) Insertion of nuchal muscles into occiput;

(2) Upper border of trapezius-mid-portion;

(3) Muscle attachments to upper medial border of scapula;

(4) Anterior aspects of the C5, C7 intertransverse spaces;

(5) 2nd rib space - about 3 cm lateral to the sternal border;

(6) Muscle attachments to lateral epicondyle;

(7) Upper outer quadrant of gluteal muscles;

(8) Muscle attachments just posterior to greater trochanter;

(9) Medial fat pad of knee proximal to joint line;

A total of eleven or more tender points in conjunction with a history of widespread pain is characteristic of the fibromyalgia syndrome.

Figure 24-1. The American College of Rheumatology Criteria recommended tender point locations. Locations of 18 (9 pairs) tender points as recommended in the American College of Rheumatology 1990 Criteria. (From Bennett RM, Kelly WN, Harris ED, Ruddy S, Sledge CB, eds. *Textbook of Rheumatology.* Philadelphia: WB Saunders Co; 1997;511–519.)

The most important physical examination for a diagnosis of fibromyalgia is to systematically palpate the 18 sites suggested by the American College of Rheumatology criteria shown in Figure 24-1:

- Bilateral occiput (at the suboccipital muscle insertion)
- Bilateral low cervical (at the anterior aspect of the intertransverse spaces between C5 and C7)
- Bilateral trapezius (midpoint of the upper border)
- Bilateral supraspinatus (origin of this muscle above the scapular spine near the border)
- Bilateral second rib (lateral to the costochondral junctions on the upper surface)
- Bilateral lateral epicondyle (2 cm distal to the epicondyle)
- Bilateral gluteal (at the upper outer quadrant of the buttock)
- Bilateral greater trochanter (posterior to the trochanter)
- Bilateral knee (medial fat pad proximal to the joint line)

A moderate and consistent amount of pressure should be applied using the thumb of the dominant hand. The amount of force applied should be 8.8 lbs (4.0 kg), which should just blanch the examiner's thumbnail. This amount of pressure does not produce significant tenderness or pain in patients without fibromyalgia.

Additional items in the physical examination include:

Vital signs

General appearance

Affect

Head and neck examination for dry mouth or evidence of temporomandibular joint dysfunction

Examination of the thyroid gland

Examination for lymphadenopathy

Abdominal examination

Examination of the extremities for joint swelling or other evidence of connective tissue disease

Neurologic examination for cranial nerves, reflexes, muscle strength, sensory functions, and cerebellar signs

Suggested Work-Up

Fibromyalgia is a clinical diagnosis, so laboratory or radiologic testing is not necessary for making a diagnosis of fibromyalgia. Testing may be performed to exclude an associated disease or another illness that may mimic fibromyalgia. Routine testing for rheumatoid factor or antinuclear antibodies is not recommended. Sleep and mood evaluations should be considered in all patients with symptoms suggestive of fibromyalgia.

Complete blood count	To evaluate for anemia or cytopenia
Erythrocyte sedimentation rate and/or C-reactive protein	Normal acute phase reactants make an underlying inflammatory disorder unlikely
Thyroid-stimulating hormone	To evaluate for hypothyroidism

Additional Work-Up

Creatine kinase	If inflammatory muscle disease is suspected
Antinuclear antibodies and rheumatoid factor	Should be obtained only if an inflammatory, rheumatologic process is suspected
Electrolytes, blood urea nitrogen, creatinine	If an underlying metabolic disorder is suspected
Sleep study	May be considered if the history suggests a primary sleep disorder, such as sleep apnea, rapid eye movement sleep behavioral disorder, periodic limb movement disorder, or narcolepsy

Further Reading

Chakrabarty S, Zoorob R. Fibromyalgia. *Am Fam Physician.* 2007;76:247–254.

McCain GA. A cost-effective approach to the diagnosis and treatment of fibromyalgia. *Rheum Dis Clin North Am.* 1996;22:323–349.

Millea PJ, Holloway RL. Treating fibromyalgia. *Am Fam Physician.* 2000;62:1575–1582.

Winfield JB. Pain in fibromyalgia. *Rheum Dis Clin North Am.* 1999;25:55–79.

Wolfe F, Clauw DJ, Fitzcharles MA, et al. The American College of Rheumatology preliminary criteria for fibromyalgia and measurement of symptom severity. *Arthritis Care Res.* 2010;62:600–610.

Yunus MB. A comprehensive medical evaluation of patients with fibromyalgia syndrome. *Rheum Dis Clin North Am.* 2002;28:201–217.

25 GALACTORRHEA

General Discussion

Galactorrhea is the inappropriate production of milk from the breast in the absence of pregnancy or beyond 6 to 12 months after pregnancy and cessation of breastfeeding. The discharge of milk may be unilateral or bilateral, may be intermittent or persistent, and may vary in terms of volume. Galactorrhea may also occur in males and in infants and teenage girls.

Distinguishing galactorrhea from other forms of nipple discharge is usually straightforward. The discharge in galactorrhea has the appearance of milk, occurs from multiple ducts in the nipple, most commonly occurs bilaterally, and is usually spontaneous.

When nipple discharge is consistent with galactorrhea, the medical history often will reveal the etiology. Important elements of the history and physical examination are outlined in the following.

Medications and Substances Associated with Galactorrhea

Amphetamines
Antipsychotics
Butyrophenones
Calcium channel blockers
Cimetidine
Cocaine
Codeine
Methyldopa
Metoclopramide
Morphine
Oral contraceptives
Phenothiazines
Prochlorperazine
Reserpine
Risperdone
Selective serotonin reuptake inhibitors
Tricyclic antidepressants
Verapamil

Causes of Galactorrhea

Acromegaly
Bronchogenic carcinoma
Chronic renal failure
Estrogen withdrawal
Heroin use

Hypothalamic and infundibular lesions
- Craniopharyngioma
- Empty sella syndrome
- Germinoma
- Histiocytosis
- Meningioma
- Pituitary stalk lesions
- Primary hypothalamic tumor
- Rathke cleft cyst
- Sarcoidosis
- Tuberculosis

Hypothyroidism

Idiopathic

Medications

Neonatal galactorrhea

Neurogenic causes
- Breast/nipple stimulation
- Burns
- Chest surgery
- Shingles
- Spinal cord injury
- Trauma

Physiologic causes of transient hyperprolactinemia
- Physical stress
- Pregnancy
- Vigorous exercise

Pituitary adenoma (usually prolactinoma)

Thoracic neoplasms

Key Historical Features

- ✓ Duration of galactorrhea
- ✓ Unilateral or bilateral
- ✓ Associated breast mass
- ✓ Medications
- ✓ Medical history, particularly thyroid disorders or renal failure
- ✓ Surgical history, especially recent chest surgery
- ✓ Family history, especially thyroid disorders or multiple endocrine neoplasia increases the risk for these processes
- ✓ Reproductive history
  - Oral contraceptives are the most common medication-related cause of galactorrhea
  - Oligomenorrhea, amenorrhea, infertility, decreased libido, or impotence suggest hyperprolactinemia
  - Amenorrhea may indicate pregnancy or pituitary tumor

✓ Constitutional symptoms
  - Fatigue and cold intolerance suggest hypothyroidism
  - Nervousness, heat intolerance, unusual sweating, and weight loss despite a normal or increased appetite suggest thyrotoxicosis
  - Polyuria and polydipsia suggest pituitary or hypothalamic disease
✓ Skin symptoms
  - Dry skin suggests hypothyroidism
  - Acne and hirsutism suggest hyperandrogenism
✓ Gastrointestinal symptoms
  - Constipation suggests hypothyroidism
✓ Neurologic symptoms
  - Headache, visual disturbance, and seizure suggest pituitary or hypothalamic disease

Key Physical Findings

✓ Vital signs
✓ Poor growth or short stature suggestive of hypothyroidism, hypopituitarism, or chronic renal failure
✓ Acromegaly or gigantism suggestive of pituitary tumor
✓ Breast examination for nodules and discharge, including determination of whether the discharge is from one duct or multiple ducts
✓ Cardiac examination for bradycardia suggestive of hypothyroidism
✓ Skin examination for dry skin, coarse hair, and myxedema suggestive of hypothyroidism; hirsutism and acne suggesting hyperandrogenism
✓ Head and neck examination for goiter suggesting hypothyroidism
✓ Eye examination for visual field defect or papilledema suggestive of a pituitary tumor or intracranial mass
✓ Neurologic examination for hand tremor suggestive of thyrotoxicosis or a cranial neuropathy suggestive of a pituitary tumor or intracranial mass

Suggested Work-Up

The evaluation of galactorrhea should proceed in a stepwise fashion and be guided by findings from the history and physical examination.

Serum prolactin	To evaluate for pituitary adenoma
Pregnancy test	To evaluate for pregnancy in women of childbearing age

Additional Work-Up

If hyperprolactinemia is confirmed, medications that may cause elevated prolactin levels should be withheld if possible. The prolactin level should then be repeated.

Thyroid-stimulating hormone	To evaluate for hypo- or hyperthyroidism

Blood urea nitrogen and creatinine	To evaluate renal function

If true hyperprolactinemia is found, magnetic resonance imaging (MRI) with gadolinium enhancement should be performed to evaluate the pituitary fossa. A serum prolactin level greater than 200 ng/ml is strongly suggestive of pituitary adenoma.

MRI of brain with gadolinium	When no other causes are identified with the stepwise laboratory evaluation outlined previously, or when an intracranial mass is suggested by history and physical examination
Follicle-stimulating hormone, luteinizing hormone, dehydroepiandrosterone	To evaluate for hyperandrogenism when it is suggested by history and physical examination

Further Reading

Benjamin F. Normal lactation and galactorrhea. *Clin Obstet Gynecol.* 1994;37:887–897.

Falkenberry SS. Nipple discharge. *Obstet Gynecol Clin North Am.* 2002;29:21–29.

Huang W, Molitch ME. Evaluation and management of galactorrhea. *Am Fam Physician.* 2012;85:1073–1080.

Jardines L. Management of nipple discharge. *Am Surg.* 1996;62:119–122.

Leung AKC, Pacaud D. Diagnosis and management of galactorrhea. *Am Fam Physician.* 2004;70:543–550.

Luciano AA. Clinical presentation of hyperprolactinemia. *J Reprod Med.* 1999;44(12 suppl):1085–1090.

Serri O, Chik CL, Ur E, Ezzat S. Diagnosis and management of hyperprolactinemia. *CMAJ.* 2003;169:575–581.

Spack NP, Neinstein LS. Galactorrhea. In: Neinstein LS, ed. *Adolescent Health Care: A Practical Guide.* 4th ed. Philadelphia: Lippincott Williams & Wilkins; 2002:1045–1051.

General Discussion

Polypoid lesions of the gallbladder, or gallbladder polyps, are a common, sometimes incidental, finding on imaging and affect an estimated 5% of the adult population. The incidence of polyps varies widely, and studies disagree on whether males or females are more commonly affected. These polyps are most often asymptomatic, but they may be associated with symptoms of right upper quadrant or epigastric pain, dyspepsia, nausea, or vomiting. The clinical significance of gallbladder polyps is unclear, although malignant transformation is postulated and of concern.

Gallbladder polyps are characterized as immobile elevated mucosal echoes that protrude into the gallbladder lumen. Most incidentally discovered gallbladder polyps are benign, and these can be further broken down into pseudopolyps (inflammatory polyps, cholesterol polyps, and adenomyomatosis) and true polyps (adenomas, lipomas, and leiomyomas). Unfortunately, imaging studies alone cannot often distinguish benign from malignant lesions.

Clinical findings and features predictive of malignancy vary in published studies. Risk factors for malignancy are size greater than 10 mm, associated symptoms, an isolated polyp, rapid growth, the concurrent presence of gallstones, a sessile polyp, and associated gallbladder wall thickening. Large size (>10 mm) and symptomatic polyps are the most cited risk factors.

Patients with gallbladder polyps that have characteristics associated with malignancy are recommended to undergo cholecystectomy because of the overall safety of the procedure balanced against the danger of potentially missed gallbladder malignancy. For polyps without these features, serial imaging with abdominal ultrasound every 3 to 6 months is preferred, with focus on changes in size, location, and number. Newer imaging modalities used to study gallbladder polyps include endoscopic ultrasound and computed tomographic imaging, although the role of these studies remains to be defined.

Key Historical Features

✓ Age >50 to 60 years
✓ Nausea and vomiting
✓ Epigastric and/or right upper quadrant abdominal pain
✓ Dyspepsia
✓ History of gallstones

Key Diagnostic Findings

✓ Polyp size (>10 mm)
✓ Isolated versus multiple polyps

✓   Sessile or adenomatous polyps
✓   Presence of gallstones
✓   Presence of gallbladder wall thickening
✓   Rapidly growing polyp

Suggested Management

Management of gallbladder polyps primarily relies on the size of the lesion. A size greater than 10 mm is the best indicator of malignancy and warrants cholecystectomy. Likewise, patients with gallbladder polyps that have characteristics associated with malignancy (as outlined in the General Discussion) are recommended to undergo cholecystectomy. In addition, any gallbladder polyp that is believed to be symptomatic should be removed from a patient otherwise fit for surgery.

There is controversy regarding the risk for malignancy in asymptomatic polyps that measure 6 to 10 mm. For asymptomatic patients with polyps 6 to 10 mm in size, follow-up ultrasound imaging in 3 to 6 and 12 months is appropriate. If the polyp size is stable, annual follow-up ultrasound is appropriate.

Management of polyps that measure 5 mm or less is not clearly established. A recent large study suggested that polyps of this size have no malignant potential and may be ignored. Many authors suggest that pedunculated polyps smaller than 5 mm do not require follow-up. However, other factors, such as the presence of gallstones, patient age older than 50 years, a wide polyp base, and focal gallbladder wall thickening of more than 3 mm warrant surgical consultation.

Further Reading

Corwin MT, Siewert B, Sheiman RG, et al. Incidentally detected gallbladder polyps: is follow-up necessary? Long-term clinical and US analysis of 346 patients. *Radiology.* 2011;258:277–282.

Gallahan WC, Conway JD. Diagnosis and management of gallbladder polyps. *Gastroenterol Clin N Am.* 2010;39:359–367.

Ito H, Hann LE, D'Angelica M, et al. Polypoid lesions of the gallbladder: diagnosis and follow-up. *J Am Coll Surg.* 2009;208:570–575.

Mellnick VM, Menias CO, Sandrasegaran K. Polypoid lesions of the gallbladder: disease spectrum with pathologic correlation. *RadioGraphics.* 2015;35:387–399.

Myers RP, Shaffer EA, Beck PL. Gallbladder polyps: epidemiology, natural history, and management. *Can J Gastroenetrol.* 2002;16:187–194.

27 GYNECOMASTIA

General Discussion

Gynecomastia, which is the excessive development of the male mammary glands, occurs when there is a disturbance in the normal circulating androgens-to-estrogen ratio in men. Gynecomastia usually presents bilaterally, and may be either physiologic or nonphysiologic. The overall prevalence of gynecomastia is estimated to be approximately 40%.

Physiologic gynecomastia has a trimodal age distribution, with the incidence peaking in newborns, adolescents, and men older than 50 years. One-half of adolescent males experience gynecomastia, typically at approximately a Tanner stage 3 or 4. Adolescent physiologic gynecomastia should resolve 6 to 24 months after onset. If the gynecomastia persists after 2 years or past 17 years of age, further evaluation is warranted. Adolescents may also experience nonphysiologic gynecomastia because of medication, substance, or supplement use or as the result of underlying genetic conditions.

After persistent pubertal gynecomastia, medication use and substance use are the most common causes of nonphysiologic gynecomastia. There is a progressive increase in the prevalence of gynecomastia with advancing age, with a final peak in incidence in men older than 50 years. This final peak results from decreasing free testosterone levels. Nonphysiologic gynecomastia can occur at any age as a result of the medications and conditions outlined in the following.

The central issue is to distinguish true gynecomastia from fatty enlargement of the breasts (pseudogynecomastia or lipomastia) and also to exclude breast carcinoma. Palpable, firm glandular tissue in a concentric mass around the nipple areolar complex is most consistent with gynecomastia. A hard, immobile mass or masses associated with skin changes, nipple retraction, nipple discharge, or enlarged lymph nodes should be considered breast carcinoma until proven otherwise. When this distinction is in doubt after careful physical examination, mammography or ultrasonography may be performed.

It is important to remember that a diagnosis is made in less than half of patients referred for gynecomastia. As such, not all cases of gynecomastia require extensive evaluation. Indications for further workup include a negative medication and drug history, breast tenderness, a mass more than 4 cm in diameter, or any findings suggestive of malignancy.

Medications and Supplements Associated with Gynecomastia

Amiodarone
Amlodipine
Anabolic steroids
Angiotensin-converting enzyme inhibitors

Antiretroviral agents
- Didanosine
- Efavirenz

Atorvastatin
Bicalutamide
Calcium channel blockers
Chemotherapy agents
- Alkylating agents
- Busulfan
- Cisplatin
- Imatinib
- Nitrosoureas
- Vincristine

Cimetidine
Clomiphene
Diazepam
Diethylstilbestrol
Digoxin
Diltiazem
Dong quai
Estrogen agonists
Estrogens
Ethionamide
Etomidate
Fenofibrate
Finasteride
Fluoxetine
Flutamide
Furosemide
Gonadotropin-releasing hormone agonists
Growth hormone
Haloperidol
Human chorionic gonadotropins
Isoniazid
Ketoconazole
Lavender
Melatonin
Methadone
Methotrexate
Methyldopa
Metoclopramide
Metronidazole
Minocycline
Minoxidil

Mirtazapine
Nifedipine
Nilutamide
Omeprazole
Paroxetine
Pencicillamine
Phenothiazines
Phenytoin
Phytoestrogens
Progesterones
Ranitidine
Reserpine
Risperidone
Rosuvastatin
Soy
Spironolactone
Sulindac
Tea tree oil
Theophylline
Tribulus terrestris
Tricyclic antidepressants
Venlafaxine
Verapamil

Causes of Gynecomastia

Adrenal disease
Alcohol abuse
Amphetamine use
Chronic renal insufficiency
Cirrhosis
Cystic fibrosis
Familial gynecomastia
Hermaphroditism
Heroin use
HIV infection
Hyperthyroidism
Idiopathic
Increased estrogen production
Malnutrition
Marijuana use
Medications
Physiologic gynecomastia

Primary hypogonadism
- 5α-reductase deficiency
- Androgen insensitivity syndrome
- Castration
- Congenital anorchia
- Hemochromatosis
- Klinefelter syndrome
- Testicular torsion
- Testicular trauma
- Viral orchitis

Secondary hypogonadism
- Kallman syndrome

Tumors
- Adrenal tumors
- Gastric carcinoma producing human chorionic gonadotropin (hCG)
- Large cell lung cancer producing hCG
- Pituitary tumors
- Renal cell carcinoma producing hCG
- Testicular tumors

Ulcerative colitis

Key Historical Features

✓ Age
✓ Onset and duration
✓ Rate of growth
✓ Pain/tenderness
✓ Nipple discharge
✓ Skin changes
✓ Systemic symptoms such as weight loss
✓ Medical history
✓ Medications
✓ Supplements
✓ Drug history

Key Physical Findings

✓ Height and weight
✓ Thyroid examination
✓ Breast examination to differentiate fatty tissue from true gynecomastia
✓ Abdominal examination to assess the liver
✓ Lymph node examination

✓ Examination of the testes
✓ Skin examination for evidence of adrenal disease

Suggested Work-Up

Aspartate aminotransferase, alanine aminotransferase, γ-glutamyl transpeptidase, total bilirubin	To evaluate liver function
Serum creatinine	To evaluate renal function
Thyroid-stimulating hormone	To evaluate for hyperthyroidism

Additional Work-Up

Serum beta hCG	If testicular tumor or retroperitoneal histologic unmixed seminoma is suspected
Serum dehydroepiandrosterone sulfate	If adrenal tumor is suspected
Urinary 17-ketosteroids	If adrenal or testicular tumor is suspected
Total testosterone, free testosterone, estradiol, luteinzing hormone, and follicle-stimulating hormone	If primary or secondary hypogonadism is suspected
Serum prolactin	If prolactinoma is suspected
Mammogram or ultrasound	If breast malignancy is suspected
Fine-needle aspiration of mass	If malignancy is suspected
Chromosomal karyotype	If both testes are small, to evaluate for Klinefelter syndrome
Testicular ultrasound	If a palpable testicular mass is present, if the gynecomastia is larger than 5 cm, if the serum hCG level is elevated, if the estradiol is high with a low level of luteinizing hormone, or if the gynecomastia is otherwise unexplained
Magnetic resonance imaging of the brain	If prolactin level is elevated

Further Reading

Braunstein GD. Gynecomastia. *N Engl J Med.* 1993;328:490–495.

Derkacz M, Chmiel-Perzynska I, Nowkowski A. Gynecomastia—a difficult diagnostic problem. *Enkokrynol Pol.* 2011;62:191.

Eckman A, Dobs A. Drug-induced gynecomastia. *Expert Opin Drug Saf.* 2008;7:691–702.

Henley DV, Lipson N, Korach KS, Bloch CA. Prepubertal gynecomastia linked to lavender and tea tree oils. *N Engl J Med.* 2007;356:479–485.

Jameel JK, Kneeshaw PJ, Rao VS, Drew PJ. Gynaecomastia and the plant product "*Tribulis terrestris.*" *Breast.* 2004;13:428–430.

Munoz CR, Alvarez Benito M, Munoz Gomariz E, et al. Mammography and ultrasound in the evaluation of male breast disease. *Eur Radiol.* 2010;20:2797–2805.

Wilson JD. Endocrine disorders of the breast. In: Isselbacher KJ, Braunwald E, Wilson JD, eds. *Harrisons's Textbook of Internal Medicine.* 13th ed. New York: McGraw-Hill; 1994:2037–2039.

Wise GJ, Roorda AK, Kalter R. Male breast disease. *J Am Coll Surg.* 2005;200:255–269.

General Discussion

Hair loss, or alopecia, can be classified in various ways, but the most common classification distinguishes nonscarring from scarring alopecia. The hair loss of scarring alopecia is permanent, whereas nonscarring alopecia usually is reversible. When patients present with hair loss, it is important to determine if they are experiencing hair shedding, which is significant amounts of hair coming out, or hair thinning, which is more visible scalp without noticeable amounts of hair falling out.

Every hair follicle goes through three phases: anagen (growth), catagen (transition between growth and resting), and telogen (resting). At any given time, approximately 85% of scalp follicles are in the anagen phase, and follicles remain in this phase for an average of 3 years. The catagen phase affects 2% to 3% of hair follicles at a time. The telogen phase occurs last, during which 10% to 15% of hair follicles undergo a rest period for approximately 3 months. At the end of telogen, the dead hair is ejected from the skin, and the cycle is repeated.

Alopecia areata is patchy hair loss of autoimmune origin. It usually occurs in well-circumscribed patches, but also may involve the entire scalp (alopecia totalis) or body (alopecia universalis). The involved scalp may be normal or show subtle erythema or edema. Short hairs that taper as they approach the scalp surface, known as exclamation mark hairs, are characteristic of alopecia areata. Alopecia areata may be associated with thyroid disease, vitiligo, or atopy. If a patient does not have any of these medical conditions and is otherwise well, no laboratory tests are necessary.

Androgenic alopecia, the most common form of alopecia in men and women, is also known as male-pattern balding, female-pattern balding, and common balding. Most patients with androgenic alopecia complain of thinning hair rather than shedding of hair. In some women, androgenic alopecia may be a manifestation of hyperandrogenism, so the history should focus on related signs (e.g., menstrual irregularities, infertility, hirsutism, and acne). No laboratory testing is required in an otherwise healthy woman with slowly progressive androgenic alopecia and no signs or symptoms of hyperandrogenism. Men with androgenic alopecia do not require a laboratory evaluation.

Cicatricial alopecia results from a condition that damages the scalp and hair follicle. Examination typically reveals plaques of erythema with or without scaling. Syphilis, tuberculosis, AIDS, herpes zoster, discoid lupus erythematosus, sarcoidosis, radiation therapy, and scalp trauma (e.g., burns) have been associated with cicatricial alopecia. If the cause of the disorder is not apparent, a punch biopsy of the scalp may be helpful in making the diagnosis.

Scarring alopecia represents a heterogeneous group of diseases manifested by erythematous papules, pustules, or scaling centered around hair follicles, resulting in eventual obliteration of follicular orifices.

Senescent (senile) alopecia is the steady decrease in the density of scalp hair that occurs in all persons as they age. Patients will note a slow, steady, diffuse pattern of thinning hair beginning at approximately age 50 years.

Syphilitic alopecia should be considered in every patient with unexplained hair loss. Hair loss may be rapid or slow and insidious and may be patchy (moth-eaten in appearance) or diffuse. Syphilic alopecia is a noninflammatory, nonscarring alopecia without erythema, scaling, or induration. However, in symptomatic syphilic alopecia, the patchy or diffuse alopecia is associated with the papulosquamous lesions of secondary syphilis on the scalp or elsewhere.

Telogen effluvium occurs when an abnormally high percentage of normal hairs from all areas of the scalp enter telogen, the resting phase of hair growth. Many factors can precipitate telogen effluvium, especially stress. This disorder also may develop because of normal physiologic events, such as the postpartum state or because of medications or endocrinopathies. Telogen effluvium usually begins 2 to 6 months after the causative event and lasts for several months. Hair loss is diffuse and may also affect pubic and axillary hair. Telogen effluvium is noninflammatory, and the scalp surface appears normal. The hair pull test is positive, although the telogen count usually does not exceed 50%.

Tinea capitis is a common condition caused by dermatophytes. Tinea capitis presents with one or several patches of alopecia, as well as scalp inflammation. Broken-off hair shafts may create a black dot appearance on the scalp. Fungal organisms can be displayed in a potassium hydroxide (KOH) preparation or may be cultured after adequate scraping of hair stubs from the periphery of the lesion.

Traction alopecia is a form of traumatic alopecia associated with certain methods of hair styling, including braiding, tight curlers, and ponytails. The outermost hairs are subjected to the most tension, and a zone of alopecia develops between braids and along the margin of the scalp.

Trichotillomania is a psychiatric impulse-control disorder in which the patient plucks the hairs. The pattern of hair loss often suggests the diagnosis. One or more well-circumscribed areas of hair loss may be present, often in a bizarre pattern with incomplete areas of clearing. The scalp may be normal or may show areas of erythema or pustule formation. Laboratory testing is not required, although psychiatric consultation may be considered.

Medications Associated with Hair Loss

Anticonvulsants
Antithyroid agents
Chemotherapy agents
Heparin
Hormones

Causes of Hair Loss

Alopecia areata
Androgenetic alopecia
Scarring (cicatricial) alopecia
- AIDS
- Discoid lupus erythematosus of the scalp
- Dissecting cellulitis
- Folliculitis decalvans
- Herpes zoster
- Lichen planopilaris
- Pseudopelade
- Radiation therapy
- Sarcoidosis
- Scalp trauma (burns, injuries)
- Syphilis
- Tuberculosis

Senescent (senile) alopecia
Syphilitic alopecia
Telogen effluvium
- Drugs
- Early stages of androgenetic alopecia
- Heavy metals
- High fever
- Hypothyroidism
- Major surgery
- Medications
- Physiologic effluvium of the newborn
- Postpartum effluvium
- Severe chronic illness
- Severe diets (crash or liquid protein diets)
- Severe infection
- Severe psychological stress

Tinea capitis
Traction alopecia
Traumatic alopecia and cosmetic alopecia
Trichotillomania

Key Historical Features

✓ Shedding versus thinning
✓ Duration of the problem
✓ Whether hair is broken or shed at the roots
✓ Grooming practices (chemical treatments, such as relaxers, bleaching, coloring, or blow drying on high heat)

- ✓ Menstrual irregularities, infertility, hirsutism, or acne in women suspected of having hyperandrogenism
- ✓ Diet
- ✓ Physical or emotional stressors within the previous 3 to 6 months
- ✓ Medical history
- ✓ Medications
- ✓ Family history of hair loss, including maternal relatives, paternal relatives, siblings, and children

Key Physical Findings

- ✓ Pattern of hair loss (patterned vs. diffuse hair loss)
- ✓ Examination of the scalp for erythema, scaling, pustules, edema, bogginess, sinus tract formation, or obliteration of follicular openings
- ✓ Examination of the hair shaft for caliber, shape, length, and fragility
- ✓ Thyroid examination
- ✓ Pubic or axillary hair loss
- ✓ Evidence of hirsutism

Suggested Work-Up

Hair pull test	Fifty to 60 hairs are grasped between the thumb and the index and middle fingers, then the hairs are gently but firmly pulled. A negative test is six or fewer hairs obtained. A positive test is more than six hairs obtained and indicates a process of active hair shedding. Microscopic evaluation of the hairs may be performed. The hair pull test is helpful in suspected cases of telogen effluvium, tinea capitis, systemic diseases, alopecia areata, alopecia totalis, alopecia universalis, and environmental factors.
Serologic test for syphilis	Recommended for all patients with unexplained hair loss to rule out syphilis

Additional Work-Up

KOH prep for fungal elements or fungal culture of skin	In patchy forms of alopecia to rule out fungal infection
Total testosterone, free testosterone, dehydroepiandrosterone sulfate, and prolactin level	In women suspected of having hyperandrogenism

Thyroid-stimulating hormone, rapid plasma reagin (RPR), prolactin, complete blood count (CBC), chemistry profile, erythrocyte sedimentation rate (ESR), antinuclear antibody (ANA), rheumatoid factor, and hair pluck test for telogen:anagen ratio	In patients with telogen effluvium
CBC, ESR, ANA, rheumatoid factor	In patients with alopecia areata
KOH examination or culture swab	In suspected cases of tinea capitis
Scalp biopsy	If the etiology is unclear or if the patient fails to improve after appropriate treatment

Further Reading

Sperling LC, Mezebish DS. Hair diseases. *Med Clin North Am.* 1998;82:1155–1169.

Springer K, Brown M, Stulberg DL. Common hair loss disorders. *Am Fam Physician.* 2003;68:93–102.

Thiedke CC. Alopecia in women. *Am Fam Physician.* 2003;67:1007–1014.

General Discussion

More than 28 million Americans have some degree of hearing impairment, and 25% to 40% of those ages 65 years or older are hearing impaired. The differential diagnosis of hearing loss can be simplified by determining whether the hearing loss is conductive or sensorineural. Conductive hearing loss is caused by imperfect function of the external canal, tympanic membrane, or ossicles, which are located in the outer and middle ear. Sensorineural hearing loss is caused by injury to the cochlea or the auditory nerve in the inner ear. A mixed hearing loss may also occur, which involves both conductive and sensorineural loss.

More than 90% of hearing loss is sensorineural. Presbycusis, which is sensorineural loss related to aging, is the most common cause of hearing loss in the United States. This type of hearing loss is typically gradual, bilateral, and characterized by high-frequency hearing loss.

The physician may be faced with a patient with sudden hearing loss. Idiopathic sudden sensorineural hearing loss develops in less than 72 hours, and usually is unilateral. The etiology is not yet clear, although a variety of mechanisms, such as viral infections, microcirculatory injuries, and immune-mediated disorders, have been proposed. A viral infection of the cochlea is believed to be the most common cause of sudden sensorineural hearing loss.

Meniere disease is characterized by the tetrad of unilateral fluctuating hearing loss, a sensation of aural fullness, tinnitus, and vertigo. Sudden, low-frequency hearing loss is a hallmark of Meniere disease, although higher frequencies are affected as the disease progresses. Hearing loss is typically associated with episodic and recurrent paroxysms of vertigo.

The evaluation of hearing loss begins with a thorough history and physical examination followed by audiography. The goal of the audiologic evaluation is to determine the laterality, severity, and site of lesion of hearing loss. Patients with sudden sensorineural hearing loss require magnetic resonance imaging (MRI) of the brain with gadolinium to rule out acoustic neuroma and other cerebellopontine angle tumors.

Medications Associated with Hearing Loss

Aminoglycosides
Chemotherapeutics agents
- Carboplatin
- Cisplatin
- Vincristine sulfate

Diuretics
- Ethacrynic acid
- Furosemide

Erythromycin
Quinine
Salicylates (especially aspirin)
Vancomycin

Causes of Hearing Loss

Conductive hearing loss
- Cerumen impaction
- Cholesteatoma
- Cyst
- Exostoses
- Foreign body
- Glomus tumor
- Middle ear effusion
- Osteomas
- Otitis externa
- Otosclerosis
- Tumor (adenoma, carcinoma, fibroma, melanoma, papilloma, sarcoma)
- Tympanic membrane perforation
- Tympanosclerosis

Sensorineural hearing loss
Bilateral hearing loss
- Autoimmune processes
- Medication
- Noise trauma
- Ototoxin exposure
- Presbycusis

Unilateral hearing loss
- Acoustic neuroma
- Infection (meningitis, labyrinthitis, cochleitis)
- Meniere disease
- Neoplasm
- Perilymph fistula
- Temporal bone fracture
- Vascular occlusive disease

Key Historical Features

✓ Onset of hearing loss
✓ Progression of hearing loss (sudden or gradual)
✓ Involvement of one or both ears
✓ Dizziness or vertigo
✓ Tinnitus

✓ Sensation of aural fullness
✓ Ear or head trauma
✓ Recent infection
✓ Ear discharge
✓ Ear pain
✓ Medical history, especially history of ear infections or ear injury. Also note history of atherosclerotic disease.
✓ Medications
✓ Family history of hearing loss
✓ Exposure to loud noises
✓ Tobacco use

Key Physical Findings

✓ Visualization and palpation of the auricle and periauricular tissues
✓ Otoscopic examination of the external auditory canal for cerumen, foreign bodies, and abnormalities of the canal skin. The mobility, color, and surface anatomy of the tympanic membrane should be noted. A pneumatic bulb may be used to assess the tympanic membrane and the aeration of the middle ear.
✓ Weber test
✓ Rinne test
✓ Head and neck examination
✓ Cranial nerve examination

Suggested Work-Up

Audiography	To determine the laterality, severity, and site of lesion of hearing loss
MRI of the brain with gadolinium enhancement	For patients with asymmetric sensorineural hearing loss to rule out acoustic neuroma and other cerebellopontine angle tumors

Additional Work-Up

Serum immunoglobulin-E, erythrocyte sedimentation rate, antinuclear antibodies, anticardiolipin antibody, and cytoplasmic antineutrophil cytoplasmic antibodies	If an autoimmune process is suspected

Further Reading

Isaacson JE, Vora NM. Differential diagnosis and treatment of hearing loss. *Am Fam Physician.* 2003;68:1125–1132.

Jerger J, Chmiel R, Wilson N, Luchi R. Hearing impairment in older adults: new concepts. *J Am Geriatr Soc.* 1995;43:928–935.

Marcincuk MC, Roland PS. Geriatric hearing loss: understanding the causes and providing appropriate treatment. *Geriatrics.* 2002;57:44–59.

Palmer CV, Ortmann A. Hearing loss and hearing aids. *Neurol Clin.* 2005;23:901–918.

Walling AD, Dickson GM. Hearing loss in older adults. *Am Fam Physician.* 2012;85:1150–1156.

Yueh B, Shapiro N, MacLean CH, Shekelle PG. Screening and management of adult hearing loss in primary care. *JAMA.* 2003;289:1976–1985.

General Discussion

Hematospermia, or blood in the ejaculate, may result from many different causes. Most men with hematospermia are young, with infections or inflammatory disorders accounting for 39% of cases. Malignancies and trauma each account for 2% of cases. Up to 46% of cases are labeled idiopathic, whereas a variety of other conditions account for the remaining cases.

For most patients, no significant workup is needed, but for a minority of patients, hematospermia may be a sign of serious urologic disease. Patients with risk factors or associated symptoms, patients 40 years and older, and patients with persistent or recurrent hematospermia require more extensive evaluation and may need urological evaluation.

The history should focus on infection and trauma. The medical history may play a role if there is a history of a bleeding disorder, hypertension, or previous malignancy. A sexual history should be included. Important elements of the physical examination are outlined in the following.

Causes of Hematospermia

Bladder sources
- Bladder tumor
- Cystitis (interstitial, eosinophilic, proliferative)

Infectious sources
- *Chlamydia trachomatis*
- Cytomegalovirus
- *Echinococcus*
- Epididymitis
- Gram-positive and gram-negative uropathogens
- Herpes simplex virus
- Hydatid disease
- *Neisseria gonorrhoeae*
- Schistosomiasis
- Seminal vesiculitis
- Tuberculosis

Prostatic sources
- Benign prostatic hyperplasia
- Bleeding following prostate biopsy, radiation therapy, brachytherapy
- Calculi/stones
- Inflammation (prostatitis)
- Malignancy
- Polyps
- Vascular lesions

Seminal vesicle sources
- Seminal vesicle cyst
- Seminal vesicle malignancy

Systemic disorders
- Amyloidosis
- Bleeding diatheses
- Chronic liver disease
- Hypertension (severe uncontrolled)
- Lymphoma

Trauma
- Excessive sex or masturbation
- Following hemorrhoidal injection
- Interrupted sex
- Penile injection
- Peyronie disease
- Prolonged sexual abstinence
- Testicular injury
- Urethral instrumentation

Urethral sources
- Condylomata
- Urethral cyst
- Urethral polyp
- Urethral stent migration
- Urethral stricture
- Urethritis (see infectious sources in the following)

Vascular
- Arteriovenous malformation
- Bladder neck and prostatic varices
- Hemangioma
- Submucosal bleeding
- Telangiectasias

Other
- Intraprostatic Müllerian duct remnants
- Seminal vesicular amyloidosis
- Seminal vesiculovenous fistula

Key Historical Features

✓ Rule out pseudo-hematospermia (make sure the bleeding is not from hematuria or blood from the sexual partner)
✓ Duration of symptoms
✓ Associated symptoms (e.g., pain, voiding symptoms, fever)
✓ Risk factors
✓ Sexual history
✓ Constitutional symptoms

- ✓ History of iatrogenic injury
- ✓ Travel history
- ✓ Medication history

Key Physical Findings

- ✓ Vital signs to evaluate for hypertension, fever, or tachycardia
- ✓ Abdominal examination
- ✓ Inspection of the penis
- ✓ Palpation of the vasa for swelling, induration, or nodularity
- ✓ Palpation of the testes
- ✓ Digital rectal examination of the prostate gland

Suggested Work-Up

Urinalysis and urine culture (preferably 72 hours after ejaculation)	To evaluate for hematuria
Prostate-specific antigen	To evaluate for prostate cancer
Urethral swabs or urine evaluation for gonorrhea and chlamydia	To evaluate for gonococcal or chlamydial urethritis in younger men or those at risk

Additional Work-Up

If the initial workup demonstrates abnormalities or if the patient has persistent hematospermia after empiric treatment with antibiotics, urologic evaluation should be considered. Additional studies may include:

Urine cytology	If tumor is suspected
Purified protein derivative	If the history suggests exposure to tuberculosis
Prothrombin time, partial thromboplastin time, complete blood count	If bleeding diathesis is suspected
Transrectal ultrasound or cystourethroscopy	May help identify the possible etiology when it is not clear from initial workup
Magnetic resonance imaging	May be helpful when seminal vesicle or prostate hemorrhage is suspected

Further Reading

Fletcher MS, Herzberg Z, Prior JR. The aetiology and investigation of hemospermia. *Br J Urol.* 1981;53:669–671.

Ganabathi K, Chadwick D, Feneley RC, Gingell JC. Hemospermia. *Br J Urol.* 1992;69:225–230.

Jones DJ. Hemospermia: a prospective study. *Br J Urol.* 1991;67:88–90.

Leary FJ, Aguilo JJ. Clinical significance of hemospermia. *Mayo Clin Proc.* 1974;49:815–817.

Mulhall JP, Albertsen PC. Hemospermia: diagnosis and management. *Urology.* 1995;46:463–467.

Papp G, Molnar J. Causes and differential diagnosis of hematospermia. *Andrologia.* 1981;13:474–478.

Stefanovic KB, Gregg PC, Soung M. Evaluation and treatment of hematospermia. *Am Fam Physician.* 2009;80:1421–1427.

General Discussion

The American Urological Association (AUA) has issued guidelines for the evaluation of microscopic hematuria in adults, and it defines clinically significant microscopic hematuria as three or more red blood cells per high-power field on microscopic evaluation of urinary sediment from two of three properly collected urinalysis specimens. However, each laboratory establishes its own thresholds based on the method of detection used.

Gross hematuria conveys a much higher risk of malignancy than microscopic disease, and little debate surrounds the need for a thorough evaluation. Visible blood in the urine is the presenting symptom in up to 85% of patients with bladder cancer and 40% of patients with renal cell carcinoma. As such, virtually all cases of hematuria as defined by AUA guidelines need a complete workup.

Dipstick testing for heme lacks specificity, because the presence of myoglobin or hemoglobin may result in a positive test when the urine contains no red cells. If the dipstick test is positive, the presence of red cells should be confirmed by microscopic examination of the urine. If the urine dipstick reveals blood, as well as leukocyte esterase, nitrites, and bacteria consistent with urinary tract infection, treatment with antibiotics is appropriate. If the hematuria resolves with treatment, no additional evaluation is necessary, but serum creatinine should be measured.

Transient microscopic hematuria may be caused by vigorous exercise, mild trauma, sexual intercourse, or menstrual contamination. If transient microscopic hematuria is suspected, urinalysis should be repeated 48 hours after discontinuation of these activities. Persistent microscopic hematuria warrants further evaluation.

Causes of microscopic hematuria may be classified as either glomerular or nonglomerular in origin. Immunoglobulin-A nephropathy is the most common glomerular cause. Nonglomerular causes involving the kidney and upper urinary tract include nephrolithiasis, neoplasm, polycystic kidney disease, medullary sponge kidney, papillary necrosis, hypercalciuria, and hyperuricosuria. Causes involving the lower urinary tract include disorders of the bladder, urethra, and prostate (e.g., bladder and prostate cancer).

Urinalysis is the most important test in the evaluation of hematuria, because it often distinguishes glomerular from nonglomerular bleeding. If proteinuria is detected on dipstick testing, total urinary protein excretion should be quantified. Twenty-four–hour urinary protein excretion greater than 300 mg suggests the kidney as a source of microscopic hematuria. Other findings that support a glomerular etiology include renal insufficiency, red cell casts, or dysmorphic red blood cells. When glomerular bleeding is suggested, no urologic evaluation is necessary. Proteinuria or renal insufficiency with microscopic hematuria warrants referral to a nephrologist for evaluation and possible renal biopsy.

If a glomerular source is ruled out or considered unlikely, the upper urinary tract should be imaged. Multiphasic computed tomography (CT) urography (without and with intravenous contrast) is the imaging procedure of choice, because it has the highest sensitivity and specificity for imaging the upper tracts. Alternatives to multiphase CT urography for patients with contraindications are outlined in the following.

Cystoscopy should be performed on all patients ages 35 years and older who present with asymptomatic hematuria. A cystoscopy should be performed on all patients who present with risk factors for urinary tract malignancies (e.g., irritative voiding symptoms, current or past tobacco use, chemical exposures), regardless of age.

The use of urine cytology and urine markers is not recommended as a part of the routine evaluation of the asymptomatic patient with microscopic hematuria. However, cytology may be useful in patients with persistent microscopic hematuria following a negative workup or those with other risk factors for carcinoma in situ (e.g., those with a smoking history; those with occupational exposure to benzenes or aromatic amines; age older than 40 years; individuals with a history of gross hematuria, urologic disease, irritative voiding symptoms, urinary tract infection, or pelvic irradiation; or those with analgesic abuse).

A thorough evaluation of the urinary system may fail to identify a source of microscopic hematuria in 19% to 68% of patients. For persistent asymptomatic microscopic hematuria after a negative urologic workup, yearly urinalyses should be conducted. If a patient has two consecutive negative annual urinalyses after negative urologic workup, then no further urinalyses are necessary. If gross hematuria, abnormal urinary cytology, or irritative voiding symptoms in the absence of infection develop, re-evaluation should be undertaken.

Medications Associated with Hematuria

Aminoglycosides
Amitriptyline
Anticonvulsants
Aspirin
Busulfan
Captopril
Cephalosporins
Chlorpromazine
Ciprofloxacin
Cyclophosphamide
Diuretics
Furosemide

Heparin
Indinavir
Mirtazapine
Nonsteroidal anti-inflammatory drugs
Omeprazole
Oral contraceptives
Penicillins
Quinine
Rifampin
Ritonavir
Triamterene
Trimethoprim-sulfamethoxazole
Vincristine
Warfarin

Causes of Microscopic Hematuria

Glomerular causes
- Fabry disease
- Goodpasture syndrome
- Hemolytic uremic syndrome
- Henoch-Schonlein purpura
- Hereditary nephritis (Alport syndrome)
- Immunoglobulin-A nephropathy
- Lupus nephritis
- Membranoproliferative glomerulonephritis
- Mesangial proliferative glomerulonephritis
- Mild focal glomerulonephritis of other causes
- Nail-patella syndrome
- Polyarteritis
- Postinfectious glomerulonephritis (endocarditis or viral)
- Poststreptococcal glomerulonephritis
- Thin basement membrane disease
- Wegener granulomatosis

Nonglomerular causes
Upper urinary tract causes
- Cytomegalovirus
- Epstein-Barr virus
- Hereditary nephritis
- Hypercalciuria
- Hyperuricosuria
- Loin pain hematuria syndrome
- Lymphoma
- Malignant hypertension

- Medications
- Medullary sponge kidney
- Multicystic kidney disease
- Nephrolithiasis
- Papillary necrosis
- Polycystic kidney disease
- Pyelonephritis
- Renal arteriovenous malformation
- Renal cell carcinoma
- Renal infarction
- Renal trauma
- Renal tuberculosis
- Renal vein thrombosis
- Sarcoidosis
- Schistosomiasis
- Sickle cell trait or disease
- Sjögren syndrome
- Solitary renal cyst
- Syphilis
- Toxoplasmosis
- Tuberculosis
- Ureteral stricture
- Ureteral transitional cell carcinoma

Lower urinary tract causes

- Benign bladder polyps and tumors
- Benign prostatic hypertrophy
- Benign ureteral polyps and tumors
- Bladder cancer
- Calculi
- Coagulopathy
- Congenital abnormalities
- Cystitis
- Endometriosis
- Epididymitis
- Foreign bodies
- Perineal irritation
- Posterior ureteral valves
- Prostate cancer
- Prostatitis
- Radiation-induced inflammation
- Schistosomiasis
- Transitional cell carcinoma of ureter or bladder
- Trauma (catheterization, blunt trauma)
- Urethral and meatal strictures
- Urethritis

Other causes
- Benign hematuria
- Exercise hematuria
- Factitious hematuria
- Menstrual contamination
- Over-anticoagulation with warfarin
- Sexual intercourse

Key Historical Features

✓ Irritative voiding
✓ Medical history, especially urologic history or pelvic irradiation
✓ Medications
✓ Cigarette smoking
✓ Travel history
✓ Occupational exposure to benzene or aromatic amines

Key Physical Findings

✓ Vital signs, especially blood pressure measurement
✓ General examination
✓ Cardiac examination for irregular rhythm that suggests atrial fibrillation or new murmur that suggest endocarditis
✓ Abdominal examination for bruits, masses, organomegaly, or aortic aneurysm
✓ Back examination for costovertebral angle tenderness
✓ Genital examination
✓ Urethral and vaginal examination in women
✓ Prostate examination in men
✓ Extremity examination for peripheral edema or petechiae

Suggested Work-Up

Urinalysis	To evaluate for bacteriuria and pyuria
Urine culture	Should be obtained if the urinalysis reveals evidence of infection
Serum creatinine	To evaluate for renal insufficiency
Multiphasic CT urography (without and with intravenous contrast)	To evaluate the upper urinary tract for renal cell carcinoma, transitional cell carcinoma, urolithiasis, cystic disease, and obstructive lesions
Cystoscopy	Recommended for all persons with asymptomatic microscopic hematuria who are 35 years and

older, as well as those who are younger but have risk factors for bladder cancer

Additional Work-Up

Urinary protein-to-creatinine concentration ratio or 24-hour urine collection	If proteinuria is detected on dipstick testing to determine total protein excretion
Urine cytology	May be useful in patients with persistent microscopic hematuria following a negative workup or those with other risk factors for carcinoma in situ

Magnetic resonance urography is an acceptable alternative imaging approach for patients with contraindications to using CT (renal insufficiency, contrast allergy, pregnancy).

Retrograde pyelogram may be added to magnetic resonance imaging (MRI) if collecting system detail is deemed imperative. For patients with contraindications to the use of multiphase CT and MRI in whom collecting system details is deemed imperative, combining noncontrast CT or renal ultrasound with retrograde pyelograms provides alternative evaluation of the entire upper tracts.

Further Reading

Ahmed Z, Lee J. Hematuria and proteinuria. *Med Clin North Am.* 1997;81:641–652.

Choyke PL. Radiologic evaluation of hematuria: guidelines from the American College of Radiology's appropriateness criteria. *Am Fam Physician.* 2008;78:347–352.

Cohen RA, Brown RS. Microscopic hematuria. *N Engl J Med.* 2003;348:2330–2338.

Davis R, Jones S, Barocas DA, et al. Diagnosis, evaluation, and follow-up of asymptomatic microhematuria (AMH) in adults: AUA guideline: American Urologic Association. *J Urol.* 2012;188(6 suppl):2473–2481.

Grossfeld GD, Carroll PR. Evaluation of asymptomatic microscopic hematuria. *Urol Clin North Am.* 1998;25:661–676.

Grossfeld GD, Wolf JS, Litwin MS, et al. Asymptomatic microscopic hematuria in adults: summary of the AUA best practice policy recommendations. *Am Fam Physician.* 2001;63:1145–1154.

Harper M, Arya M, Hamid R, Patel HR. Haematuria: a streamlined approach to management. *Hosp Med.* 2001;62:696–698.

Mazhari R, Kimmel PL. Hematuria: an algorithmic approach to finding the cause. *Cleve Clin J Med.* 2002;69:870–876.

McDonald MM, Swagerty D. Assessment of microscopic hematuria in adults. *Am Fam Physician.* 2006;73:1748–1754.

Sokolosky MC. Hematuria. *Emerg Med Clin North Am.* 2001;19:621–632.

Thaller TR, Wang LP. Evaluation of asymptomatic microscopic hematuria in adults. *Am Fam Physician.* 1999;60:1143–1154.

Yun EJ, Meng MV, Carroll PR. Evaluation of the patient with hematuria. *Med Clin North Am.* 2004;88:329–343.

General Discussion

Hemoptysis, the coughing up of blood from the respiratory tract, must be differentiated from hematemesis (the vomiting of blood) and pseudohemoptysis (the spitting of blood that originates in the nasopharynx or oropharynx). Blood in the lungs may originate from bronchial arteries, pulmonary arteries, bronchial capillaries, and alveolar capillaries. This discussion focuses on nonmassive hemoptysis, which is generally considered to be less than 200 ml/day.

Tuberculosis is the most common cause of hemoptysis worldwide. However, bronchitis, bronchiectasis, and bronchogenic carcinoma represent the most common causes of hemoptysis in the United States. In the United States, acute and chronic bronchitis account for 26% of cases, whereas primary lung cancers account for 23% of cases. The underlying cause is never found in 7% to 34% of cases of hemoptysis.

The appearance of the blood and the clinical history can offer clues to the cause of hemoptysis. Red, frothy blood mixed with purulent sputum usually is associated with an underlying pulmonary infection. Weight loss raises concern for cancer, especially in a smoker aged older than 40 years who has had hemoptysis lasting longer than 1 week. Night sweats, fever, and generalized illness may suggest tuberculosis as the cause. Persons who have recently travelled to Asia, South America, or the Middle East may present with hemoptysis as a result of parasitic infections (e.g., schistosomiasis). A monthly pattern of bleeding in a menstruating woman suggests pulmonary endometriosis. Goodpasture syndrome should be considered if the urinalysis reveals hematuria.

Medications Associated with Hemoptysis

Anticoagulants
Nonsteroidal anti-inflammatory drugs
Penicillamine

Causes of Hemoptysis

Anticoagulation therapy
Bioterrorism
- Pneumonic plague
- T2 mycotoxin
- Tularemia

Bronchiectasis
Broncholithiasis

Coagulopathy
- Hemophilia
- von Willebrand disease
- Thrombocytopenia

Cocaine use
Cystic fibrosis
Foreign body
Goodpasture syndrome
Heart failure
Idiopathic hemoptysis
Idiopathic pulmonary hemosiderosis
Infection
- Ascariasis
- Bronchitis
- Fungal infections (aspergilloma)
- Hydatid cyst
- Lung abscess
- Mycobacteria, especially tuberculosis
- Necrotizing pneumonia
- Paragonimiasis
- Pneumonia
- Schistosomiasis
- Tuberculosis

Lupus pneumonitis
Lymphangioleiomyomatosis
Neoplasm
- Adenoma
- Bronchial carcinoid
- Bronchogenic carcinoma
- Kaposi sarcoma
- Metastatic lung cancer

Pulmonary endometriosis
Trauma to the airway
Vascular
- Arteriovenous malformation
- Broncho-arterial fistula
- Mitral stenosis
- Pulmonary embolism/infarct
- Rupture of pulmonary artery by balloon-tipped catheter
- Ruptured thoracic aneurysm

Vasculitis
- Behçet disease
- Wegener granulomatosis

Key Historical Features

- ✓ Color of blood
- ✓ Patterns of bleeding
- ✓ Quantity of blood loss
- ✓ Association of hemoptysis with menstruation
- ✓ Medical history (especially history of lung disease, malignancy, immunosuppression, or bleeding disorders)
- ✓ Medications, especially anticoagulants or NSAIDs
- ✓ Family history
- ✓ History of smoking
- ✓ Alcohol use
- ✓ Recent travel
- ✓ Environmental exposures to asbestos, arsenic, chromium, nickel, and ethers
- ✓ Complete review of systems
  - Fever
  - Weight loss
  - Night sweats
  - Fatigue
  - Productive cough
  - Generalized illness
  - Chest pain
  - Dyspnea on exertion
  - Orthopnea
  - Paroxysmal nocturnal dyspnea
  - Hematuria
  - Nausea/vomiting
  - Changes in color of stool
  - Calf tenderness

Key Physical Findings

- ✓ Vital signs
- ✓ Pulse oximetry
- ✓ General examination for signs of cachexia or patient distress
- ✓ Inspection of the nose and oropharynx for evidence of bleeding
- ✓ Evaluation for lymphadenopathy
- ✓ Cardiovascular examination (especially for congestive heart failure)
- ✓ Examination of the thorax for trauma or other abnormalities
- ✓ Pulmonary examination (auscultation for stridor, wheezing, crackles, or diminished breath sounds)
- ✓ Abdominal examination for evidence of hepatic congestion or masses
- ✓ Examination of the extremities for cyanosis, clubbing, or edema

Suggested Work-Up

Pulse oximetry	To evaluate oxygenation status
Chest x-rays	To evaluate for underlying pathology such as tumors, infiltrates, atelectasis, and cavitary lesions
Computed tomography (CT) scan with intravenous contrast enhancement	Useful in many cases of hemoptysis when chest x-ray is normal. Useful for diagnosing bronchiectasis, peripheral masses, alveolar consolidation, and abnormal enhancing vessels.
Sputum for gram stain and acid-fast stain. Sputum culture for bacteria, fungus, and mycobacterium	If an infectious etiology is suspected
Sputum smear for cytology	If cancer is suspected by history, if the patient is a smoker, if the patient is older than 40 years, or if the patient has suspicious findings on chest x-ray
Complete blood count	To quantify blood loss, detect evidence of infection, and detect thrombocytopenia
Prothrombin time and partial thromboplastin time	If coagulopathy is suspected

Additional Work-Up

Bronchoscopy	Should be considered in high-risk patients to rule out malignancy. May be used to visualize the origin of bleeding and to control the bleeding. Bronchoscopy permits tissue biopsy, bronchial lavage, and brushings for pathologic diagnosis.
CT scan or ventilation-perfusion scan	Useful in patients suspected of having hemoptysis due to pulmonary embolism or infarct
Pulmonary arteriography	Selective angiography may locate the site of bleeding, and bronchial artery embolization may be used to control bleeding in cases of massive hemoptysis
Test of sputum for occult blood	If there is doubt that the sputum contains blood

| Arterial blood gases | To assess oxygenation, ventilation, and circulation in patients with signs of hemodynamic instability or respiratory impairment |
| Urinalysis | If vasculitis or Goodpasture syndrome is suspected |

Further Reading

Bidwell JL, Pachner RW. Hemoptysis: diagnosis and management. *Am Fam Physician.* 2005;72:1253–1260.

Corder R. Hemoptysis. *Emerg Med Clin North Am.* 2003;21:421–435.

Jean-Baptiste E. Clinical assessment and management of massive hemoptysis. *Crit Care Med.* 2000;28:1642–1647.

Reisz G, Stevens D, Boutwell C, Nair V. The causes of hemoptysis revisited. A review of the etiologies of hemoptysis between 1986 and 1995. *Mo Med.* 1997;94:633–635.

Tasker AD, Flower CDR. Imaging the airways: hemoptysis, bronchiectasis, and small airways disease. *Clin Chest Med.* 1999;20:761–773.

33 HIRSUTISM

General Discussion

Hirsutism is defined as the presence of excessive terminal hair in a pattern not normal in the female in areas such as the face, chest, or upper abdomen. This disorder is a sign of increased androgen action on hair follicles, which may result from increased levels of endogenous or exogenous androgens or from increased sensitivity of hair follicles to normal levels of circulating androgens.

Hirsutism should be distinguished from hypertrichosis, which is generalized excessive hair growth not caused by androgen excess. Hypertrichosis may be congenital or caused by metabolic disorders such as anorexia nervosa, thyroid dysfunction, and porphyria.

The most common triggering factor for hirsutism is excess androgen production. Although androgens may come from an exogenous source, androgen excess is most commonly endogenous. The two primary sources of endogenous androgens are the adrenal glands and the ovaries. Adrenal causes include congenital adrenal hyperplasia, Cushing syndrome, or tumor. Ovarian causes include polycystic ovary syndrome (the most common cause of hirsutism) and tumors.

When evaluating hirsutism, it is important to determine whether hirsutism exists alone or whether virilization is also present. This distinction is important because virilization may reflect a serious underlying pathologic condition (e.g., malignancy). Virilization presents with a wide range of signs of androgen excess, such as acne, hirsutism, frontotemporal balding, amenorrhea, oligomenorrhea, deepening of the voice, and clitoromegaly.

Medications Associated with Hirsutism

Anabolic steroids
Aripiprazole
Bimatoprost
Bupropion
Carbamazepine
Clonazepam
Corticosteroids
Cyclosporine
Danazol
Dantrolene
Diazoxide
Donepezil
Estrogens
Eszopiclone

Fluoxetine
Interferon alfa
Isotretinoin
Lamotrigine
Leuprolide
Methyldopa
Metoclopramide
Mycophenolate
Olanzapine
Paroxetine
Phenothiazines
Pregabalin
Progestins (especially levonorgestrel, norethindrone, and norgestrel)
Reserpine
Selegiline
Tacrolimus
Testosterones
Tiagabine
Trazodone
Venlafaxine
Zonisamide

Medications Associated with Hypertrichosis

Acitretin
Azelaic acid
Cetirizine
Citalopram
Corticosteroids (topical)
Cyclosporine
Etonogestrel implant
Phenytoin

Causes of Hirsutism

Acromegaly
Adrenal hyperplasia (congenital or late-onset form)
Cushing syndrome
Exogenous pharmacologic source of androgens
Familial hirsutism
Hyperprolactinemia
Iatrogenic hirsutism
Idiopathic hirsutism
Idiopathic hyperandrogenemia

Medications
Polycystic ovary syndrome
Thyroid dysfunction
Tumor (ovarian, adrenal, or pituitary)

Key Historical Features

✓ Onset and extent of hair growth
✓ Medical history
✓ Menstrual and reproductive history
✓ Hair patterns of family members (idiopathic hirsutism is often familial)
✓ Medications
✓ Supplements
✓ Family history
✓ Weight gain or change in muscle mass
✓ Changes in voice
✓ Abdominal symptoms
✓ Breast discharge or galactorrhea
✓ Skin symptoms, such as acne, dryness, or striae
✓ Virilization symptoms

Key Physical Findings

✓ Blood pressure, height, weight
✓ Evaluation of hair distribution and characteristics
✓ Skin evaluation (for acanthosis nigricans, acne, striae, hyperpigmentation)
✓ Breast examination for nipple discharge or galactorrhea
✓ Abdominal examination for masses
✓ Pelvic examination for masses
✓ Signs of Cushing syndrome
✓ Signs of virilization

Suggested Work-Up

Early morning total testosterone	To evaluate for hyperandrogenism
Serum prolactin	To evaluate for pituitary tumors
Thyroid-stimulating hormone	To evaluate for thyroid dysfunction

Additional Work-Up

If early morning total testosterone level is ≤200 ng/dl:

Thyroid-stimulating hormone	To evaluate thyroid function
Prolactin level	To evaluate for hyperprolactinemia
17-hydroxyprogesterone (17-OHP)	To evaluate for adrenal hyperplasia

Corticotropin stimulation test	If 21-hydroxylase deficiency/late-onset adrenal hyperplasia is suspected based upon the results of the 17-OHP level
Dexamethasone suppression test or 24-hour urinary cortisol measurement	If Cushing syndrome is suspected
Fasting serum glucose	To evaluate for insulin resistance in patients suspected of having polycystic ovary syndrome

If early morning total testosterone level is more than 200 ng/dl or if patient has signs and/or symptoms of androgen-secreting tumor, such as virilization, rapid onset of hirsutism, palpable abdominal or pelvic mass:

Serum testosterone, serum 17-OHP, and dehydroepiandosterone sulfate	To evaluate for ovarian and adrenal tumors
Computed tomography of the abdomen and pelvis	To assess the adrenal glands and ovaries in patients whose history, physical, or laboratory evaluation suggest the presence of a virilizing tumor

Further Reading

Bode D, Seehusen DA, Baird D. Hirsutism in women. *Am Fam Physician.* 2012;85:373–380.

Deplewski D, Rosenfield RL. Role of hormones in pilosebaceous unit development. *Endocr Rev.* 2000;21:363–392.

Gilchrist VJ, Hecht BR. A practical approach to hirsutism. *Am Fam Physician.* 1995;52:1837–1846.

Hunter MH, Carek PJ. Evaluation and treatment of women with hirsutism. *Am Fam Physician.* 2003;67:2565–2572.

Leung AK, Robson WL. Hirsutism. *Int J Dermatol.* 1993;32:773–777.

Physicians' Desk Reference Web site. Available at: http://www.pdr.net. Accessed 02.09.14.

Plouffe L. Disorders of excessive hair growth in the adolescent. *Obstet Gynecol Clin North Am.* 2000;27:79–99.

Redmond GP, Bergfeld WF. Diagnostic approach to androgen disorders in women: acne, hirsutism, and alopecia. *Cleve Clin J Med.* 1990;57:423–427.

Speroff L, Glass RH, Kase NG, eds. *Clinical Gynecologic Endocrinology and Infertility.* 6th ed. Baltimore, MD: Lippincott Williams & Wilkins; 1999:529–556.

General Discussion

The three pathophysiological mechanisms for hypercalcemia are increased bone resorption, increased gastrointestinal absorption of calcium, and decreased renal excretion of calcium. Increased bone resorption accounts for most cases of hypercalcemia and is seen in both primary hyperparathyroidism and malignancy. Increased gastrointestinal absorption of calcium is usually mediated by vitamin D through an increase in the production of 1,25 dihydroxyvitamin D, a mechanism seen in lymphomas and granulomatous disease. Decreased renal excretion of calcium is rare but may be caused by medications such as diuretics and lithium, which affect the renal handling of calcium.

Concentrations of calcium are highly modulated through the actions of parathyroid hormone (PTH), calcitonin, and vitamin D acting on target organs, such as bones, the kidneys, and the gastrointestinal tract. Primary hyperparathyroidism represents the leading cause of hypercalcemia, and malignancy is the second leading cause. Together, they account for more than 90% of the cases of hypercalcemia.

Primary hyperparathyroidism is usually caused by a single adenoma of the gland. Glandular hyperplasia, multiple adenomas, and parathyroid malignancy are less common. The hypercalcemia of malignancy is caused by increased bone resorption from skeletal metastases or the production of PTH-related peptide, which stimulates osteoclasts.

Because low albumin levels can affect the total calcium level, the evaluation of hypercalcemia begins with the calculation of the corrected calcium level using the following formula:

$$\text{Corrected calcium} = [4.0\,\text{g/dl} - (\text{plasma albumin})] \times 0.8 + (\text{serum calcium})$$

If the patient is on any medications known to be associated with hypercalcemia, the causative medications should be stopped, and the calcium levels rechecked. If the patient is not on any of these medications, or if the calcium level remains high, the workup for hypercalcemia may begin. The serum PTH level helps guide the evaluation of hypercalcemia. PTH is elevated in primary hyperparathyroidism and suppressed in malignancy-associated hypercalcemia. The remainder of the diagnostic evaluation is outlined in the following.

Medications and Ingestions Associated with Hypercalcemia

Betelnuts
Calcium

Calcium and vitamin D (milk-alkali syndrome)
Dialysate calcium
Ganciclovir
Growth hormone therapy
Lithium
Manganese
Parenteral nutrition
Tamoxifen
Theophylline
Thiazide diuretics
Thyroid hormone excess
Vitamin A
Vitamin D

Causes of Hypercalcemia

Endocrine/metabolic disorders
- Familial hypocalciuric hypercalcemia
- Hyperthyroidism
- Hypoadrenalism
- Hypophosphatasia
- Lactase deficiency
- Multiple endocrine neoplasia types I and IIa
- Pheochromocytoma
- Primary hyperparathyroidism
- Vipoma
- William syndrome

Granulomatous disease
- Bartonella (cat-scratch disease)
- Berylliosis
- Blastomyces
- Candidiasis
- Coccidioidomycosis
- Cryptococcus
- Cytomegalovirus
- Histoplasmosis
- HIV/AIDS-associated
- Leprosy
- Nocardia
- Pneumocystis
- Pulmonary eosinophilic granuloma
- Sarcoidosis
- Silicone injections
- Talc

- Tuberculosis
- Wegener granulomatosis

Immobilization

- Guillan-Barré syndrome
- Paget disease
- Thyrotoxicosis
- Whole-body cast

Inflammatory disease

- Acute rheumatic fever
- Crohn disease
- Richter syndrome
- Systemic lupus erythematosis
- Wegener granulomatosis

Malignancy

- Leukemia
- Lymphoma
- Multiple myeloma
- Solid tumors (lung cancer, breast cancer, renal cell carcinoma, prostate cancer, cholangiocarcinoma, colon cancer, and squamous cell carcinoma of the head and neck)

Medications (see the preceding)

Milk-alkali syndrome

PTH-related

Renal disease

- Renal failure (recovery phase, rhabdomyolysis)
- Tertiary hyperparathyroidism

Key Historical Features

✓ Age
✓ Sex
✓ Risk factors for malignancy
✓ Medical history
✓ Medications
✓ Family history (especially of hypercalcemia-associated conditions)
✓ Constitutional symptoms
  - Fatigue
  - Itching
  - Muscle weakness
  - Polydipsia
  - Polyuria
✓ Gastrointestinal symptoms
  - Abdominal pain
  - Anorexia

- • Constipation
- • Nausea and vomiting
- ✓ Neurologic symptoms
  - • Coma
  - • Confusion
  - • Impaired concentration and memory
  - • Lethargy
  - • Seizure

Key Physical Findings

- ✓ Blood pressure for evidence of hypertension
- ✓ General examination, especially for evidence of depression
- ✓ Head and neck examination, focusing on the thyroid and parathyroid glands
- ✓ Abdominal examination, especially for the possibility of ulcer, pancreatic tumor, or pancreatitis
- ✓ Neurological examination to test for proximal muscle weakness, easy fatigability, and muscle atrophy

Suggested Work-Up

Serum calcium	To determine the calcium level
Serum albumin	Used to calculate the corrected calcium
Serum ionized calcium	To determine the calcium level
PTH	Increased in primary hyperparathyroidism and suppressed in malignancy-associated hypercalcemia
Serum phosphorus	To evaluate for hyperphosphatemia
Serum electrolytes	To assess metabolic status
Blood urea nitrogen and creatinine	To evaluate renal function
Vitamin D	To evaluate for mineral and bone disorder
Magnesium	To evaluate for hypomagnesemia
Electrocardiogram	To evaluate for shortened QTc intervals and the presence of the Osborn wave (J wave)

Additional Work-Up

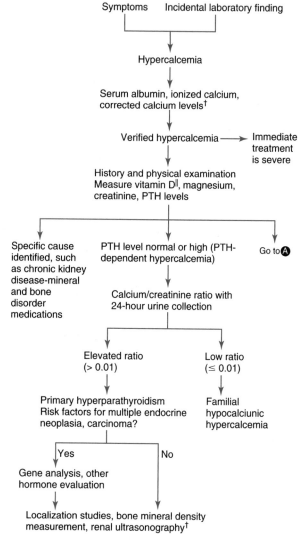

Symptoms   Incidental laboratory finding

↓

Hypercalcemia

↓

Serum albumin, ionized calcium, corrected calcium levels†

↓

Verified hypercalcemia ⟶ Immediate treatment is severe

↓

History and physical examination
Measure vitamin D‖, magnesium, creatinine, PTH levels

- Specific cause identified, such as chronic kidney disease-mineral and bone disorder medications

- PTH level normal or high (PTH-dependent hypercalcemia)

  ↓

  Calcium/creatinine ratio with 24-hour urine collection

  - Elevated ratio (> 0.01)

    ↓

    Primary hyperparathyroidism
    Risk factors for multiple endocrine neoplasia, carcinoma?

    - Yes ↓
      Gene analysis, other hormone evaluation

    - No

    ↓

    Localization studies, bone mineral density measurement, renal ultrasonography†

  - Low ratio (≤ 0.01)

    ↓

    Familial hypocalciunic hypercalcemia

- Go to Ⓐ

†—*Choice of localization studies is institution-specific; sestamibi scans and ultrasonography are most commonly used. Renal imaging with plain radiography or ultrasonography is indicated only when nephrolithiasis is suspected.*

‖—*Vitamin D deficiency: 25-hydroxyvitamin D level < 20 ng per mL (50 nmol per L).*

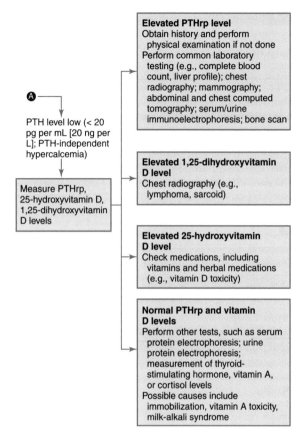

Figure 34-1. Adapted from Michels TC, Kelly KM. Parathyroid disorders. *Am Fam Physician.* 2013;88:249–257.

Further Reading

Ariyan CE, Sosa JA. Assessment and management of patients with abnormal calcium. *Crit Care Med.* 2004;32(4 suppl):S146–S154.

Barri YM, Knochel JP. Hypercalcemia and electrolyte disturbances in malignancy. *Hematol Oncol Clin North Am.* 1996;10:775–790.

Carroll MF, Schade DS. A practical approach to hypercalcemia. *Am Fam Physician.* 2003;67:1959–1966.

Deftos LJ. Hypercalcemia in malignant and inflammatory diseases. *Endocrinol Metab Clin North Am.* 2002;31:141–158.

Michels TC, Kelly KM. Parathyroid disorders. *Am Fam Physician.* 2013;88:249–257.

Taniegra ED. Hyperparathyroidism. *Am Fam Physician.* 2004;69:333–339.

35 HYPERCOAGULABLE STATES

General Discussion

Hypercoagulability, or thrombophilia, describes a group of hereditary and acquired conditions that confer a propensity to develop thrombi in the veins, arteries, or both. Antiphospholipid antibody syndrome is the most common hypercoagulable state, followed by factor V Leiden mutation. Individuals with a personal or family history of thrombosis have a higher risk of thrombosis than the general population.

Diagnostic thrombophilia testing is indicated in patients with idiopathic or recurrent venous thromboembolism (VTE), first VTE at age younger than 40 years, VTE in the setting of a strong family history, VTE in an unusual vascular site (e.g., cerebral, hepatic, mesenteric, or renal veins), neonatal purpura fulminans, warfarin-induced skin necrosis, and recurrent pregnancy loss. Diagnostic tests should be performed at least 4 to 6 weeks after an acute thrombotic event or discontinuation of anticoagulant or thrombolytic therapies, including warfarin, heparin, direct thrombin inhibitors, direct factor Xa inhibitors, and fibrinolytic agents.

Testing generally should be performed in a step-wise manner, beginning with high-yield screening tests followed by appropriate specific confirmatory tests, as outlined in the following.

Acquired Risk Factors for Thrombophilia

Major surgery, orthopedic surgery, or trauma
Immobilization
Solid or hematologic malignancy
Pregnancy
Oral contraceptive use
Estrogen replacement therapy
Antiphospholipid antibody syndrome (includes lupus anticoagulant and
    anticardiolipin antibodies)
Heparin-induced thrombocytopenia
Paroxysmal nocturnal hemoglobinuria
Obesity
Nephrotic syndrome
Polycythemia vera
Smoking

Hereditary Risk Factors for Thrombophilia

Activated protein C resistance/factor V Leiden
Prothrombin gene G20210A mutation
Protein C deficiency

Protein S deficiency
Antithrombin deficiency
Hyperhomocysteinemia
Elevated factor VIII activity
Dysfibrinogenemia

Key Historical Features

✓   Site of thrombosis
✓   Recent immobilization
✓   Previous bleeding or thrombotic events
✓   Medical history, especially liver, autoimmune, or cardiovascular disease
✓   Pregnancy history
✓   Family history
✓   Medications
✓   Tobacco use

Suggested Work-Up

Complete blood count	To screen for myeloproliferative disease
Prothrombin time (international normalized ratio) and activated prothrombin time (aPTT)	To screen for lupus anticoagulant
Lupus anticoagulant (hexagonal phase phospholipid neutralization)	To screen for lupus anticoagulant
Anticardiolipin antibody	To screen for anticardiolipin antibody
Protein C functional assay	To screen for protein C deficiency
Protein S functional assay	To screen for protein S deficiency
Antithrombin III functional assay	To screen for antithrombin deficiency
Activated protein C resistance assay	To screen for factor V Leiden (activated protein C resistance)
Factor VIII level	To screen for elevated factor VIII level
Fibrinogen	To screen for dysfibrinogenemia
Homocysteine level	To screen for hyperhomocysteinemia
Prothrombin G20210A single nucleotide polymorphism	To screen for prothrombin G20210A gene mutation

Additional Work-Up

Dilute Russell Viper Venom test, platelet neutralization procedure, incubated aPTT mixing study	If screening for lupus anticoagulant is positive
B2GPI antibody assay	If screening for anticardiolipin antibody is positive
Protein C, protein S, or antithrombin antigenic assay	If the functional assays for any of these anticoagulants are positive
Factor V Leiden single nucleotide polymorphism analysis	If activated protein C resistance assay is positive

Further References

Alpert MA. Homocysteine, atherosclerosis, and thrombosis. *South Med J.* 1999;92:858–865.

Bande BD, Bande SB, Mohite S. The hypercoagulable states in anaesthesia and critical care. *Indian J Anaesth.* 2014;58:665–671.

Barger AP, Hurley R. Evaluation of the hypercoagulable state: whom to screen, how to test and treat. *Postgrad Med.* 2000;108:59–66.

DeStefano V, Finazzi G, Mannucci PM. Inherited thrombophilia: pathogenesis, clinical syndromes, and management. *Blood.* 1996;87:5331–5344.

Faioni EM, Valsecchi C, Palla A, et al. Free protein S deficiency is risk factor for venous thrombosis. *Thromb Haimost.* 1997;78:1343–1346.

Federman DG, Kirsner RS. An update on hypercoagulable disorders. *Arch Intern Med.* 2001;161:1051–1056.

Koster T, Blann AD, Briet E, et al. Role of clotting factor VIII in effect of von Willebrand factor on occurrence of deep-vein thrombosis. *Lancet.* 1995;345:152–155.

Nakashima MO, Rogers HJ. Hypercoagulable states: an algorithmic approach to laboratory testing and update on monitoring of direct oral anticoagulants. *Blood Research.* 2014;49:85–94.

Poort SR, Rosendaal FR, Reitsma PH, et al. A common genetic variant in the 3′-untranslated region of the prothrombin gene is associated with elevated plasma prothrombin levels and an increase in thrombosis. *Thromb Haimost.* 1997;78:1430–1433.

Tait RC, Walker ID, Retsma PH, et al. Prevalence of protein C deficiency in the healthy population. *Thromb Haimost.* 1995;73:87–93.

36 HYPERKALEMIA

General Discussion

Hyperkalemia is defined as a serum potassium concentration greater than 5.0 or 5.5 mEq/L, depending on the laboratory assay. Hyperkalemia can become life-threatening when the potassium concentration rises to greater than 6.5 mEq/L. Hyperkalemia is often asymptomatic, but it may affect normal cardiac conduction, producing characteristic electrocardiographic (ECG) changes that are outlined in the following. Although there is no clear correlation between the degree of hyperkalemia and the likelihood of life-threatening arrhythmias, an arrhythmia is more likely to occur if the serum potassium concentration increases rapidly. All patients with a serum potassium concentration greater than 6.0 mEq/L should be considered at risk for cardiac arrhythmias.

All disorders of potassium occur because of abnormal handling of potassium in one of three ways: problems with potassium intake; problems with potassium excretion; or problems with distribution of potassium between the intracellular and extracellular spaces. Renal disorders are the most common cause of hyperkalemia, followed by cell lysis. Patients with acute renal failure are at greater risk for life-threatening complications from hyperkalemia because the potassium level rises more rapidly.

The primary source of potassium intake is through food. Fruits and vegetables have the highest concentrations of potassium. Salt substitutes represent a commonly overlooked source of dietary potassium. Under normal circumstances, 80% to 90% of dietary potassium is eliminated via renal excretion.

The organs affected by hyperkalemia are the cardiac, neuromuscular, and gastrointestinal systems. Symptoms may include generalized malaise and fatigue, palpitations, paresthesias, muscle cramps, or muscle weakness that can progress to a flaccid paralysis. Nausea, vomiting, and diarrhea can also occur.

Medications and Supplements Associated with Hyperkalemia

Alpha-blockers
Amino acids
- Arginine
- Epsilon-aminocaproic acid
- Lysine
Angiotensin-converting enzyme inhibitors
Angiotensin receptor blockers
Azole antifungals
Beta-blockers (nonselective)
Cyclosporine

Digoxin

Eplerenone

Ethinyl estradiol/drospirenone

Herbal remedies and nutritional supplements

- Alfalfa
- Dandelion
- Hawthorn berries
- Horsetail
- Lily of the valley
- Milkweed
- Nettle
- Noni juice
- Siberian ginseng

Heparin

Nonsteroidal anti-inflammatory drugs

Penicillin G potassium

Pentamidine

Potassium-sparing diuretics

- Amiloride
- Spironolactone
- Triamterene

Potassium supplements

Succinylcholine

Suxamethonium

Tacrolimus

Trimethoprim-sulfamethoxazole

Causes of Hyperkalemia

Acidosis

Adrenal insufficiency (Addison disease)

AIDS

Amyloidosis

Burns

Congenital adrenal hyperplasia

Diabetes mellitus

Familial hyperkalemic periodic paralysis

Fluoride toxicity

Heart failure

Hematoma reabsorption

Hereditary enzyme deficiencies

Hypertonicity (hyperglycemia, hypernatremia)

Infusion of packed red blood cells (massive blood transfusion)

Insulin deficiency or resistance

Low renin level
Medications
Obstructive uropathy
Poisoning/ingestion
Prolonged fasting
Pseudohyperkalemia
- Fist clenching with tourniquet in place
- Hemolysis
- Leukocytosis (white blood cell count $>100,000/mm^3$)
- Thrombocytosis (platelets $>1,000,000/mm^3$)

Pseudohypoaldosteronism
Renal failure (acute and chronic)
Renal insufficiency
Renal transplantation
Rhabdomyolysis
Selective hypoaldosteronism
Sickle cell anemia
Systemic lupus erythematosus
Trauma
Tumor lysis syndrome
Type 4 renal tubular acidosis

Key Historical Features

✓ Fatigue/malaise
✓ Palpitations
✓ Muscle cramps
✓ Muscle weakness
✓ Paresthesias
✓ Gastrointestinal symptoms
✓ History of salt substitute intake
✓ Medical history, especially renal insufficiency
✓ Medications
✓ Herbal and dietary supplement use
✓ Diet history
✓ Family history

Key Physical Findings

✓ Cardiac examination for bradycardia or arrhythmias
✓ Gastrointestinal examination
✓ Neurologic examination for muscle weakness or decreased deep tendon reflexes

Suggested Work-up

ECG

To evaluate the effect of hyperkalemia on the myocardium. May reveal peaked T waves, widened QRS complexes, increased PR interval, atrioventricular conduction blockade with a slow idioventricular rhythm, and ventricular fibrillation.

Serum electrolytes

To measure electrolytes and evaluate for acidosis

Blood urea nitrogen and creatinine

To evaluate renal function

Spot urine for potassium, creatinine, and osmoles

To calculate the fractional excretion of potassium (FEK):

$$\frac{U_K \times S_{Cr}}{S_K \times U_{Cr}} \times 100$$

(where K = potassium and Cr = creatinine):
FEK less than 10% indicates renal etiology.
FEK greater than 10% indicates extrarenal etiology

Morning serum cortisol level

To assess for adrenal insufficiency

Additional Work-up

Adrenocorticotrophic hormone stimulation test

If the morning serum cortisol level is low, to evaluate for adrenal insufficiency

Measurement of plasma and serum potassium concentrations

If pseudohyperkalemia is suspected

Further Reading

Gennari FJ. Disorders of potassium homeostasis; hypokalemia and hyperkalemia. *Crit Care Clin.* 2002;18:273–288.

Hollander-Rodriguez JC, Calvert JF. Hyperkalemia. *Am Fam Physician.* 2006;73:283–290.

Mandal AK. Hypokalemia and hyperkalemia. *Med Clin North Am.* 1997;81:611–639.

Medford-Davis L, Rargique Z. Derangements of potassium. *Emerg Med Clin N Am.* 2014;32:329–347.

Schaefer TJ, Wolford RW. Disorders of potassium. *Emerg Med Clin North Am.* 2005;23:723–747.

Weiner ID, Wingo CS. Hyperkalemia: a potential silent killer. *J Am Soc Nephrol.* 1998;9:1535–1543.

General Discussion

Hypernatremia is defined as a serum sodium concentration greater than 145 mEq/L. In contrast to hyponatremia, which usually results from a defect in renal water handling, the primary defect in hypernatremia is impaired water intake. Hypernatremia represents a deficit of water in relation to the body's sodium stores, which may result from a net water loss or a hypertonic sodium gain. Unlike hyponatremia, hypernatremia always represents a hyperosmolar state. The majority of cases of hypernatremia result from a net water loss.

Hypernatremia is rarely found in an alert patient who has access to water and a normal thirst mechanism. Sustained hypernatremia occurs when thirst is impaired or access to water is limited; therefore, the groups at highest risk are patients with altered mental status, intubated patients, older adults, and infants. In older adults, hypernatremia is usually associated with infirmity or febrile illness. Hypernatremia is also more common after age 60 years because increased age is associated with decreased osmotic stimulation of thirst and decreased maximal urinary concentration.

Signs and symptoms of hypernatremia reflect central nervous system dysfunction and are most prominent when the increase in the serum sodium concentration is large and occurs rapidly. Patients may present with lethargy, weakness, or restlessness. Consequences of hypernatremia include decreased left ventricular contractility, hyperventilation, impaired glucose use, muscle cramps, and rhabdomyolysis. Older adult patients generally have few symptoms until the serum sodium concentration exceeds 160 mmol/L. Brain shrinkage induced by hypernatremia can cause vascular rupture, with cerebral bleeding and permanent neurologic damage or death.

The initial step in evaluating a patient with hypernatremia is to determine the volume status of the patient. Hypovolemic hypernatremia is usually caused by an inability to detect or respond to the sensation of thirst. Hypervolemic hypernatremia is usually the result of iatrogenic complications (e.g., administration of sodium bicarbonate during the treatment of acidosis), or accidental or intentional poisoning. Euvolemic hypernatremia is most often caused by diabetes insipidus.

Central diabetes insipidus results from deficient vasopressin secretion, whereas nephrogenic diabetes insipidus results from end organ hyporesponsiveness to vasopressin. Diabetes insipidus is associated with variable degrees of polyuria and an inability to concentrate urine maximally.

Medications Associated with Hypernatremia

Amphotericin B
Demeclocycline
Foscarnet
Lactulose
Lithium
Loop diuretics
Methoxyflurane
Vasopressin receptor antagonists

Causes of Hypernatremia*

Net water loss
- Burns
- Excessive sweating
- Gastrointestinal losses (vomiting, diarrhea, nasogastric suctioning, enterocutaneous fistula, lactulose)
- Hypothalamic disorder (primary hypodipsia, re-setting of osmostat)
- Insensible losses
- Intrinsic renal disease
- Loop diuretics
- Nephrogenic diabetes insipidus (hypercalcemia, hypokalemia, medications, medullary cystic disease)
- Neurogenic diabetes insipidus (trauma, encephalopathy, tumor, cyst, tuberculosis, sarcoidosis, histiocytosis, idiopathic, aneurysm, meningitis, encephalitis, Guillain-Barré syndrome, ethanol ingestion)
- Osmotic diuresis with glucose, urea, or mannitol
- Third space fluid losses (bowel obstruction, ileus, pancreatitis)

Hypertonic sodium gain
- Cushing syndrome
- Hypertonic dialysis
- Hypertonic feeding
- Hypertonic sodium chloride infusion
- Intrauterine injection of hypertonic saline
- Primary hyperaldosteronism
- Sea water ingestion
- Sodium bicarbonate infusion
- Sodium chloride ingestion

---

*Adapted from Table 1 in Adrogue HJ, Madias NE. Hypernatremia. *New England Journal of Medicine* 2000;342:1493–1499.

Key Historical Features

✓ Symptoms of hypernatremia (muscle weakness, lethargy, irritability, restlessness, confusion, coma)
✓ Fever
✓ Nausea or vomiting
✓ Presence of thirst
✓ Polyuria and polydipsia
✓ Recent fluid losses
✓ Recent intravenous or intrauterine fluid administration
✓ Medical history, especially any neurologic disease
✓ Medications
✓ Functional status and ability to obtain drinking water

Key Physical Findings

✓ Vital signs
✓ Assessment of volume status
✓ Head and neck examination to evaluate for dry mucous membranes
✓ Cardiac examination for tachycardia
✓ Neurologic examination for hyper-reflexia, spasticity, or weakness

Suggested Work-Up

Urine osmolality and low urine sodium and a maximally concentrated urine sodium (>700 mmol/kg) suggests extrarenal hypotonic fluid losses.

Concentration

When losses are renal in origin, the urine osmolality is inappropriately low. With diuretics, osmotic diuresis, or salt wasting, the urine osmolality is isotonic at approximately 300 mmol/kg. Patients with urine osmolality of less than 200 mmol/kg usually have some form of diabetes insipidus.

A urine osmolality of less than 150 mmol/kg in the setting of hypertonicity and polyuria is diagnostic of diabetes insipidus.

Additional Work-Up

Vasopressin administration	If diabetes insipidus is suspected, to differentiate the hypothalamic and nephrogenic forms
Serum potassium and serum calcium	If nephrogenic diabetes insipidus is suggested by the previously outlined diagnostic evaluation

Further Reading

Adrogue HJ, Madias NE. Hypernatremia. *N Engl J Med*. 2000;342:1493–1499.

Fall PJ. Hyponatremia and hypernatremia: a systematic approach to causes and their correction. *Postgrad Med*. 2000;107:75–82.

Fried LF, Palevsky PM. Hyponatremia and hypernatremia. *Med Clin North Am*. 1997;81:585–609.

Harring TR, Deal NS, Kuo DC. Disorders of sodium and water balance. *Emerg Med Clin North Am*. 2014;32:379–401.

Kumar S, Berl T. Sodium. *Lancet*. 1998;352:220–228.

38 HYPERTENSION

General Discussion

The relationship between blood pressure and the risk of cardiovascular disease is continuous, consistent, and independent of other risk factors. As blood pressure rises, so does the risk of myocardial infarction, heart failure, stroke, and kidney disease. For individuals 40 to 70 years of age, each increment of 20 mm Hg in systolic blood pressure or 10 mm Hg in diastolic blood pressure doubles the risk of cardiovascular disease across the entire blood pressure range from 115/75 to 185/115 mm Hg.

Normal blood pressure is defined as less than 120/80 mm Hg. The term "prehypertension" is used for blood pressures ranging from 120 to 139 mm Hg systolic and/or 80 to 89 mm Hg diastolic.

The evaluation of patients with hypertension has three objectives. First, the patient's lifestyle and cardiovascular risk factors should be assessed. Second, identifiable causes of hypertension should be identified. Third, the presence or absence of target organ damage and cardiovascular disease should be assessed.

Five percent to 10% of patients with hypertension have an underlying, potentially correctable etiology that can be identified. Whenever a patient is diagnosed with hypertension, the initial assessment should be directed at excluding secondary causes. Indications for further investigation into a possible secondary cause include resistant hypertension, early- or late-onset hypertension, a severe or accelerated course, or specific drug intolerances. Signs and symptoms that may suggest a secondary cause include vascular bruits, symptoms of catecholamine excess, or unprovoked hypokalemia.

Medications and Herbal Supplements Associated with Hypertension

Adrenal steroids
Buspirone
Carbamazepine
Clozapine
Cyclosporin
Decongestants
Diet pills
Ephedra
Erythropoietin
Fluoxetine
Ginseng
Lithium
Ma huang
Methylprednisolone

Nonsteroidal anti-inflammatory drugs
- Cyclooxygenase-2 inhibitors
- Ibuprofen
- Naproxen

Oral contraceptives (estrogen)
Over-the-counter medicines (bitter orange, ephedra, ma haung)
Prednisone
Tacrolimus
Tricyclic antidepressants

Identifiable Causes of Hypertension

Aldosteronism
Chronic kidney disease
Chronic steroid therapy
Coarctation of the aorta
Cushing syndrome
Illicit drug use
- Amphetamines
- Cocaine

Obstructive sleep apnea
Parathyroid disease
Pheochromocytoma
Renal artery stenosis
- Due to fibromuscular dysplasia, especially in young adults, particularly women

Renovascular disease (renal artery stenosis)
Thyroid disease

Suggested Work-Up

Electrocardiography	To evaluate for end-organ damage
Urinalysis	To evaluate for end-organ damage
Serum potassium	To evaluate for secondary hypertension
Serum creatinine	To evaluate for secondary hypertension
Serum calcium	To evaluate for secondary hypertension
Hemoglobin and hematocrit	To evaluate for hypertension-induced hemoconcentration
Fasting blood glucose	To evaluate for glucose intolerance or diabetes
Fasting lipid panel	To evaluate for hyperlipidemia

Additional Work-Up

More extensive testing for identifiable causes is not generally indicated unless blood pressure control is not achieved or the clinical and routine laboratory evaluation strongly suggests a secondary cause of hypertension.

Magnetic resonance imaging with gadolinium (generally preferred) or computed tomography (CT) of the renal arteries (renal Doppler can be used, but accuracy may be affected by body recurrent flash pulmonary edema, renal habitus, and operator skill)	If renal artery stenosis is suspected (early onset of hypertension, abdominal bruit, accelerated hypertension, failure of uncertain etiology, or acute renal failure precipitated by therapy with an angiotensin-converting enzyme inhibitor or angiotensin receptor blocker)
Renal ultrasound	In patients with elevated creatinine or abnormal urinalysis on initial screening
Thyroid-stimulating hormone	If thyroid dysfunction is suspected
Aldosterone/renin ratio (measured in the morning at least 2 hours after waking and in the upright position)	If hyperaldosteronism (primary aldosteronism) is suspected (e.g., presence of nonmedication-induced hypokalemia or of nonmedication-induced hypokalemia or resistant hypertension). Ratio greater than 20 and accompanied by aldosterone level greater than 15 ng/dL is indicative. Refer patient to endocrinology.
Dexamethasone suppression test or 24-hour urinary free cortisol or late-night salivary cortisol test	In patients suspected of having Cushing disease (truncal obesity, glucose intolerance, striae)
Drug screening	In patients suspected of having drug-induced hypertension
24-hour urinary metanephrine and normetanephrine	In patients suspected of having pheochromocytoma (typically only indicated in patients with labile hypertension or paroxysms of hypertension accompanied by headache, palpitations, pallor, and perspiration)
Sleep study (polysomnography)	If sleep apnea is suspected

| CT angiogram | In patients suspected of having coarctation of the aorta (decreased pressure in the lower extremities or delayed or absent femoral arterial pulses) |
| Serum parathyroid hormone | If parathyroid disease is suspected (hypercalcemia on initial screen) |

Further Reading

James PA, Oparil S, Carter BL, et al. 2014 evidence-based guideline for the management of high blood pressure in adults. Report from the panel members appointed to the Eight Joint National Committee (JNC 8). *JAMA.* 2014;311:507–520.

Lewington S, Clarke R, Qizilbash N, et al. Age-specific relevance of usual blood pressure to vascular mortality: a meta-analysis of individual data for one million adults in 61 prospective studies. *Lancet.* 2002;360:1903–1913.

Philips LS, Branch WT, Cook CB, et al. Clinical inertia. *Ann Intern Med.* 2001;135:825–834.

Viera AJ. Diagnosis of secondary hypertension: an age-based approach. *Am Fam Physician.* 2010;82:1471–1478.

General Discussion

Hyperthyroidism is the excess production and release of thyroid hormone by the thyroid gland, which results in inappropriately high serum levels. The overall incidence of subclinical and overt hyperthyroidism is estimated to be 1.2% in the general population. Hyperthyroidism occurs in all age groups and is more common in women than in men.

Graves disease is the most common cause of hyperthyroidism, causing 60% to 80% of cases. Graves disease is an autoimmune condition in which antibodies against the thyroid-stimulating hormone (TSH) receptor cause unopposed stimulation of the thyroid gland. Toxic multinodular goiter, the most common cause of hyperthyroidism in those older than age 50 years, is caused by unwarranted release of thyroid hormones from multiple autonomously functioning nodules in the thyroid gland. Toxic adenoma tends to present at a younger age and is a single hyperfunctioning nodule in the thyroid gland that produces a surplus of thyroid hormone. Subacute thyroiditis is inflammation of the thyroid gland that typically follows a viral upper respiratory infection and results in additional release of preformed thyroid hormone.

Hyperthyroidism may present as a spectrum from asymptomatic, subclinical hyperthyroidism to a life-threatening thyroid storm. Serious complications of undiagnosed hyperthyroidism include altered mental status, delirium, insomnia, anorexia, muscle weakness, osteoporosis, atrial fibrillation, congestive heart failure, thromboembolism, cardiovascular collapse, and death. Thyroid storm is a true endocrine emergency that needs to be identified rapidly and treated aggressively.

Subclinical hyperthyroidism is diagnosed in asymptomatic patients with low TSH but who have normal free T_4 and free T_3. Clinical hyperthyroidism presents with the typical signs and symptoms outlined in the following.

Older adult patients often present a diagnostic challenge because they may present with lone symptoms or atypical presentations. They may present with negative symptoms, such as depressive symptoms, lethargy, or apathetic facies. Older adult patients may also present with only a small goiter, weight loss, worsening of underlying cardiovascular disease, or new-onset atrial fibrillation.

Medications Associated with Hyperthyroidism

Amiodarone
Campath 1-H monoclonal antibody

Highly active antiretroviral therapy
Interferon-α
Levothyroxine
Lithium
Tyrosine kinase inhibitors

Causes of Hyperthyroidism

Beta-human chorionic gonadotropin (high levels as found in molar
hydatidiform pregnancies and choriocarcinoma)
Factitious hyperthyroidism
Follicular thyroid carcinoma
Graves disease
Iodine-induced hyperthyroidism (iodine ingestion, radiographic contrast,
amiodarone)
Lymphocytic thyroiditis (Hashimoto thyroiditis)
Medication-induced thyroiditis
Ovarian tumors (struma ovarii)
Pituitary adenoma–secreting TSH
Postpartum thyroiditis
Subacute thyroiditis
Suppurative thyroiditis
Toxic adenoma
Toxic multinodular goiter
Trophoblastic tumor

Key Historical Features

✓ Constitutional symptoms
- Anxiety
- Excessive perspiration
- Fatigue
- Heat intolerance
- Nervousness
- Pruritis
- Thirst
- Weight loss

✓ Cardiac symptoms
- Anginal symptoms
- Exertional dyspnea
- Orthopnea
- Palpitations
- Reduced exercise tolerance

✓ Pulmonary symptoms
  - Dyspnea
✓ Gastrointestinal symptoms
  - Difficulty swallowing
  - Dyspepsia
  - Frequent bowel movements
  - Nausea and vomiting
  - Rapid intestinal transit time
✓ Genitourinary symptoms
  - Erectile dysfunction
  - Nocturia
  - Urinary frequency
✓ Ophthalmologic symptoms
  - Diplopia
  - Eye irritation or dryness
  - Excessive tearing
  - Pain with eye movements
  - Visual blurring
✓ Reproductive symptoms
  - Amenorrhea
  - Decreased libido
  - Gynecomastia
  - Infertility
  - Menometrorrhagia
  - Oligomenorrhea
  - Spider angiomas
✓ Neuromuscular symptoms
  - Fatigability
  - Generalized weakness
  - Proximal muscle weakness
✓ Psychiatric symptoms
  - Altered mental status
  - Emotional lability
  - Insomnia
  - Memory loss
  - Nightmares and vivid dreams
  - Poor attention span
  - Restlessness
✓ Medical history
✓ Medications
✓ Recent pregnancy
✓ Smoking
✓ Family history

Key Physical Findings

✓ Vital signs, especially tachycardia or hypertension
✓ Skin and hair
- Warm, smooth, velvety skin
- Skin hyperpigmentation
- Palmar erythema
- Pretibial myxedema
- Fine, brittle scalp hair
- Diffuse alopecia
- Nail changes (onycholysis)

✓ Eyes
- Exophthalmos
- Proptosis
- Lid lag
- Infrequent blinking
- Vasodilation of the conjunctiva
- Lid or periorbital edema
- Papilledema

✓ Thyroid
- Diffuse enlargement
- Single nodule
- Multinodular goiter
- Bruit

✓ Cardiovascular
- Tachycardia
- Bounding pulses
- Rapid and brisk carotid upstroke
- Systolic flow murmurs
- Atrial arrhythmias, such as atrial fibrillation or atrial flutter

✓ Pulmonary
- Tachypnea

✓ Musculoskeletal
- Decreased muscle strength
- Decreased muscle volume
- Muscle atrophy
- Muscle weakness, especially proximal

✓ Neurologic
- Brisk reflexes
- Fidgeting
- Nervousness
- Hyperactivity and rapid speech

Suggested Work-Up

TSH and free T_4	To evaluate thyroid function
Radioactive iodine thyroid scan and update test	To distinguish Graves disease (diffuse distribution of tracer), toxic multinodular goiter (localized distribution of tracer), toxic adenoma (localized distribution of tracer), subacute thyroiditis (decreased uptake), and exogenous thyroid hormone ingestion (decreased uptake)

Additional Work-Up

Thyroglobulin level	May help distinguish Graves disease (elevated thyroglobulin), subacute thyroiditis (elevated thyroglobulin) from factitious thyrotoxicosis (decreased thyroglobulin)
Thyroid peroxidase antibodies	Elevated in many cases of Graves disease and lymphocytic thyroiditis
C-reactive protein and erythrocyte sedimentation rate	Often increased in subacute thyroiditis

Further Reading

Devereaux D, Tewelde SZ. Hyperthyroidism and thyrotoxicosis. *Emerg Med Clin N Am.* 2014;32:277–292.

Donangelo I, Braunstein GD. Update on subclinical hyperthyroidism. *Am Fam Physician.* 2011;83:933–938.

Ginsberg J. Diagnosis and management of Graves' disease. *Can Med Assoc J.* 2003;168:575–585.

McKeown NJ, Tews MC, Gossain VV, Shah SM. Hyperthyroidism. *Emerg Med Clin North Am.* 2005;23:669–685.

Reid JR, Wheeler SF. Hyperthyroidism: diagnosis and treatment. *Am Fam Physician.* 2005;72:623–630.

Vaidya B, Pearce SHS. Diagnosis and management of thyrotoxicosis. *BMJ.* 2014;249:g5128.

40 HYPOCALCEMIA

General Discussion

Hypocalcemia is defined as a total calcium concentration of less than 8.5 mg/dL or an ionized calcium concentration of less than 4.5 mg/dL (1.1 mmol/L). Half of serum calcium is bound to albumin; therefore, serum calcium levels must be corrected for the albumin level before confirming the diagnosis of hypercalcemia or hypocalcemia. Hypocalcemia ranges in presentation from asymptomatic in mild cases to acute life-threatening crises in severe cases.

Serum calcium levels are regulated by three main calcium-regulating hormones: parathyroid hormone (PTH), vitamin D, and calcitonin through their effects on the bowel, kidneys, and skeleton. Hypocalcemia is most commonly a consequence of vitamin D deficiency or hypoparathyroidism, or a resistance to these hormones. Inadequate vitamin D levels lead to a reduction in gastrointestinal calcium absorption. Low PTH levels result in excessive urinary calcium losses, decreased bone remodeling, and reduced intestinal calcium absorption. Hypoparathyroidism is most commonly seen following inadvertent removal of or damage to the parathyroid glands or their vascular supply during total thyroidectomy. Autoimmune hypoparathyroidism is less common and can present alone or as part of a polyglandular endocrinopathy.

Symptoms of hypocalcemia are outlined in the following. In addition to these symptoms, hypocalcemia can result in prolonged QT intervals and electrocardiographic changes that mimic myocardial infarction or heart failure.

Medications Associated with Hypocalcemia

Aminoglycosides
Antiepileptics
Bisphosphonates
Chemotherapeutic agents, especially cisplatin
Cisplatin
Diuretics
Foscarnet
Histamine-2 receptor blockers
Proton pump inhibitors
Sodium phosphate preparations

Causes of Hypocalcemia

Citrated blood transfusion
Congenital abnormalities (DiGeorge syndrome)

Critical illness

Fanconi syndrome

Heavy metal (iron, copper) infiltration of the parathyroid gland

Hypermagnesemia

Hypomagnesemia

Hypoparathryoidism (following surgery or due to autoimmune disease, genetic causes, or metastatic infiltration)

Liver disease (end stage)

Pancreatitis

Phosphate infusion

Pseudohypoparathyroidism

Radiation of parathyroid glands

Renal disease (secondary hyperparathyroidism)

Sclerotic metastases

Tumor lysis

Vitamin D deficiency

Vitamin D resistance

Key Historical Features

- ✓ Paresthesias
- ✓ Perioral numbness
- ✓ Muscle cramping or spasms
- ✓ Muscle twitching
- ✓ Tetany
- ✓ Seizures
- ✓ Headache
- ✓ Impaired vision
- ✓ Neuropsychiatric symptoms
- ✓ Cognitive impairment
- ✓ Personality changes
- ✓ Dysphagia
- ✓ Dyspnea
- ✓ Edema
- ✓ Palpitations
- ✓ Syncope
- ✓ Growth or mental retardation, or hearing loss suggesting genetic abnormality
- ✓ Medical history
- ✓ Previous head or neck surgery

Key Physical Findings

✓ Head and neck examination for poor dentition
✓ Cardiopulmonary examination for laryngeal stridor, bronchospasm, or evidence of congestive heart failure
✓ Neurologic examination for Chvostek and Trousseau signs
✓ Skin examination for dry skin, brittle nails, or coarse hair

Suggested Work-Up

Serum calcium	To determine the serum calcium concentration
Albumin	Used to correct the calcium concentration for hypoalbuminemia
Ionized calcium	To help determine true serum calcium concentration
Phosphorus	Phosphorus level can differentiate vitamin D deficiency from pseudohypoparathyroidism if PTH level is elevated
Magnesium	To evaluate for hyper- or hypomagnesemia
Creatinine	To evaluate renal function
PTH	To evaluate for hypoparathyroidism
25-hydroxyvitamin D	To evaluate for vitamin D deficiency

Additional Work-Up

24-hour urinary collection for calcium, calcium/creatinine ratio	To differentiate calcium-sensing receptor abnormality from hypoparathyroidism if PTH level is normal or low
1,25-dihydroxyvitamin D	Can be useful in diagnosing hypoparathyroidism
Alkaline phosphatase	If renal osteodystrophy or other bone disorder is suspected
Renal ultrasound	To assess for nephrolithiasis
DNA sequencing	If genetic mutation is suspected

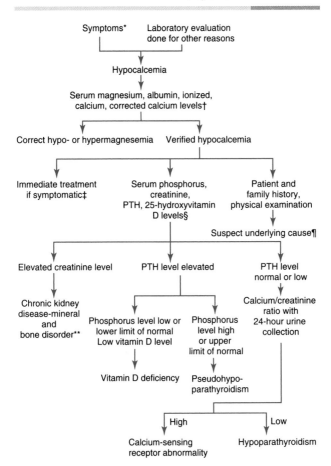

†—Ideal laboratory testing should be performed with the patient fasting and with minimal venous occlusion. Corrected serum calcium = measured serum calcium + 0.8(4 – measured serum albumin); calcium is measured in mg per dL, and albumin is measured in g per dL.
‡—Calcium gluconate, 1 to 2 g intravenously slowly over 10 minutes, with clinical and electrocardiographic monitoring, followed by slow infusion (10 g of calcium gluconate in 1 L of dextrose 5% at 1 to 3 mg per kg per hour).
**—Includes renal osteodystrophy and other disorders of mineralization.

Figure 40-1. Evaluation of Hypocalcemia. *PTH*, Parathyroid hormone. (From Michels TC, Kelly KM. Parathyroid disorders. *American Family Physician* 2013;88:249–257.)

Further Reading

Chang WTW, Radin B, McCurdy MT. Calcium, magnesium, and phosphate abnormalities in the emergency department. *Emerg Med Clin North Am*. 2014;32:349–366.

Fong J, Khan A. Hypocalcemia. *Can Fam Physician*. 2012;58:158–162.

Michels TC, Kelly KM. Parathyroid disorders. *Am Fam Physician*. 2013;88:249–257.

General Discussion

Symptoms of hypoglycemia begin at plasma glucose levels of approximately 60 mg/dL, and impairment of nervous system function begins at approximately 50 mg/dL. Clinical hypoglycemia is confirmed when the Whipple triad is present: (1) symptoms or signs consistent with hypoglycemia; (2) a simultaneous low blood glucose level (typically defined as a blood glucose level of less than 55 mg/dL); and (3) resolution of symptoms after raising the plasma glucose level.

Symptoms consistent with hypoglycemia are broadly categorized as autonomic or neuroglycopenic. Adrenergic symptoms consist of palpitations, tremor, and anxiety. Cholinergic symptoms include hunger, sweating, and paresthesia. Neuroglycopenic symptoms arise due to central nervous system glucose deprivation. Neuroglycopenic symptoms include confusion, amnesia, blurred vision, diplopia, dysarthria, seizure, and loss of consciousness.

The causes of hypoglycemia may be categorized into three main groups for the purposes of evaluation. These categories are medication- or toxin-induced hypoglycemia, disorders associated with fasting hypoglycemia, and disorders associated with postprandial hypoglycemia. Each of these categories is outlined in detail in the following. The list of medications associated with hypoglycemia are also listed in the following. An alternative classification system considers whether the patient is seemingly well or has a concurrent illness when considering possible causes of hypoglycemia.

Four simultaneous criteria should be present to establish the diagnosis of insulinoma:

1. Blood glucose less than 40 mg/dL
2. Symptoms of neuroglycopenia
3. Plasma insulin greater than 5 μU/mL
4. Plasma C-peptide greater than 0.6 ng/mL

Medications Associated with Hypoglycemia*

Angiotensin-converting enzyme inhibitors
Acetazolamide
Acetohexamide
Aspirin
Azapropazone
Benzodiazepines
Buformin

---

*Medication list from Marks V, Teale JD. Drug-induced hypoglycemia. *Endocrinology and Metabolism Clinics* 1999;28:555–577.

Carbutamide
Chloroquine
Chlorpromazine
Chlorpropamide
Cibenzoline
Cimetidine
Ciprofloxacin
Clipizide
Cycloheptolamide
Dicumarol
Diphenhydramine
Disopyramide
Doxepin
Ecstasy (MDMA)
Etomidate
Ethionamide
Enflurane
Fenoterol
Fluoxetine
Formestane
Furosemide
Gatifloxacin
Glibenclamide
Gliclazide
Glimepiride
Glipizide
Glyburide
Haloperidol
Halothane
Herbal extracts
Insulin-like growth factor-1
Imipramine
Indomethacin
Insulin
Interferon-α
Isoniazid
Isoxsuprine
Lidocaine
Lithium
Maprotiline
Mefloquine
Metahexamide
Metoprolol
Monoamine oxidase inhibitors

Nadolol
Nateglinide
Nefazodone
Octreotide
Orphenadrine
Oxytetracycline
Para-aminobenzoic acid
Para-aminosalicylic acid
Paracetamol
Pentamidine
Perhexiline
Phenindione
Phenformin
Phenytoin
Phenylbutazone
Pindolol
Propoxyphene
Propranolol
Quinine
Ranitidine
Repaglinide
Ritodrine
Salicylates
Selegiline
Sulfixasol
Sulfonylureas
Sulfadiazine
Sulfadimidine
Sulfamethoxazole
Sulfaphenazole
Terbutaline
Tolazamide
Tolbutamide
Trimethoprim/sulfamethoxazole
Warfarin

Causes of Hypoglycemia

Medications and toxins

- Alcohol
- Factitious hyperinsulinism
- Hypoglycin (present in Caribbean akee fruit)
- Insulin-induced hypoglycemia (excessive insulin dose, severe exercise, or inadequate food intake)
- Medications as listed previously

- Toadstool
- Vacor (a rodenticide)

Disorders associated with fasting hypoglycemia

- Adrenal insufficiency
- Cardiac failure
- Chronic kidney disease
- Gastric tumors
- Growth hormone deficiency
- Hepatocellular carcinoma
- Insulin autoantibodies
- Insulin receptor antibodies
- Insulinoma
- Liver disease
- Noninsulinoma pancreatogenous hypoglycemia syndrome
- Non-islet cell tumors
- Pituitary insufficiency
- Renal failure
- Sarcoma

Disorders associated with postprandial hypoglycemia

- Early type 2 diabetes
- Galactosemia
- Hereditary fructose intolerance
- Idiopathic postprandial hypoglycemia
- Postgastrectomy or postgastric bypass hypoglycemia

Key Historical Features

- ✓ Headaches
- ✓ Fatigue
- ✓ Diaphoresis
- ✓ Weakness
- ✓ Confusion
- ✓ Difficulty speaking
- ✓ Blurred vision
- ✓ Palpitations
- ✓ Neuromuscular symptoms
- ✓ Nervousness
- ✓ Slurred speech
- ✓ Difficulty concentrating
- ✓ Aberrant behavior
- ✓ Focal neurologic signs and symptoms
- ✓ Seizures
- ✓ Coma
- ✓ Medical history
- ✓ Medications

Key Physical Findings

✓ Vital signs
✓ Abdominal examination
✓ Neurologic examination

Suggested Work-Up

Measurement of plasma glucose during a symptomatic episode	To establish hypoglycemia as the cause of the patient's symptoms
Meal tolerance test	To determine whether the patient has postprandial hypoglycemia
Measurement of glucose, insulin C-peptide, pro-insulin, β-hydroxybutyrate, and insulin antibodies during a hypoglycemic event or during a prolonged fast	To evaluate for a hyperinsulinism, including insulinoma. Endogenous hyperinsulinism is confirmed by plasma insulin concentration of at least 3 μU/mL, plasma C-peptide concentration of at least 0.2 nmol/L, and plasma proinsulin concentration of at least 5.0 pmol/L. This is a state of apparent hypoglycemia, confirmed by a plasma glucose of less than 55 mg/dL.

Additional Work-Up

Computed tomography (CT) or magnetic resonance imaging	To localize an insulinoma once the diagnosis has been established. Detection rates of 70% and 85%, respectively.
Endoscopic pancreatic ultrasonography with fine needle aspiration	To localize an insulinoma once the diagnosis has been established
Combination CT with endoscopic pancreatic ultrasonography	To localize an insulinoma once the diagnosis has been established. Localization rate approaches 100%.

Further Reading

Marks V, Teale JD. Drug-induced hypoglycemia. *Endocrinol Metabol Clin.* 1999;28:555–577.

Marks V, Teale JD. Hypoglycemia: factitious and felonious. *Endocrinol Metabol Clin.* 1999;28:579–601.

Martens P, Tits J. Approach to the patient with spontaneous hypoglycemia. *Eur J Intern Med.* 2014;25:415–421.

Noone TC, Hosey J, Firat Z, Semelka RC. Imaging and localization of islet-cell tumours of the pancreas on CT and MRI. *Best Pract Res Clin Endocrinol Metab.* 2005;19:195–211.

Pourmotabbed G, Kitabchi AE. Hypoglycemia. *Obstet Gynecol Clin.* 2001;28:383–400.

Service FJ. Hypoglycemia. *Endocrinol Metabol Clin.* 1997;26:937–955.

General Discussion

Hypokalemia is defined as a serum potassium of less than 3.6 mEq/L. Hypokalemia has been associated with an increased risk of hypertension, ischemic stroke, hemorrhagic stroke, dysrhythmias, and hospital admissions and deaths due to heart failure and cardiovascular events. Even mild or moderate hypokalemia increases the risk of cardiac arrhythmia in patients with cardiac ischemia, heart failure, or left ventricular hypertrophy, particularly in the presence of digoxin.

Hypokalemia primarily affects the cardiac, skeletal muscle, gastrointestinal, and renal organ systems. However, patients with hypokalemia often have no symptoms, particularly when the disorder is mild (serum potassium 3.0–3.5 mEq/L). Nonspecific symptoms such as fatigue, muscle weakness, and constipation may be reported as the hypokalemia becomes more severe. Muscle necrosis can occur when serum potassium decreases to less than 2.5 mEq/L, and an ascending paralysis can develop at serum concentrations of less than 2.0 mEq/L.

The etiology of hypokalemia falls into three broad categories: insufficient potassium intake; transcellular shift of potassium from the extracellular to intracellular compartments; or excessive potassium loss. Diuretics are the most common drug-related cause of hypokalemia. Potassium losses via the gastrointestinal tract, which are usually the result of diarrhea, are the second most common cause of hypokalemia in developed countries. Inadequate potassium intake is rarely a cause of hypokalemia.

Medications and Substances Associated with Hypokalemia

Albuterol
Aminoglycosides
Amphotericin B
Ampicillin
Caffeine
Carbenicillin
Carbenoxolone
Chloroquine overdose
Cisplatin
Diuretics
- Acetazolamide
- Bumetanide
- Chlorthalidone
- Ethacrynic acid
- Furosemide
- Indapamide

- Metolazone
- Quinethazone
- Thiazides
- Torsemide

Ephedrine
Epinephrine
Fludrocortisone
Foscarnet
Gentamicin
Glucocorticoids (in high doses)
Gossypol
Hydrocortisone
Insulin overdose
Isoproterenol
Licorice
Loop diuretics
- Bumetanide
- Furosemide
- Torsemide

Mineralocorticoids
- Fludrocortisone

Penicillin
Phenolphthalein
Phenylpropanolamine
Pseudoephedrine
Ritodrine
Sodium polystyrene sulfonate
Terbutaline
Theophylline
Verapamil overdose

Causes of Hypokalemia

Adrenocorticotrophic hormone–producing bronchogenic tumor
Alcoholism
Barium poisoning
Bartter syndrome
Caffeine intake
Chewing tobacco containing glycyrrhizic acid
Chloride depletion (metabolic alkalosis)
Chloroquine overdose
Congenital adrenal hyperplasia
- 11β-hydroxysteroid deficiency
- 17α-hydroxylase deficiency

Cushing syndrome
Delirium tremens

Diarrhea
Gastric suctioning
Gitelman syndrome
Hyperthyroidism
Hypokalemic familial periodic paralysis
Inadequate potassium intake (rare)
Insulin overdose
Laxative abuse
Leukemia
Licorice ingestion containing glycyrrhizic acid
Liddle syndrome
Magnesium depletion
Malignant hypertension
Medications
Osmotic diuresis (uncontrolled diabetes)
Primary hyperaldosteronism
- Adrenal adenoma
- Adrenal carcinoma
- Bilateral adrenal hyperplasia

Renal tubular acidosis types I and II
Renin-secreting tumor
Renovascular hypertension
Secondary hyperaldosteronism
Trauma
Vomiting
Vasculitis

Key Historical Features

✓ Muscle weakness
✓ Paralysis
✓ Worsening of weakness with exercise
✓ Vomiting
✓ Diarrhea
✓ Laxative abuse
✓ Licorice intake
✓ Medical history
✓ Medications
✓ Alcohol abuse
✓ Chewing tobacco use

Key Physical Findings

✓ Vital signs (particularly heart rate and blood pressure)
✓ Cardiovascular examination for arrhythmias
✓ Neurologic examination for muscle weakness, especially proximal

Suggested Work-Up

Electrocardiogram	May reveal U waves, prolonged PR interval, T-wave inversion, ST-segment depression, and QT interval prolongation
Serum electrolytes	To evaluate for acidosis and hyperchloremia
Blood urea nitrogen and creatinine	To evaluate renal function
Serum magnesium	To evaluate for magnesium depletion

Additional Work-Up

Basal plasma renin activity and plasma aldosterone level	If hypertension is present, to evaluate for primary or secondary hyperaldosteronism
Morning urinary pH and ammonium chloride test	To evaluate for type I renal tubular acidosis if hypokalemia and hyperchloremic metabolic acidosis are present
24-hour urinary calcium	To evaluate for hypercalciuria
Plain film of the abdomen or renal ultrasound	To evaluate for nephrocalcinosis or nephrolithiasis
Plasma renin activity, plasma aldosterone level, urinary chloride, and urinary prostaglandin E_2 levels	If Bartter syndrome is suspected (short stature, failure to thrive, muscle weakness/cramps, polyuria, and nocturia)

Further Reading

Gennari FJ. Disorders of potassium homeostasis: hypokalemia and hyperkalemia. *Crit Care Clin.* 2002;18:273–288.

Gennari FJ. Hypokalemia. *New Engl J Med.* 1998;339:451–458.

Mandal AK. Hypokalemia and hyperkalemia. Renal disease. *Med Clin North Am.* 1997;81:611–639.

Schaefer TJ, Wolford RW. Disorders of potassium. *Emerg Med Clin North Am.* 2005;23:723–747.

Webster A, Brady W, Morris F. Recognising signs of danger: ECG changes resulting from an abnormal serum potassium concentration. *Emerg Med J.* 2002;19:74–77.

43 HYPONATREMIA

General Discussion

Hyponatremia is generally defined as a plasma sodium level of less than 135 mEq/L. Hyponatremia may lead to significant morbidity and mortality. Most patients with hyponatremia are asymptomatic, and symptoms usually do not appear until the plasma sodium level drops to less than 125 mEq/L. Symptoms of hyponatremia are usually nonspecific and include headache, nausea, and lethargy. However, neurologic and gastrointestinal symptoms may be present in cases of severe hyponatremia, with the risk of seizure and coma increasing as the sodium level decreases. If the sodium level decreases quickly, symptoms may be present at sodium levels greater than 120 mEq/L.

The evaluation of hyponatremia begins with a targeted history to evaluate for causes of hyponatremia, such as congestive heart failure, renal impairment, liver disease, malignancy, hypothyroidism, or Addison disease. Hyponatremia is then classified according to the volume status of the patient as hypovolemic, hypervolemic, or euvolemic.

Hypervolemic hyponatremia results in increased total body water and the presence of edema. The three main causes of hypervolemic hyponatremia are congestive heart failure, liver cirrhosis, and renal impairment (e.g., renal failure and nephrotic syndrome).

Differentiating between hypovolemia and euvolemia may be difficult clinically. An elevated hematocrit or a blood urea nitrogen-to-creatinine ratio greater than 20 may suggest hypovolemia, but these levels are not always present. If the patient's volume status is not clear, the measurement of plasma osmolality and urinary sodium concentration are useful for evaluating euvolemic or hypovolemic patients.

Normal plasma osmolality (280–300 mOsm/kg of water) can be caused by pseudohyponatremia or by the absorption of large volumes of hypotonic irrigation fluid during transurethral resection of the prostate. Pseudohyponatremia may occur in the presence of severe hypertriglyceridemia and hyperproteinemia. Increased plasma osmolality (greater than 300 mOsm/kg of water) in a patient with hyponatremia is caused by severe hyperglycemia. Decreased plasma osmolality (less than 280 mOsm/kg of water) may occur in a patient who is hypovolemic or euvolemic. The urinary sodium excretion is used to further refine the differential diagnosis.

A high urinary sodium concentration (greater than 30 mmol/L) may result from renal disorders, the syndrome of inappropriate antidiuretic hormone secretion (SIADH), reset osmostat syndrome, endocrine deficiencies, medications, or drugs. A low urinary sodium concentration (less than 30 mmol/L) may result from vomiting, diarrhea, severe burns, acute water overload, or psychogenic polydipsia.

SIADH occurs when antidiuretic hormone is secreted independently of the body's need to conserve water. SIADH is a diagnosis of exclusion, but it should be suspected when hyponatremia is accompanied by a low serum osmolality with an inappropriately high urine osmolality. The diagnostic criteria for SIADH are:

- Hypotonic hyponatremia
- Urine osmolality greater than 100 mmol/kg
- Absence of extracellular volume depletion
- Normal thyroid and adrenal function
- Normal cardiac, hepatic, and renal function

Medications Associated with Hyponatremia

Acetaminophen
Amiodarone
Angiotensin-converting enzyme inhibitors
Antidiuretic hormone
Barbiturates
Beta-blockers
Carbamazepine
Carboplatin
Chlorpromazine
Chlorpropamide
Cisplatin
Clofibrate
Colchicine
Cyclophasphamide
Cytoxan
Desmopressin
Haloperidol
Indapamide
Interferon-α and -γ
Isoproterenol
Loop diuretics
Methotrexate
Monoamine oxidase inhibitors
Monoclonal antibodies
Morphine
Nicotine
Nonsteroidal anti-inflammatory drugs
Opiates
Oxcarbazepine
Oxytocin
Phenothiazines
Proton pump inhibitors

Psychotropic medications
Selective serotonin reuptake inhibitors
Sodium valproate
Sulfonylureas
Theophylline
Thiazide diuretics
Tolbutamide
Tricyclic antidepressants
Vasopressin
Vinca alkaloids
Vincristine

Causes of Hyponatremia

Acute intermittent porphyria
Acute psychosis
Addison disease
Congestive heart failure
Gastrointestinal disorders
- Diarrhea
- Vomiting
Ecstasy ingestion
HIV/AIDS
Hyperproteinemia
Hypertriglyceridemia (severe)
Hypothyroidism
Liver disease
Neoplasms
- Bronchogenic carcinoma
- Duodenal carcinoma
- Lymphoma
- Mesothelioma
- Pancreatic carcinoma
- Prostate carcinoma
- Thymoma
Neurologic disorders
- Alcohol withdrawal (delirium tremens)
- Brain abscess
- Cerebrovascular accident
- Encephalitis
- Guillain-Barré syndrome
- Hydrocephalus
- Meningitis
- Subarachnoid hemorrhage
- Subdural hematoma

- Trauma
- Tumors

Pre-eclampsia

Psychogenic polydipsia

Pulmonary/chest disorders

- Aspergillosis
- Bronchiectasis
- Bronchogenic carcinoma
- Cystic fibrosis
- Empyema
- Pneumonia (viral and bacterial)
- Positive pressure ventilation
- Tuberculosis

Renal disorders

- Chronic pyelonephritis
- Nephrotic syndrome
- Polycystic kidney
- Renal artery stenosis or occlusion
- Renal failure
- Salt-losing nephropathies

Reset osmostat syndrome

SIADH

Third space losses

- Burns
- Ileus
- Pancreatitis
- Peritonitis

Key Historical Features

✓ Symptoms of hyponatremia
  - Headache
  - Nausea/vomiting
  - Lethargy/malaise
  - Cramps
  - Dizziness
  - Falls
  - Confusion
  - Seizure activity
  - Psychosis
  - Coma
✓ Medical history
✓ Surgical history
✓ Psychiatric history
✓ Medications
✓ Drug use

Diagnostic Algorithm for Hyponatremia

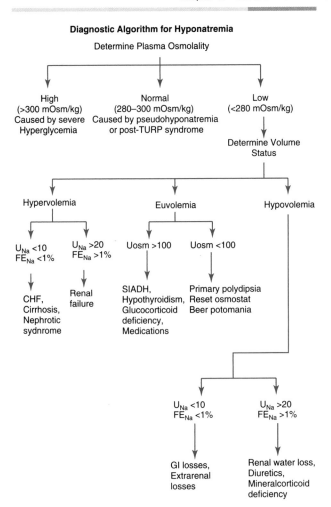

Figure 43-1. Diagnostic algorithm for hyponatremia.
CHF, Congestive heart failure; *GI*, gastrointestinal; *SIADH*, syndrome of inappropriate antidiuretic hormone secretion; *TURP*, transurethral resection of the prostate.

Suggested Work-Up

Serum osmolality	To help evaluate euvolemic or hypovolemic patients
Urine osmolality	To help evaluate for SIADH
Urinary sodium excretion	To help refine the diagnosis in a patient with low plasma osmolality
Serum electrolytes	To evaluate for hyperkalemia or bicarbonate abnormalities
Serum creatinine	To evaluate renal function
Thyroid-stimulating hormone	To evaluate for hypothyroidism
Cortisol and adrenocorticotrophic hormone	To evaluate for Addison disease

Additional Work-Up

24-hour urine collection for protein or spot urine protein/creatinine ratio	If nephrotic syndrome is suspected (greater than 3 g of protein are present in nephrotic syndrome)
Serum triglycerides and protein levels	If pseudohyponatremia is suspected

Further Reading

Fried LF, Palevsky PM. Hyponatremia and hypernatremia. *Med Clin North Am.* 1997;81:585–609.

Goh KP. Management of hyponatremia. *Am Fam Physician.* 2004;69:2387–2394.

Harring TR, Deal NS, Kuo DC. Disorders of sodium and water balance. *Emerg Med Clin North Am.* 2014;32:379–401.

Milonis HJ, Liamis GL, Elisaf MS. The hyponatremic patient: a systematic approach to laboratory diagnosis. *Can Med Assoc J.* 2002;166:1056–1062.

Sterns RH. Disorders of plasma sodium—causes, consequences, and correction. *N Engl J Med.* 2015;372:55–65.

Yeates KE, Singer M, Morton AR. Salt and water: a simple approach to hyponatremia. *Can Med Assoc J.* 2004;170:365–369.

General Discussion

Hypothyroidism usually results from decreased thyroid hormone production and secretion by the thyroid gland. Hypothyroidism is far more common in women and in the elderly. The prevalence of overt hypothyroidism is approximately 2% in women who are age 70 years or older.

Hypothyroidism may occur from primary gland failure or insufficient thyroid gland stimulation by the pituitary gland (secondary hypothyroidism) or hypothalamus (tertiary hypothyroidism). Primary gland failure can result from many causes, including autoimmune destruction (Hashimoto disease), congenital abnormalities, iodine deficiency, and infiltrative disease. In the United States, the most common cause of hypothyroidism is autoimmune disease. Central causes of hypothyroidism usually present with other manifestations of pituitary or hypothalamic dysfunction and are characterized by inappropriately normal or low levels of thyroid-stimulating hormone (TSH) relative to insufficient thyroid hormone.

Untreated hypothyroidism can contribute to hypertension, dyslipidemia, decreased cardiac output, infertility, cognitive impairment, neuromuscular dysfunction, and sleep apnea. The most common symptoms of hypothyroidism are fatigue and cold intolerance. Other symptoms of hypothyroidism include weight gain, constipation, depression, difficulty concentrating, memory impairment, weakness, arthralgias, myalgias, dry skin, menorrhagia, and hair loss.

All patients with symptoms of hypothyroidism should be evaluated for thyroid dysfunction. Screening for asymptomatic adults is controversial, with some guidelines not recommending routine screening, whereas other guidelines recommend screening after a certain age. Screening in asymptomatic adults may also be considered in those with risk factors for hypothyroidism, such as a history of autoimmune disease, family history of thyroid disease, presence of goiter, history of head or neck irradiation, previous radioactive iodine therapy, or treatment with drugs associated with thyroid dysfunction.

Myxedema coma refers to severe complications of hypothyroidism, involving hypothermia and stupor or coma. Myxedema coma can be precipitated by mild illnesses, cold exposure, myocardial infarction, and medications that affect the central nervous system.

Medications Associated with Hypothyroidism

Amiodarone
Ethionamide
Interferon-α
Interleukin-2
Iodine excess
Lithium

Methimazole
Propylthiouracil
Sulfonamides
Tyrosine kinase inhibitors

Causes of Hypothyroidism

Primary hypothyroidism
- Agenesis and dysgenesis of the thyroid
- External irradiation
- Hashimoto disease (autoimmune thyroiditis)
- Infections
  - *Mycobacterium tuberculosis*
  - *Pneumocystis carinii*
- Infiltrative disorders
  - Amyloidosis
  - Hemochromatosis
  - Leukemia
  - Lymphoma
  - Sarcoidosis
  - Scleroderma
- Invasive fibrous thyroiditis
- Iodine deficiency
- Medications
- Postpartum thyroiditis
- Radioactive iodine therapy
- Silent thyroiditis
- Subacute thyroiditis
- Thyroid hormone resistance
- Thyroidectomy

Secondary/tertiary hypothyroidism (central hypothyroidism)
- Chronic lymphocytic hypophysitis
- Congenital abnormalities (defects in thyrotropin-releasing hormone, TSH, or both)
- Infections
- Infiltrative disorders
- Other brain tumors (nonpituitary)
- Pituitary disorders (tumors, metastasis, hemorrhage, necrosis, and aneurysms)
- Surgery
- Trauma

Key Historical Features

✓ Associated symptoms
- Fatigue
- Weakness
- Depression

- • Sleep disturbances
- • Decreased appetite
- • Memory loss
- • Cold intolerance
- • Decreased sweating
- • Weight gain
- • Muscle cramps
- • Dry skin
- • Brittle nails
- • Coarse hair
- • Hair loss
- • Hearing loss
- • Hoarseness
- • Swelling of the face
- • Pretibial swelling
- • Menorrhagia
- • Infertility
- • Constipation
- • Paresthesias
- • Changes in taste and smell
✓ Medical history (especially head and neck irradiation, as well as diseases associated with hypothyroidism, such as diabetes mellitus, hyperlipidemia, Sjögren syndrome, pernicious anemia, systemic lupus erythematosus, rheumatoid arthritis, primary biliary cirrhosis, chronic hepatitis, vitiligo, and carpal tunnel syndrome)
✓ Surgical history
✓ Family history
✓ Medications

Key Physical Findings

✓ Vital signs
✓ Head and neck examination for:
  - • Thyroid nodules or goiter. Note any thyroidectomy scars.
  - • Ophthalmopathy (proptosis, periorbital edema, conjunctival injection, abnormal extraocular muscle function)
  - • Pemberton sign (facial plethora, raised jugular vein pressure, and inspiratory stridor when patients raise their arms above their head) indicates a neck mass (e.g., goiter).
✓ Cardiovascular examination for bradycardia or evidence of pericardial effusion
✓ Pulmonary examination for evidence of pleural effusion
✓ Abdominal examination for ascites
✓ Neurologic examination for proximal weakness, peripheral neuropathy, and a slow return phase of deep tendon reflexes

Suggested Work-Up

Serum TSH and free thyroxine (T_4)	Elevated TSH and low free T_4 indicates primary hypothyroidism. Elevated TSH and normal T_4 indicates subclinical hypothyroidism. Low free T_4 with a low or inappropriately normal serum TSH level is consistent with secondary central hypothyroidism.

Additional Work-Up

Total triiodothyronine (T_3)	Less useful than T_4 because it may be normal in patients with hypothyroidism
Thyroid peroxidase (TPO) autoantibodies	Often detectable in patients with Hashimoto thyroiditis (may be useful in patients with subclinical hypothyroidism)
Thyroglobulin autoantibodies	Usually present with Hashimoto thyroiditis, although less commonly present than TPO autoantibodies
Magnetic resonance imaging of the brain and pituitary gland	If central hypothyroidism is present
Thyroid ultrasound	If a thyroid nodule is detected on examination
Fine needle aspiration	If a thyroid nodule is detected, to determine if the nodule is malignant
Luteinizing hormone, follicle-stimulating hormone, cortisol level, prolactin, insulin-like growth factor-I	If central hypothyroidism is diagnosed (to evaluate for hypopituitarism)
Electrolytes	Severe hypothyroidism may result in hyponatremia
Lipid panel	Hypothyroidism is associated with elevated triglycerides and elevated low-density lipoprotein cholesterol

Complete blood count	Hypothyroidism is associated with anemia
Fasting blood sugar	To evaluate for diabetes (because of the relationship between autoimmune conditions)

Further Reading

American Association of Clinical Endocrinologists. Medical guidelines for clinical practice for the evaluation and treatment of hyperthyroidism and hypothyroidism. *Endocr Pract.* 2002;8:458–469.

Bensenor IM, Olmos RD, Lotufo PA. Hypothyroidism in the elderly: diagnosis and management. *Clin Interv Aging.* 2012;7:97–111.

Devdhar M, Ousman YH, Burman KD. Hypothyroidism. *Endocrinol Metabol Clin North Am.* 2007;36:595–615.

Gaitonde DY, Rowley KD, Sweeney LB. Hypothyroidism: an update. *Am Fam Physician.* 2012;86:244–251.

Helfand M. U.S. Preventive Services Task Force. Screening for subclinical thyroid dysfunction in nonpregnant adults: a summary of the evidence for the U.S. Preventive Services Task Force. *Ann Intern Med.* 2004;140:128–141.

Wartofsky L, Van Nostrand D, Burman KD. Overt and 'subclinical' hypothyroidism in women. *Obstet Gynecol Surv.* 2006;61:535–542.

General Discussion

Infertility affects 10% to 15% of couples and becomes more common with increasing age. Clinical evaluation of infertility is indicated if a pregnancy has not occurred after 1 year of regular unprotected intercourse. An infertility workup should also be initiated on female patients who complain of infertility and have any of the following abnormalities: irregular menses or amenorrhea; bleeding between periods; dyspareunia; history of upper genital tract infection; and history of a ruptured appendix or other abdominal surgery. They should also have a workup if they are older than 35 years of age.

Because men account for approximately 40% of all infertility, the male partner should be evaluated early in the infertility workup. Historical factors affecting the male partner should also be considered in determining when to begin an infertility evaluation. The following historical factors in the male partner warrant an early investigation: difficulty achieving or maintaining an erection; inability to ejaculate during intercourse; history of testicular injury; history of mumps; history of an undescended testicle; or history of infection in the prostate gland, epididymis, or testicles.

There are several tests that every infertile couple should have performed. The first is a semen analysis of the male partner, regardless of how many pregnancies he has caused, because sperm counts can change over time. The second test is a hysterosalpingogram (HSG), which helps determine whether the uterine cavity is normal in size and shape, and whether the fallopian tubes are patent. Although the HSG is the initial test to evaluate tubal patency, patients at high risk for infection, such as those with a history of clinically diagnosed pelvic inflammatory disease, are best evaluated initially via laparoscopy and hysteroscopy. Laparoscopy is more invasive than HSG, but it remains the best test to identify endometriosis and peritubal adhesions.

Routine hormonal assessment, especially in a young, apparently ovulatory patient, is controversial. There is less disagreement about performing a hormonal assessment in women aged 35 years and older. The suggested workup is outlined in the following.

Approximately 5% to 10% of infertile couples proceed through a complete infertility evaluation without a cause identified and are said to have unexplained infertility. Additional specialized testing may be performed by infertility clinics, such as ultrasound, antisperm antibodies, and sperm function assays. Empiric treatment regimens have been designed to treat subtle disorders that may not be diagnosed.

Causes of Female Infertility

Endometriosis
Male factors

Ovulatory dysfunction
- Adrenal disease
- Aging
- Diminished ovarian reserve
- Hyperprolactinemia
- Hypothalamic amenorrhea
- Oligomenorrhea
- Polycystic ovary syndrome
- Thyroid disease
- Tobacco use

Tubal disease (obstruction from causes such as tubal surgery or pelvic inflammatory disease)

Uterine causes
- Congenital uterine anomaly
- Intrauterine synechiae (Asherman syndrome)
- Polyps
- Poor cervical mucus quantity or quality
- Septate uterus
- Uterine fibroids

Unexplained infertility

Key Historical Features

✓ Patient age
✓ Duration of infertility
✓ Timing of sexual intercourse
✓ Galactorrhea
✓ History of dyspareunia
✓ Age at menarche
✓ Intermenstrual bleeding
✓ Determination of whether the woman is currently having regular, monthly menstrual cycles
✓ Previous contraceptive use
✓ Reproductive history, especially previous pregnancies with the same male partner
✓ Medical history, especially thyroid disorders and diabetes mellitus
✓ Surgical history, especially appendectomy or other abdominal surgery
✓ Gynecologic history, especially sexually transmitted diseases, pelvic inflammatory disease, uterine fibroids, pelvic irradiation, or previous use of an intrauterine device
✓ Medications, especially oral contraceptives
✓ Family history, especially genetic diseases
✓ Cigarette smoking
✓ Caffeine use
✓ Alcohol use
✓ Illicit drug use

Key Physical Findings

✓ Height and weight
✓ Skin examination for acne or hirsutism
✓ Breast examination for breast formation and the presence of galactorrhea
✓ Pelvic examination for evidence of infection, uterine fibroids, ovarian cysts, or endometriosis
✓ Genital examination of the male partner for phimosis, balanitis, testicular size, or evidence of testicular tumor

Suggested Work-Up

Semen analysis	To evaluate for a male factor for infertility
HSG	To evaluate the uterine cavity and determine whether the fallopian tubes are patent
Thyroid-stimulating hormone	To evaluate for thyroid disorders
Prolactin level	To evaluate for hyperprolactinemia
Follicle-stimulating hormone (FSH)	Low or normal FSH levels are most common in patients with polycystic ovary syndrome and hypothalamic amenorrhea
Estradiol and FSH level on cycle day 3 of the menstrual cycle	May be useful in women aged older than 35 years to assess ovarian reserve. An FSH level of less than 10 mIU/mL combined with an estradiol level of less than 80 pg/mL suggests favorable follicular potential. Elevated basal FSH levels suggest declining fertility potential, and a concentration greater than 20 mIU/mL virtually excludes the chance of a spontaneous pregnancy.
Serum progesterone on cycle day 21	A level greater than 10 ng/mL confirms that ovulation has occurred.

Additional Work-Up

Serum 17α-hydroxyprogesterone and serum testosterone	To evaluate patients with signs of hyperandrogenism for late-onset congenital adrenal hyperplasia and androgen-secreting tumors

Urinary luteinizing hormone kit	Can be used to predict ovulation
Basal body temperature measurement	May be used to help predict the timing of ovulation, but it is no longer recommended as part of the routine investigation of the infertile couple
Clomiphene citrate challenge	May be used to increase the sensitivity of a basal test
FSH determination	The FSH level is measured both before and after the administration of 100 mg of clomiphene citrate during day 5 through day 9 of the menstrual cycle. Elevation in the serum FSH level after the clomiphene citrate challenge indicates decreased ovarian reserve.
Transvaginal ultrasound	Obtaining an antral follicle count can be useful in evaluating ovarian reserve and predicting responsiveness to gonadotropin stimulation
Total testosterone and dehydroepiandrosterone sulfate levels	If signs of androgen excess are found on physical examination
Hysteroscopy and/or laparoscopy	Generally indicated in women with otherwise unexplained infertility and when there is evidence or suspicion of endometriosis, intrapelvic adhesions, or fallopian tube disease, particularly if the HSG suggests tubal disease that may be amenable to surgical repair.
Serum antibody to *Chlamydia trachomatis*	May be used as a screening tool for tubal pathologic conditions in infertile women
Cervical cultures	Routine cervical cultures to identify active current infection with chlamydia or gonorrhea in low-risk populations tend to be unrevealing.

Endometrial biopsy	Provides an indirect measure of ovulation and evaluates the cumulative effect of progesterone on the endometrium. However, there is little role for routine endometrial biopsy as part of a general infertility evaluation.
Sonohysterography	May be used as an alternative to HSG to evaluate the uterine cavity, but it provides little information about the patency of the fallopian tubes
Magnetic resonance imaging	May be helpful in visualizing the uterine cavity and determining tubal patency

Further Reading

Brugh VM, Nudell DM, Lipshultz LI. What the urologist should know about the female infertility evaluation. *Urol Clin North Am.* 2002;29:983–992.

Hargreave TB, Mills JA. Investigating and managing infertility in general practice. *Br Med J.* 1998;316:1438–1441.

Illions EH, Valley MT, Kaunitz AM. Infertility: a clinical guide for the internist. *Med Clin North Am.* 1998;82:271–295.

Jose-Miller AB, Boyden JW. Infertility. *Am Fam Physician.* 2007;75:849–856.

Penzias AS. Infertility: contemporary office-based evaluation and treatment. *Obstet Gynecol Clin.* 2000;27:473–486.

Smith S, Pfeifer SM, Collins JA. Diagnosis and management of female infertility. *JAMA.* 2003;290:1767–1770.

Taylor A. ABC of subfertility: extent of the problem. *Br Med J.* 2003;327:434–436.

General Discussion

Infertility, which is defined as the inability to conceive after 1 year of frequent, unprotected intercourse, affects 10% to 15% of couples. Half of these couples have a component of male factor infertility, and 20% to 30% are caused solely by a male factor. The most common male factor is a varicocele. Evaluation of male fertility should be a routine part of the evaluation of an infertile couple, because 50% of male infertility is potentially correctable.

Endocrine disorders remain an important etiology of male infertility and may be associated with significant medical pathology, which may have important implications both for the male and for his potential offspring. Testicular failure or dysfunction (primary hypogonadism) is the most common identifiable cause.

The etiology of male infertility remains unclear in nearly one-half of cases.

Medications Associated with Male Infertility

Chemotherapy
Cimetidine
Colchicine
Methotrexate
Narcotics
Nitrofurantoin
Spironolactone
Sulfasalazine

Causes of Male Infertility

Abnormal spermatogenesis
Absent epididymis or obstruction
Absent vas deferens or obstruction
Alcohol abuse
Anabolic steroid use
Androgen excess state
  • Exogenous administration
  • Tumor
Androgen resistance
Anorchia
Caffeine excess
Chemotherapy
Congenital adrenal hyperplasia
Cryptorchidism

Cushing syndrome
Cystic fibrosis
Diabetes mellitus
Erectile dysfunction
Estrogen excess state (tumor)
Gonadotoxin exposure (organic solvents, pesticides, excessive heat, heavy
   metals)
Hypogonadotropic hypogonadism
Klinefelter syndrome
Marijuana use
Medications
Multiple sclerosis
Obstruction
Orchitis
Pelvic injury/surgery
Prader-Willi syndrome
Primary hypogonadism
Prolactinoma
Radiation exposure
Retrograde ejaculation
Sarcoidosis
Sexually transmitted disease
Testicular torsion
Testicular trauma
Thyroid dysfunction
Tobacco use
Tuberculosis
Unknown cause
Varicocele
Y chromosome defect

Key Historical Features

✓ Duration of the infertility
✓ Previous evaluation and treatment for infertility
✓ Previous pregnancies for either partner
✓ Frequency and timing of intercourse
✓ Sexual dysfunction
✓ Use of lubricants during intercourse
✓ Previous testicular disorders, such as cryptorchidism or torsion
✓ Medical history, especially diabetes or thyroid disorders
✓ Surgical history, especially inguinal, scrotal, or retroperitoneal surgery
✓ Family history
✓ Medications
✓ Alcohol

✓ Tobacco use
✓ Caffeine intake
✓ Use of illicit drugs, especially anabolic steroids
✓ History of sexually transmitted disease
✓ Exposure to environmental toxins or radiation exposure
✓ Review of systems
  • Anosmia suggests a hypothalamic or pituitary etiology
  • Frequent respiratory infections suggests Young syndrome or Kartagener syndrome
  • Headaches, galactorrhea, and visual field disturbances suggest a central nervous system tumor

Key Physical Findings

✓ Signs of androgen deficiency (decreased facial and body hair, increased body fat, decreased muscle mass, small testes, Tanner stage <5)
✓ Examination for gynecomastia
✓ Position and size of the urethral meatus
✓ Testicular size
✓ Presence of varicocele
✓ Presence and contour of vasa deferentia and epididymides
✓ Prostate examination

Suggested Work-Up

Semen analysis (two samples taken 2 weeks apart)	To evaluate semen variables
Serum testosterone	To evaluate for underlying endocrine disorders
Follicle-stimulating hormone	Low level suggests hypogonadism
Luteinizing hormone	Low level with low testosterone suggests hypogonadotropic hypogonadism
Prolactin	To evaluate for hyperprolactinemia

Additional Work-Up

Fasting blood glucose	If diabetes mellitus is suspected
Complete blood count	If infection is suspected
Gonorrhea and chlamydia cultures or urine polymer chain reaction	If genital infection is suspected
Thyroid-stimulating hormone	If hypo- or hyperthyroidism is suspected

Renal and liver function studies	If renal or liver function abnormalities are suspected
Scrotal ultrasonography	If testicular abnormality, such as tumor or hydrocele, is suspected
Transrectal ultrasonography	To evaluate for retrograde ejaculation or ejaculatory duct obstruction if the volume of ejaculate is low
24-hour urinary free cortisol level	If Cushing syndrome is suspected
Serum 17-hydroxyprogesterone	If congenital adrenal hyperplasia is suspected
Quantitation of leukocytes in semen	May help identify underlying infection or inflammation in the semen
Antisperm antibody testing	The presence of antisperm antibody correlates with lower pregnancy rates

Further Reading

Brugh VM, Lipshultz LI. Male factor infertility: evaluation and management. *Med Clin North Am.* 2004;88:367–385.

Jarow JP. Endocrine causes of male infertility. *Urol Clin North Am.* 2003;30:83–90.

Jose-Miller AB, Boyden JW, Frey KA. Infertility. *Am Fam Physician.* 2007;75:849–856.

Kolettis PN. Evaluation of the subfertile man. *Am Fam Physician.* 2000;67:2165–2172.

Spitz A, Kim ED, Lipshultz LI. Contemporary approach to the male infertility evaluation. *Obstet Gynecol Clin North Am.* 2000;27:487–516.

General Discussion

Insomnia is the subjective perception of difficulty with sleep initiation, duration, consolidation, or quality that occurs despite adequate opportunity for sleep, which results in some form of daytime impairment, such as lack of energy, fatigue, irritability, and difficulty concentrating.

Insomnia is one of the most common concerns encountered in clinical practice. Insomnia symptoms occur in approximately 33% to 50% of the adult population, whereas insomnia symptoms with distress or impairment occur in 10% to 15% of the adult population. Risk factors for insomnia include increasing age, female sex, comorbid disorders (medical, psychiatric, sleep, and substance use), shift work, and possibly unemployment and lower socioeconomic status.

Patients with insomnia may complain of difficulty falling asleep, frequent awakenings, difficulty returning to sleep, awakening too early in the morning, or sleep that does not feel restful, refreshing, or restorative. It is common for multiple types of symptoms to co-occur and for the specific presentation to vary over time. Instruments that are helpful in the evaluation and differential diagnosis of insomnia include self-administered questionnaires (e.g., Epworth Sleepiness Scale), at-home sleep logs, symptom checklists, psychological screening tests, and bed partner interviews.

Most cases of insomnia develop initially in response to a medical or psychosocial stressor. As sleeplessness persists, the patient may begin to associate the bed with wakefulness and heightened arousal rather than sleep, thus perpetuating the insomnia. In general, patients with prolonged periods of wakefulness before, after, or during sleep are likely to have a behavioral, psychiatric, or circadian disorder. In contrast, patients whose symptoms are primarily frequent and who have brief nocturnal awakenings, sleep fragmentation, or nonrefreshing sleep are more likely to have a medical or primary sleep disorder.

One model of insomnia conceptualizes predisposing, precipitating, and perpetuating factors. Predisposing factors are those that increase an individual's vulnerability to insomnia and may include personality characteristics, lifestyle, and extreme circadian rhythm tendencies. A precipitant may be any major stressor, such as situational crises, as well as medical, psychiatric, and underlying sleep disorders. Perpetuating factors include maladaptive responses to the initial sleep difficulty, such as daytime napping or the use of alcohol to help with sleep.

Medications and Substances Associated with Insomnia

Albuterol
Alpha-receptor agonists and antagonists

Amphetamine derivatives
Beta-blockers
Caffeine
Cocaine
Codeine
Dextroamphetamine
Diet pills
Diuretics
Duloxetine
Ephedrine and derivatives
Methylphenidate
Monoamine oxidase inhibitors
Nicotine
Oxycodone
Pemoline
Phenylephrine
Phenylpropanolamine
Propoxyphene
Pseudoephedrine
Quinidine
Selective serotonin reuptake inhibitors
Steroids
Theophylline
Venlafaxine

Comorbid Medical and Psychiatric Conditions Associated with Insomnia

Cardiovascular causes
- Angina
- Congestive heart failure
- Dyspnea
- Dysrhythmias

Endocrine causes
- Diabetes mellitus
- Hyperthyroidism
- Hypothyroidism

Environmental causes
- Caffeine or alcohol intake before bedtime
- Daytime napping
- Eating or exercising before bedtime
- Noise
- Jet lag
- Shift work
- Temperature issues

Gastrointestinal causes
- Cholelithiasis
- Colitis
- Irritable bowel syndrome
- Peptic ulcer disease
- Reflux

Genitourinary causes
- Benign prostatic hypertrophy
- Enuresis
- Incontinence
- Interstitial cystitis
- Nocturia

Musculoskeletal causes
- Fibromyalgia
- Kyphosis
- Osteoarthritis
- Rheumatoid arthritis
- Sjögren syndrome

Neurologic causes
- Chronic pain disorders
- Dementia
- Headache disorders
- Neuromuscular disorders
- Parkinson disease
- Peripheral neuropathy
- Seizure disorders
- Stroke
- Traumatic brain injury

Primary sleep disorders
- Central sleep apnea
- Circadian rhythm sleep disorders
- Obstructive sleep apnea
- Parasomnias
- Periodic limb movement disorder
- Restless leg syndrome

Pulmonary causes
- Asthma
- Chronic obstructive pulmonary disease
- Emphysema
- Laryngospasm

Psychiatric causes
- Amnestic disorders
  - Alzheimer disease
  - Other dementias

- Anxiety disorders
  - Generalized anxiety disorder
  - Obsessive compulsive disorder
  - Panic disorder
  - Posttraumatic stress disorder
- Mood disorders
  - Bipolar disorder
  - Dysthymia
  - Major depressive disorder
- Other disorders
  - Adjustment disorders
  - Attention deficit disorder
  - Bereavement
  - Personality disorders
  - Stress
- Psychotic disorders
  - Schizoaffective disorder
  - Schizophrenia

Reproductive causes
- Menopause
- Menstrual cycle variations
- Pregnancy

Other causes
- Allergies
- Bruxism
- Rhinitis
- Sinusitis
- Alcohol and other substance use and/or dependence and/or withdrawal

Key Historical Features

✓ Primary insomnia complaint
  - Characterization of complaint
    - Difficulty falling asleep
    - Awakenings
    - Poor or unrefreshing sleep
  - Onset
  - Duration
  - Frequency
  - Severity
  - Course
  - Perpetuating factors
  - Past and current treatments and responses

✓ Pre-sleep conditions
  - Pre-bedtime activities
  - Bedroom environment
  - Evening physical and mental status

✓ Sleep–wake schedule
  - Time to fall asleep
  - Awakenings
    - Number, characterization, duration
    - Associated symptoms
    - Associated behaviors
  - Final awakening versus time out of bed
  - Amount of sleep obtained

✓ Nocturnal symptoms
  - Respiratory
  - Motor
  - Behavioral and psychological

✓ Daytime activities and function
  - Identify sleepiness versus fatigue
  - Napping
  - Work
  - Lifestyle
  - Travel
  - Daytime consequences
    - Quality of life
    - Mood disturbance
    - Cognitive dysfunction
    - Exacerbation of comorbid conditions

✓ Medical history
✓ Psychiatric history
✓ Medications (prescription and over-the-counter)
✓ Caffeine intake
✓ Alcohol use
✓ Tobacco use
✓ Substance use

Suggested Work-Up

The evaluation of insomnia is primarily historical, as outlined previously. Laboratory testing is not indicated for the routine evaluation of insomnia, unless there is suspicion for comorbid disorders.

It often is helpful to ask the patient to keep a sleep diary for a few weeks to record bedtime, total sleep time, time until sleep onset, number of awakenings, use of sleep medications, time out of bed in the morning, a rating of the quality of sleep, and daytime symptoms of sleep deprivation.

Additional Work-Up

Polysomnography	To establish the cause when an underlying sleep disorder, such as obstructive sleep apnea or movement disorder, is suspected by the history

Further Reading

American Academy of Sleep Medicine. *International Classification of Sleep Disorders, 2nd ed.: Diagnostic and Coding Manual.* Westchester, IL: American Academy of Sleep Medicine; 2005.

Eddy M, Walbroehl GS. Insomnia. *Am Fam Physician.* 1999;59:1911–1916.

National Heart, Lung, and Blood Institute Working Group on Insomnia. Insomnia: assessment and management in primary care. *Am Fam Physician.* 1999;59:3029–3038.

Neubauer DN. Insomnia. *Prim Care Clin Office Pract.* 2005;32:375–388.

Roth T, Roehrs T. Insomnia: epidemiology, characteristics, and consequences. *Clin Cornerstone.* 2003;5:5–15.

Schutte-Rodin S, Broch L, Buysse D, Dorsey C, Sateia M. Clinical guideline for the evaluation and management of chronic insomnia in adults. *J Clin Sleep Med.* 2008;4:487–504.

General Discussion

Leukocytosis is defined as a white blood cell (WBC) count greater than 11,000/mm^3. Circulating leukocytes consist of neutrophils, monocytes, eosinophils, basophils, and lymphocytes. Any one or all of these cell types may increase to abnormal levels in peripheral blood in response to various stimuli. An increase in neutrophils is the most common cause of leukocytosis. In most instances, elevated WBC counts are the result of normal bone marrow reacting to infection or inflammation. Leukocytosis may also occur as a result of physical or emotional stress. Causes of stress leukocytosis include anxiety, overexertion, seizures, anesthesia, and administration of epinephrine. Stress leukocytosis reverses within hours of elimination of the causative factor. Leukocytosis may also be caused by medications, malignancy, hemolytic anemia, and splenectomy.

A WBC response of more than 50,000/mm^3 associated with a cause outside the bone marrow is termed a leukemoid reaction, which is usually caused by a relatively benign process, such as infection or inflammation.

Certain clinical factors increase the suspicion that a leukocytosis may be caused by an underlying bone marrow disorder. These factors include a WBC count greater than 30,000/mm^3, concurrent anemia or thrombocytopenia, life-threatening infection or immunosuppression, lethargy, significant weight loss, bleeding, bruising, or petechiae. Evidence of enlargement of the liver, spleen, or lymph nodes also suggests an underlying bone marrow disorder. The first step in evaluating leukocytosis is to examine the WBC differential to determine which WBC type is elevated.

Neutrophilia usually reflects an inflammatory response to acute or subacute infections; therefore, it should trigger a diagnostic search for its cause. When neutrophilia occurs in the absence of evidence of acute inflammation or illness, other explanations should be considered. These include chemical effects from medications, malignancies, and chronic myeloproliferative disorders. A peripheral blood smear that shows circulating blasts suggests an acute leukemia, and leukoerythroblastic blasts suggest myelofibrosis or other marrow-infiltrating processes. In the case of a simple left-shifted neutrophilia, chronic myelogenous leukemia (CML) or another myeloproliferative disorder must be distinguished from a leukemoid reaction. Diagnostic tests are available to help make this distinction and are outlined in the following.

Monocytosis is defined as absolute peripheral blood monocyte counts greater than 0.50×10^9/L. Monocytosis is often seen in patients with tuberculosis, syphilis, sarcoidosis, fungal infections, and ulcerative colitis. Mild monocytosis is common with Hodgkin disease and a variety of cancers. Significant monocytosis is most often seen with hematopoietic malignancies. Monocytosis that persists should be considered a marker of a myeloproliferative disorder until proved otherwise by bone marrow biopsy and cytogenetic studies.

Eosinophilia occurs when the eosinophil count in the peripheral blood exceeds 0.4×10^9/L. The first diagnostic step is to exclude the possibility that eosinophilia is caused by drugs, parasite infection, asthma, allergic conditions, vasculitides, lymphoma, or metastatic cancer.

Peripheral blood basophilia is very rare and suggests chronic basophilic leukemia. Bone marrow biopsy and hematology consultation are recommended.

Lymphocytosis is defined as a lymphocyte count greater than 4.0×10^9/L. Mild to moderate lymphocytosis (lymphocyte counts less than 12×10^9/L) is most commonly caused by viral infection. With the exception of pertussis, acute bacterial infections rarely cause lymphocytosis. Most patients with lymphocytosis have signs of an underlying illness. In patients who do not have evidence of an infectious process or benign disorder, the diagnostic approach depends on establishing a tissue diagnosis to exclude malignant disease. The early phases of B-, T-, or NK-cell lymphoproliferative malignancies in adults can mimic benign polyclonal or reactive lymphocytosis.

Causes of Neutrophilia

Chemicals
- Ethylene glycol
- Histamine
- Mercury poisoning
- Venoms (reptiles, insects, jellyfish)

Drugs
- Corticosteroids
- Epinephrine
- Lithium
- Granulocyte colony stimulating factor
- Granulocyte-macrophage colony stimulating factor

Endocrine and metabolic disorders
- Ketoacidosis
- Lactic acidosis
- Thyrotoxicosis

Infections
- Bacteria
- Fungi
- Parasites
- *Rickettsia*
- Viruses

Myeloproliferative disorders
- Acute leukemia
- Agnogenic myeloid metaplasia
- CML

- Essential thrombocytosis
- Polycythemia vera

Neoplastic disorders
- Breast carcinoma
- Bronchogenic carcinoma
- Gastric carcinoma
- Lymphoma, especially Hodgkin disease
- Melanoma
- Metastatic cancer to bone marrow
- Pancreatic carcinoma
- Renal cell carcinoma

Non-neoplastic hematologic disorders
- Acute hemolytic anemias
- Acute transfusion reactions
- Postsplenectomy
- Recovery from bone marrow failure

Other disorders
- Eclampsia
- Exfoliative dermatitis
- Hypoxia
- Pregnancy
- Tissue necrosis

Rheumatologic and autoimmune disorders
- Autoimmune hemolytic anemia
- Gout
- Inflammatory bowel disease
- Rheumatoid arthritis
- Vasculitis

Trauma
- Crush injury
- Electrical injury
- Hypothermia
- Thermal injury

Causes of Eosinophilia

Adrenal insufficiency
Allergic reactions
Dermatologic conditions
Hypereosinophilic syndrome
Immunologic disorders
- Eosinophilia myalgia syndrome
- Lupus erythematosus
- Periarteritis
- Rheumatoid arthritis

Infections
- Chorea
- Genitourinary infections
- Leprosy
- Parasitic infections
- Scarlet fever

Malignancy
- Hodgkin lymphoma
- Non-Hodgkin lymphoma

Myeloproliferative disorders
- CML
- Myelofibrosis
- Polycythemia vera

Pleural and pulmonary conditions
- Loffler syndrome
- Pulmonary infiltrates

Sarcoidosis

Causes of Basophilia

Alteration of marrow and reticuloendothelial compartments
- Chronic hemolytic anemia
- Hodgkin disease
- Splenectomy

Endocrine causes
- Estrogens
- Hypothyroidism
- Ovulation

Infections
- Chronic sinusitis
- Viral infections (varicella)

Inflammatory conditions
- Chronic airway inflammation
- Chronic dermatitis
- Inflammatory bowel disease

Myeloproliferative disorders
- CML
- Myelofibrosis
- Polycythemia vera

Causes of Lymphocytosis

Infections
- Acute infectious lymphocytosis
- Adenovirus

- Babesiosis
- Brucellosis
- Cat scratch disease (*Bartonella henselae*)
- Coxsackievirus
- Cytomegalovirus infection
- Epstein-Barr virus (EBV) infection (mononucleosis)
- Hepatitis
- HIV infection
- Measles
- Mumps
- Pertussis
- Rickettsial infection
- Syphilis (secondary)
- Toxoplasmosis
- Tuberculosis
- Typhoid fever
- Varicella
- Viral infections

Neoplastic disorders
- Acute lymphocytic leukemia
- Carcinoma
- Chronic lymphocytic leukemia
- CML
- Hodgkin disease
- Thymoma

Other conditions
- Drug reactions
- Graves disease
- Hypersensitivity reactions
- Persistent polyclonal B-cell lymphocytosis
- Postsplenectomy lymphocytosis
- Sjögren syndrome
- Stress-induced lymphocytosis

Causes of Monocytosis

Gastrointestinal disorders
- Cirrhosis
- Granulomatous colitis
- Ulcerative colitis

Infections
- Brucellosis
- Endocarditis
- Fungal infections
- Paratyphoid

- • Protozoal infections
- • Recovery from acute infections
- • Syphilis
- • Tuberculosis
- • Typhoid
- • Viral infections (varicella)

Neoplastic diseases
- • Acute monocytic leukemia
- • Acute myelomonocytic leukemia
- • Chronic lymphocytic leukemia
- • Chronic myelomonocytic leukemia
- • Carcinoma
- • Hodgkin disease
- • Juvenile chronic myelomonocytic leukemia
- • Multiple myeloma
- • Myelodysplasia
- • Waldenström macroglobulinemia

Other disorders
- • Congenital neutropenia
- • Drug reactions
- • Recovery from marrow suppression
- • Sarcoidosis

Key Historical Features

✓ Fever
✓ Sweats
✓ Weight loss
✓ Easy bruising or bleeding
✓ Medical history
✓ Medications

Key Physical Findings

✓ Vital signs for evidence of fever
✓ Pallor
✓ Evidence of lymphadenopathy
✓ Abdominal examination for hepatomegaly or splenomegaly
✓ Skin and extremity examination for purpura or petechiae

Suggested Work-Up of Leukocytosis

WBC with differential	To determine which WBC type is elevated
Peripheral blood smear	To exclude the possibility of an acute leukemia and to classify the

process as granulocytosis
(neutrophilia, eosinophilia, or
basophilia), monocytosis, or
lymphocytosis

Suggested Work-Up of Neutrophilia

Leukocyte alkaline phosphatase (LAP)	LAP is usually increased when neutrophilia represents a reaction to an acute illness. LAP score is markedly decreased in cases of CML.
Peripheral blood fluorescence in situ hybridization (FISH) test for *bcr/abl*	To evaluate for CML if the patient's history does not suggest a leukemoid reaction
Hematology consultation and bone marrow aspiration	May be required to help determine the cause of neutrophilia

Suggested Work-Up of Monocytosis

Monocytosis that persists or does not obviously accompany a chronic infectious, inflammatory, or granulomatous process warrants hematology consultation.

Suggested Work-Up of Eosinophilia

Stool test for ova and parasites	To evaluate for gastrointestinal parasitic infection

For primary eosinophilia (not due to drugs, parasitic infection, asthma, allergic conditions, etc.), the following tests are suggested:

Serum tryptase	Increased levels suggest mastocytosis
T-cell immunophenotyping and TCR gene rearrangement analysis	Positive test results suggest an underlying clonal T-cell disorder
Serum interleukin-5	Elevated level requires evaluation of the bone marrow for the presence of a clonal T-cell disease
Serum immunoglobulin-E (IgE) level	Increased IgE level may decrease the risk of developing eosinophilia-associated heart disease
Bone marrow biopsy including cytogenetic studies FISH for	Recommended in all patients with primary eosinophilia to distinguish

FIPIL I-PDGFRA mutation, immunohistochemical stains for tryptase, and mast cell immunophenotyping | between clonal eosinophilia and the hypereosinophilic syndrome

Suggested Work-Up of Basophilia

Bone marrow biopsy and hematology consultation | To evaluate for chronic basophilic leukemia

Suggested Work-Up of Lymphocytosis

EBV serology	Indicated in most cases of lymphocytosis in young adults to evaluate for EBV infection
Bone marrow biopsy	Required when the peripheral blood smear shows leukoerythroblastosis or lymphoblasts. Also required if the lymphocytosis persists in a patient who has no evidence of acute or subacute infection.
Immunophenotyping by flow cytometry	To provide evidence for or against dominance of one lymphocyte type and differentiation stage
Hematology consultation	Recommended for any lymphocytosis that is not reactive

Further Reading

Abramson N, Melton B. Leukocytosis: basics of clinical assessment. *Am Fam Physician.* 2000;62:2053–2060.

Bagby GC. Leukopenia and leukocytosis. In: Goldman L, ed. *Cecil Textbook of Medicine.* 22nd ed. Philadelphia: Saunders; 2004.

Tefferi A, Hanson CA, Inwards DJ. How to interpret and pursue an abnormal complete blood cell count in adults. *Mayo Clin Proc.* 2005;80:923–936.

49 LEUKOPENIA

General Discussion

The normal peripheral white blood cell count ranges from 5.0 to 10.0×10^9/L. Leukopenia is defined as a total white blood cell count less than 4.5×10^9/L. When leukopenia is discovered, the first step is to determine which type of white blood cell is at lower levels than normal.

Neutropenia occurs when a patient's peripheral neutrophil count is less than 1.5×10^9/L, although the definition may vary among institutions. The normal range in Yemenite Jews and African-Americans is somewhat lower. The risk of bacterial infection is substantially increased when the peripheral neutrophil count falls to less than 0.5×10^9/L. The diagnostic evaluation of neutropenia must first address whether the patient has fever, sepsis, or both.

The most frequent cause of acquired neutropenia is medications. Any drug should be considered to be a potential cause until proved otherwise. Neutropenia may also occur as a manifestation of a wide variety of systemic diseases. Infection is a common cause of neutropenia, particularly viral infections and sepsis.

Normal lymphocyte counts range from 2 to 4×10^9/L, with approximately 20% B lymphocytes and 70% T lymphocytes. Lymphocytopenia is defined as a peripheral blood lymphocyte count less than 1.5×10^9/L. Protein-calorie malnutrition is the most common cause of lymphocytopenia worldwide. There generally are no specific clinical manifestations of lymphocytopenia. However, the patient may exhibit signs of immunologic deficiency depending upon the underlying cause of the lymphocytopenia, the degree of immunodeficiency, and the duration of the disease.

Medications Associated with Neutropenia

Acetazolamide
Alkylating agents
Allopurinol
Aminopyrine
Anthracyclines
Brompheniramine
Captopril
Carbamazepine
Chloramphenicol
Chlorpromazine
Chlorpropamide
Chlorthalidone
Cimetidine
Cisplatin
Clozapine

Dactinomycin
Dapsone
Deferiprone
Ethosuximide
Ganciclovir
Gold salts
Hydrochlorothiazide
Hydroxyurea
Ibuprofen
Indomethacin
Isoniazid
Levamisole
Mephenytoin
Methimazole
Methyldopa
Nitrofurantoin
Olanzapine
Para-aminosalicylic acid
Penicillamine
Penicillins
Phenylbutazone
Phenytoin
Procainamide
Prochlorperazine
Promazine
Propranolol
Propylthiouracil
Pyrimethamine
Quinidine
Quinine
Recombinant interferons
Rifampin
Rituximab
Streptokinase
Sulfasalazine
Thiouracil
Ticlopidine
Tocainide
Tolbutamide
Trimethadione
Trimethoprim-sulfamethoxazole
Tripelennamine
Vancomycin
Vinca alkaloids
Zidovudine

Medications Associated with Lymphocytopenia

Cyclophosphamide
Cyclosporine
Cytotoxic chemotherapy
Fludarabine
Glucocorticoids
Quinine

Causes of Neutropenia

Acquired aplastic anemia
Aplastic anemia
Autoimmune neutropenia (can occur with collagen and/or vascular
 disorders)
Benign ethnic neutropenia
Benzene toxicity
Chronic idiopathic neutropenia
Cocaine use
Congenital neutropenias (Kostmann syndrome and cyclic neutropenia)
Copper deficiency
Ethanol
Folate deficiency
Heroin use
Immune-mediated leukopenia
Large granular lymphocyte leukemia
Medications
Metastatic cancer (lung, breast, prostate, stomach, hematopoietic)
Myelodysplastic syndrome
Nonlymphocytic leukemia
Paroxysmal nocturnal hemoglobinuria
Postinfectious neutropenia (following bacterial, viral, parasitic, or
 rickettsial infection)
Pseudoneutropenia
Sepsis
Vitamin B_{12} deficiency

Causes of Lymphocytopenia

Alcohol abuse
Autoimmune and connective tissue diseases (lupus and rheumatoid
 arthritis)
Bacterial infections
Chronic renal failure
Chronic right ventricular failure
Congenital immunodeficiency states
 • Adenosine deaminase deficiency
 • Bruton X-linked agammaglobulinemia

- DiGeorge syndrome
- Nezelof syndrome
- Severe combined immunodeficiency
- Wiskott-Aldrich syndrome

Extracorporeal circulation
Graft versus host disease
Hemorrhage
Malignancy
- Hodgkin disease
- Multiple myeloma

Malnutrition
Medications
Older age
Postoperative state
Protein-losing enteropathy
Radiation
Sarcoidosis
Sepsis (bacterial or fungal)
Severe acute respiratory syndrome
Thoracic duct drainage or rupture
Thymoma
Trauma
Tuberculosis or other granulomatous infection
Viral infections, especially AIDS

Key Historical Features

✓ Attempt to determine the chronicity of the leukopenia
✓ Fever
✓ Recent infection
✓ Symptoms of underlying systemic disease
✓ Dietary practices
✓ Risk factors for HIV infection
✓ Medical history
✓ Surgical history, especially bariatric surgery
✓ Family history
✓ Medications
✓ Alcohol use

Key Physical Findings

✓ Vital signs, especially presence of fever
✓ Thorough examination for a source of infection, with special attention to the lungs, genitourinary system, gastrointestinal system, oropharynx, and skin

✓ Lymphatic examination for lymphadenopathy
✓ Abdominal examination for splenomegaly
✓ Skin examination for rash
✓ Joint examination for evidence of collagen and/or vascular disorder
✓ Neurologic examination for evidence of nutritional deficiency

Suggested Work-Up of Neutropenia

Examination of the peripheral blood smear and differential white blood cell count	To determine which white blood cell line is involved
Lymphocyte immunophenotyping	To evaluate for leukemia
T-cell receptor gene rearrangement studies	To evaluate for leukemia
Anti-nuclear antibody, anti-DNA antibody, complement (C3 and C4) levels, and urinalysis, including protein and/or creatinine ratio	To evaluate for collagen/vascular disease
Erythrocyte sedimentation rate and/or C-reactive protein	To evaluate for underlying infection or inflammatory process

Suggested Work-Up of Lymphocytopenia

Quantification of B-cells, CD4+, and CD8+	To evaluate the subsets of lymphocytes remaining in the circulation
Quantitative immunoglobulin levels	To detect deficiencies of cell-mediated immunity

Additional Work-Up for Leukopenias

Serum folate, homocysteine, methylmalonic acid, vitamin B_{12}, and copper levels	If folate, vitamin B_{12}, or copper deficiency is suspected

Further Reading

Bagby GC. Leukopenia and leukocytosis. In: Goldman L, ed. *Cecil Textbook of Medicine*. 22nd ed. Philadelphia: Saunders; 2004.

Tefferi A, Hanson CA, Inwards DJ. How to interpret and pursue an abnormal complete blood cell count in adults. *Mayo Clin Proc*. 2005;80:923–936.

General Discussion

The aging population has led to an increasing incidence and prevalence of memory complaints, especially in older adult patients. The prevalence of Alzheimer dementia (AD) is projected to almost triple over the next 40 years, from approximately 5 million patients in 2010 to more than 13 million patients by the year 2050. The proportion of people with AD in the United States rises for each age group, from 15% of those aged 65 to 74 years old to 44% of those aged 75 to 84 years old. Early identification allows the patient and family to plan for the disease and the physician to institute treatment earlier, which leads to a delay in institutionalization among AD patients.

It is important to remind patients and families that no one has a perfect memory. As we age, our memory might show common changes with things such as remembering the name of an actor/actress, forgetting an item at the grocery store, or needing to write more things onto lists. A memory issue truly becomes a problem when it begins to affect a person's ability to function in some way. The 2011 Alzheimer's Association guidelines divide dementia into three stages: preclinical AD, mild cognitive impairment (MCI) due to AD, and dementia due to AD.

The *Diagnostic and Statistical Manual of Mental Disorders-V* has renamed cognitive impairment as minor or major neurocognitive disorder. Minor neurocognitive disorder is similar to MCI and is defined as having evidence of modest cognitive decline with preserved function. Major neurocognitive disorder is synonymous with the diagnosis of dementia, with cognitive decline and disruption in function. Dementia is the diagnosis that requires a deficit and/or decline in memory and at least one other realm of cognitive functioning. Dementia is progressive and irreversible, and it affects how one functions in his or her daily life.

Cognitive function is typically divided into multiple categories: orientation, recall (immediate, short-term, and long-term), attention, language, executive, and visual–spatial function. The progression aspect of dementia results in a decline in the cognitive functions over time (either by history or by examination). The irreversible aspect of dementia refers to factors that can cause delirium, such as medications (e.g., benzodiazepines, anticholinergic medications, opiates), infections, electrolyte disturbances (e.g., sodium, calcium), and endocrine abnormalities (e.g., thyroid, sugar). Functional change refers to tasks that a patient used to be able to do that he or she cannot do now because of his or her cognitive function. Typically, the basic functional status is addressed by activities of daily living: bathing, dressing, feeding, grooming, toileting, and transfers. Higher level function is assessed by instrumental activities of daily living: taking medications, managing money, using the telephone, shopping, food preparation, housekeeping, laundry, and transportation.

Risk factors for dementia include a first-degree relative with AD, cardiovascular risk factors, low social and cognitive engagement, lower education, and a history of traumatic brain injury. Common questions include time frame of cognitive change (slow and gradual, rapid, stepwise) and new areas of cognitive impairment (repetitive, forgetting conversations, word finding difficulties, misplacing objects, and so on). In addition, any associated focal neurologic symptoms (balance and falling problems, urine incontinence, tremors, and hallucinations) might help in the diagnosis of the cognitive disorder or dementia type.

There are several different subtypes of dementia that are commonly diagnosed. Alzheimer-type dementia is a neurodegenerative dementia characterized by β amyloid plaques and tau tangles and is believed to include 70% to 80% of all dementias. It is a gradually progressive disease that typically starts with short-term memory decline, language issues, and mood changes. Vascular dementia exists either alone or with AD. Patients with vascular dementia typically have evidence of other vascular diseases, such as coronary artery disease or peripheral vascular disease. Vascular dementia often presents with a stepwise progression of difficulties with judgment, planning, organizing, and memory. Lewy body dementia is related to Parkinson disease. Patients with Lewy body dementia typically have early hallucinations and movement disorders, and they respond very poorly to antipsychotic medications. Frontotemporal dementia typically presents with disinhibited behaviors and memory changes. Other types of dementias include primary progressive aphasia, in which language deficits are more pronounced than memory deficits. Normal pressure hydrocephalus is a dementia characterized by symptoms of cognitive impairment, urinary incontinence, and gait disorder. Prion diseases such as Creutzfeldt-Jakob disease (CJD), although rare, present with a rapid course of memory disorder and coordination issues.

Common Causes of Dementia

AD
Frontotemporal dementia
Lewy body dementia
Mixed dementia
Normal pressure hydrocephalus
Primary progressive aphasia
Prion disease (e.g., Creutzfeldt-Jakob disease)
Vascular dementia
Other
- Depression
- Parkinson disease
- Alcohol-related dementia
- Huntington disease

- Prion disease
- Trauma
- Chronic infections (neurosyphilis, AIDS)
- Encephalitis
- Hypothyroidism
- Vitamin B_{12} deficiency

Key Historical Features

✓ Time frame of cognitive change (slow and gradual, rapid, stepwise)
✓ New areas of cognitive impairment (repetitive, forgetting conversations, word-finding difficulties, misplacing objects)
✓ First-degree relatives with AD
✓ Cardiovascular risk factors
✓ Focal neurologic symptoms (balance problems, falls, urinary incontinence, tremors, hallucinations)

Key Examination Findings

✓ Vital signs, especially blood pressure and pulse oximetry
✓ Neurologic examination for parkinsonian symptoms (tremor, masked facies, increased tone, shuffling gait) or normal pressure hydrocephalus (the triad of cognitive impairment, urinary incontinence, and magnetic gait disorder)
✓ Cardiovascular examination
✓ Depression screening, typically with the Patient Health Questionnaire 9 (PHQ-9), Geriatric Depression Scale, or other tool
✓ Memory screening with a modality such as the Mini-Cog
✓ Diagnostic tests of cognitive functioning such as the Mini Mental State Evaluation (MMSE), the Montreal Cognitive Assessment (MOCA), or the St. Louis University Memory Screen (SLUMS)

Suggested Work-Up

Electrolytes	To evaluate for electrolyte derangement
Blood urea nitrogen and creatinine	To evaluate renal function
Glucose	To evaluate for hypoglycemia or diabetes
Complete blood count	To evaluate for chronic infection
Thyroid-stimulating hormone	To evaluate for hypothyroidism
Calcium	To evaluate for hypercalcemia
Vitamin B_{12}	To evaluate for vitamin B_{12} deficiency

Folate	To evaluate for folate deficiency
Magnetic resonance imaging or noncontrast computed tomography of the brain	To evaluate for space occupying lesions and to evaluate for other intracranial pathologies, such as normal pressure hydrocephalus, intracranial vascular disease, or subdural hematoma

Additional Work-Up

The following tests should be performed when clinical suspicion warrants them:

Rapid plasma reagin (RPR)	If syphilis is suspected
Lyme disease titer	If Lyme disease is suspected
HIV	If HIV/AIDS is suspected
Urinalysis, urine culture and sensitivity	If urinary tract infection is suspected
Erythrocyte sedimentation rate	If inflammatory disease is suspected
Aspartate aminotransferase, alanine aminotransferase, bilirubin	If liver disease is suspected
Heavy metal assays	If exposure to heavy metals is suspected
Lumbar puncture	Consider for patients with suspected cerebral vasculitis, HIV infection, neurosyphilis, prion disease, or cerebral Lyme disease
Neuropsychologic testing	Can comprehensively assess multiple domains of higher cognitive functioning, including intelligence and behavioral functioning, and can be used to identify cognitive impairment in patients with higher baseline cognitive abilities. It may also reveal subtle cognitive impairment in persons with suspected cognitive impairment or dementia. Neuropsychologic testing is not recommended routinely for all patients with suspected dementia.
Electroencephalography	Indicated only if prion disease is suspected

Further Reading

Adelman AM, Daly MP. Initial evaluation of the patient with suspect dementia. *Am Fam Physician*. 2005;71:1745–1750.

Alzehimer's Association Report. 2014 Alzheimers disease facts and figures. *Alzheimers Dement*. 2014;10:e47–e92.

American Psychiatric Association. *Diagnostic and Statistical Manual of Mental Disorders*. 5th ed. Washington, DC: American Psychiatric Association; 2013.

Clarfield AM. The decreasing prevalence of reversible dementias: an updated meta-analysis. *Arch Intern Med*. 2003;163:2219–2229.

Friedland RP, Wilcock GK. Dementia. In: Evans JG, Williams TF, Beattie BL, Michel JP, Wilcock GK, eds. *Oxford Textbook of Geriatric Medicine*. 2nd ed. Oxford, UK: Oxford University Press; 2000:922–932.

Geldmacker DS, Kirson NY, Birnbaum HG, et al. Implications of early treatment among Medicaid patients with Alzheimer's disease. *Alzheimers Dement*. 2014;10:214–224.

Hebert LE, Weuve J, Scherr PA, Evans DA. Alzheimer disease in the United States (2010–2050) estimated using the 2010 Census. *Neurology*. 2013;80:1778–1783.

Howard R, McShane R, Lendesay J, et al. Donepezil and memantine for moderate-to-severe Alzheimer's disease. *N Engl J Med*. 2012;266:893–903.

Kaye JA. Diagnostic challenges in dementia. *Neurology*. 1998;51:S45–S52.

Knopman DS, DeKosky ST, Cummings JL, et al. Practice parameter: diagnosis of dementia (an evidence-based review). *Neurology*. 2001;56:1143–1153.

Leifer BP. Early diagnosis of Alzheimer's disease; clinical and economic benefits. *J Am Geriatr Soc*. 2003;51(5 suppl Dementia):S281–S288.

Lorentz WJ, Scanlon J, Brush M. The Mini-Cog: a cognitive 'vital signs' measure for dementia screening in multi-lingual elderly. *Int J Geriatr Psychiatry*. 2000;15:1021–1027.

Schwartz S, Froelich L, Burns A. Pharmacological treatment of dementia. *Curr Opin Psych*. 2012;25:542–550.

General Discussion

The first step in the evaluation of muscle weakness is differentiating true muscle weakness from fatigue and asthenia. Fatigue is the inability to continue performing a task after multiple repetitions, whereas asthenia is a sense of exhaustion in the absence of actual muscle weakness.

Peripheral nerve lesions must be distinguished from central nervous system (CNS) disease. Peripheral neuropathies and myopathies usually follow a gradual progressive deterioration, whereas central lesions are more commonly acute or subacute.

The history and physical examination represent an important part of the evaluation of muscle weakness. Details of the history and physical examination are outlined in the following. Disease onset and progression, as well as the pattern of muscle weakness, are key historical features. During the physical examination, the muscle weakness must be objectively confirmed, quantified, and localized, if possible.

The laboratory and radiographic evaluation should be guided by findings from the history and physical examination. In the absence of features suggesting a particular diagnosis, the evaluation may proceed in a stepwise fashion, beginning with a general laboratory evaluation as outlined in the following.

Medications Associated with Muscle Weakness

Amiodarone
Chemotherapeutic agents
Cimetidine
Corticosteroids
Gemfibrozil
Interferon
Laminvudine
Leuprolide acetate
Methimazole
Nonsteroidal anti-inflammatory drugs
Penicillin
Propylthiouracil
Statins
Sulfonamides
Zidovudine

Causes of Muscle Weakness

Cocaine use
Electrolyte imbalance

- Hypercalcemia
- Hyperkalemia
- Hypermagnesemia
- Hypokalemia
- Hypomagnesemia

Endocrine causes
- Acromegaly
- Hyperparathyroidism
- Hyperthyroidism
- Hypopituitarism
- Hypothyroidism
- Vitamin D deficiency

Genetic causes
- Distal myopathies
- Muscular dystrophy
- Myotonic dystrophy type 2

Infectious causes
- Diphtheria
- Epstein-Barr virus
- HIV
- Influenza
- Lyme disease
- Meningitis
- Polio
- Rabies
- Syphilis
- Tetanus
- Tick paralysis
- Toxoplasmosis

Metabolic causes
- Acid maltase deficiency
- Aldolase A deficiency
- Brancher enzyme deficiency
- Carnitine deficiency
- Carnitine palmitoyltransferase II deficiency
- Myophosphorylase deficiency
- Phosphofructokinase deficiency
- Mitochondrial defects
- Trifunctional protein deficiency

Neurologic causes
- Amyotrophic lateral sclerosis
- Botulism
- Carbamate intoxication
- Cerebrovascular accident
- Cervical spondylosis

- Degenerative disc disease
- Epidural hematoma
- Guillain-Barré syndrome
- Lambert-Eton myasthenic syndrome
- Multiple sclerosis
- Myasthenia gravis
- Neoplasm
- Organophosphate intoxication
- Spinal cord injury
- Spinal muscle atrophy
- Subdural hematoma

Rheumatologic causes
- Dermatomyositis
- Inclusion body myositis
- Polymyalgia rheumatica
- Polymyositis
- Rheumatoid arthritis
- Systemic lupus erythematosus
- Systemic sclerosis/scleroderma

Other causes
- Alcohol toxicity
- Amyloidosis
- Sarcoidosis

Key Historical Features

✓ Age
✓ Onset of symptoms
✓ Rate of progression of symptoms
✓ Pattern of muscle weakness
- Global or focal
- Proximal or distal
- Unilateral or bilateral
✓ Associated symptoms
- Abdominal pain
- Arthralgias
- Constipation
- Diarrhea
- Dysphagia
- Easy bruising
- Malaise
- Menorrhagia
- Rash
- Weakness associated with exercise or activity

✓ Medical history
✓ Medications
✓ Family history
✓ Social history
  • Alcohol consumption
  • Drug use
  • Toxin exposure

Key Physical Findings

✓ Examination of the thyroid gland
✓ Head and neck examination for ptosis or fatigable weakness
✓ Assessment of muscle strength
✓ Evaluation of ability to stand and write
✓ Neurologic examination
✓ Mental status testing
✓ Cardiac examination
✓ Pulmonary examination
✓ Skin examination for rash
✓ Extremity examination for joint inflammation

Suggested Work-Up

Complete blood count	To evaluate for infection
Electrolytes	To evaluate for potassium imbalance
Blood urea nitrogen and creatinine	To evaluate for uremia
Glucose	To evaluate for hypoglycemia or hyperglycemia
Calcium	To evaluate for hypercalcemia
Magnesium	To evaluate for hyper- or hypomagnesemia
Phosphorus	To evaluate for hypophosphatemia
Thyroid-stimulating hormone	To evaluate for thyroid-related myopathy
Creatine kinase	May be elevated in inflammatory myopathies, muscular dystrophies, sarcoidosis, alcoholism, infections, storage myopathies, and adverse drug reactions
Erythrocyte sedimentation rate and antinuclear antibody (ANA)	To evaluate for rheumatologic myopathies

Electromyelogram	To help establish the presence of a myopathy and indicate if a neuropathy or neuromuscular disease is present

Additional Work-Up

Brain computed tomography scan or magnetic resonance imaging	If cerebrovascular disease is suspected
Lumbar puncture	If meningitis, encephalitis, or multiple sclerosis is suspected
Parathyroid hormone	If hypercalcemia or uremia is present on initial screening
Rheumatoid factor	If rheumatoid arthritis is suspected
Anti-double-stranded DNA, antiphospholipid antibodies, anti-Sm antibody, anti-Ro(SSA) and anti-La(SSB) antibodies, antihistone antibody, anti-RNP antibody, C3 and C4 levels	If lupus is suspected
Anticentromere antibodies	If scleroderma is suspected
Aspartate aminotransferase, alanine aminotransferase, gamma-glutamyl transferase (GGT), and vitamin B_{12} level	If alcoholism is suspected
Adrenocorticotrophic hormone (ACTH) assay or ACTH stimulation test	If adrenal insufficiency is suspected (hypoglycemia, hyponatremia, hyperkalemia)
24-hour urinary free cortisol or dexamethasone suppression test	If Cushing disease is suspected
Growth hormone assay	If acromegaly is suspected
Vitamin D assay	If osteomalacia is suspected
Toxicologic analysis	If toxin exposure is suspected
Pulmonary function tests	If Guillain-Barré syndrome is suspected
Muscle biopsy	If the diagnosis is inconclusive after a thorough history, physical examination, laboratory, radiologic, and electromyographic evaluation

Further Reading

Anagnos A, Ruff RL, Kaminski HJ. Endocrine neuromyopathies. *Neurol Clin.* 1997;15:673–696.

LoVecchio F. Approach to generalized weakness and peripheral neuromuscular disease. *Emerg Med Clin North Am.* 1997;15:605–623.

O'Rourke KS. Myopathies in the elderly. *Rheum Dis Clin North Am.* 2000;26:647–672.

Saguil A. Evaluation of the patient with muscle weakness. *Am Fam Physician.* 2005;71:1327–1336.

Yazici Y, Kagen LJ. Clinical presentation of the idiopathic inflammatory myopathies. *Rheum Dis Clin North Am.* 2002;28:823–832.

General Discussion

Muscle pain may be the result of muscle disease, but joint and bone disease may also produce complaints of muscle pain. Pain from disease of overlying tissue, fascia, or tendons may also be referred to muscle. In addition, disease of the major peripheral nerves or of their smaller intramuscular branches may produce both muscle pain and muscle weakness. Muscle pain may be a major symptom in inflammatory, metabolic, endocrine, and toxic myopathies.

Metabolic myopathies is a term applied to a heterogeneous group of disorders that result from the inability of skeletal muscle to produce or maintain adequate levels of energy in the form of adenosine triphosphate. The metabolic myopathies are classified according to the altered area of metabolism as muscle glycogenoses, disorders of lipid metabolism, or mitochondrial myopathies. Patients with metabolic myopathies have widely variable symptoms, including premature fatigue, episodic aches, cramps, and pains occasionally accompanied by extensive rhabdomyolysis with myoglobinuria, and fixed, progressive muscle weakness. The diagnosis of a metabolic myopathy usually requires muscle biopsy with a combination of analyses, including histology, histochemistry, electron microscopy, and biochemistry.

Multiple drugs and toxins can cause myopathy. Patients at risk for developing adverse reactions are those who have reduced abilities to metabolize or excrete the drug and its metabolites. These include infants, children, older adult patients, and those who have liver or renal failure. There are several recognized mechanisms in which toxins can produce muscle damage. Toxins may cause a direct toxic or biochemical effect. Secondary effects of toxins resulting in muscle damage include immune activation with inflammation, vascular insufficiency and/or ischemia, hypokalemia, muscle overactivity, compression, or direct injury resulting from repeated injections. Because toxin-related muscle damage can be readily reversible once exposure stops, toxic myopathies should be considered early in the differential diagnosis of myalgias.

The idiopathic inflammatory myopathies are a group of disorders characterized by proximal muscle weakness and nonsuppurative inflammation of skeletal muscle, often accompanied by extramuscular manifestations. The idiopathic inflammatory myopathies include dermatomyositis, polymyositis, inclusion body myositis, and cancer-associated myositis. Patients with idiopathic inflammatory myopathy may present with a variety of nonspecific symptoms, such as fatigue, myalgias, arthralgias, malaise, and weight loss.

Medications Associated with Myalgias

Albuterol
Aminocaproic acid

Amiodarone
Amphetamines
Amphotericin B
Chloroquine
Cimetidine
Clofibrate
Colchicine
Corticosteroids (chronic use)
Cyclosporine
Danazol
Diuretics
Emetine
Enalapril
Finasteride
Gemfibrozil
Glucocorticoids
Halothane
Hydroxymethylglutaryl-CoA reductase inhibitors (statins)
Hydralazine
Hydroxychloroquine
Interferon-alfa
Isotretinoin
L-dopa
Labetalol
Lamotrigine
Laxatives
Levodopa
Leuprolide
Meperidine
Nicotinic acid
Omeprazole
Pancuronium
Penicillamine
Phenytoin
Procainamide
Propofol
Quinacrine
Rifampin
Succinylcholine
Sulfonamides
Tacrolimus
Tretinoin
L-tryptophan
Valproic acid
Vincristine

Vitamin E
Zidovudine

Causes of Myalgias

Adrenal insufficiency
Alcohol abuse
Amyopathic dermatomyositis
Amyotrophic lateral sclerosis
Antisynthetase syndrome
Cancer-associated myositis
Collagen vascular disease
Dermatomyositis
Diabetes mellitus
Disorders of lipid metabolism
Drug-induced myopathic syndromes
- Alcohol
- Cocaine
- Heroin
- Ipecac
- L-tryptophan
- Medications
- Toluene abuse

Familial periodic paralysis
Fibromyalgia
Guillain-Barré syndrome
Hyperthyroidism
Hypothyroidism
Inclusion body myositis
Infectious myositis
- Bacterial
- Coxsackie virus
- Fungal
- Influenza virus
- Parasitic

Licorice
Medications
Mitochondrial myopathies
Mixed connective tissue syndrome
Muscle glycogenoses
Myasthenia gravis
Occult or metastatic carcinoma
Osteomalacia
Overlap syndromes
Partial defects in dystrophin

Polyarteritis nodosa
Polymyalgia rheumatica
Polymyositis
Porphyria
Rheumatoid arthritis
Scleroderma
Sepsis
Systemic lupus erythematosus
Temporal arteritis
Vigorous activity

Key Historical Features

✓ Age of onset
✓ Muscle weakness
✓ Fatigue
✓ Insomnia
✓ Depressive symptoms
✓ Stiffness and pain in the hips and shoulders
✓ Joint pain
✓ Medical history
✓ Medications
✓ Alcohol use
✓ Substance abuse
✓ Review of systems

Key Physical Findings

✓ Vital signs
✓ Cardiac examination for the presence of cardiomyopathy
✓ Examination of the joints for swelling
✓ Examination of the skin for any skin changes such as rash
✓ Evaluation of muscle strength and identification of the pattern of muscle groups affected
✓ Neurologic examination to screen for the presence of neuropathy

Suggested Work-Up

Serum creatine kinase	To evaluate for muscle fiber necrosis
Urine myoglobin	Nonspecific marker of myopathy. Myoglobin is not normally detectable in urine, and myoglobinuria should be suspected when a urine sample tests positive for hemoglobin but

| | urine microscopy reveals no red blood cells. |
| Electromyography (EMG) | To help identify neuromuscular disease |

Additional Work-Up

Muscle biopsy	May be needed to confirm the diagnosis and determine the cause of the muscle dysfunction
Erythrocyte sedimentation rate	To evaluate for inflammation if rheumatologic or inflammatory conditions are suspected (e.g., polymyalgia rheumatica, temporal arteritis)
Magnetic resonance imaging	May be used as a noninvasive differential diagnostic method
Serum lactic dehydrogenase, aspartate aminotransferase, creatine kinase, and aldolase	If steroid-induced myopathy is suspected
Adrenocorticotrophic hormone stimulation test	If adrenal insufficiency is suspected

Further Reading

Anagnos A, Ruff RL, Kaminski HJ. Endocrine neuromyopathies. *Neurol Clin.* 1997;15:673–696.

O'Rourke KS. Myopathies in the elderly. *Rheum Dis Clin North Am.* 2000;26:647–672.

Wald JJ. The effects of toxins on muscle. *Neurol Clin.* 2000;18:695–718.

Walsh RJ, Amato AA. Toxic myopathies. *Neurol Clin.* 2005;23:397–428.

Wortmann RL, DiMauro S. Differentiating idiopathic inflammatory myopathies from metabolic myopathies. *Rheum Dis Clin North Am.* 2002;28:759–778.

Yazici Y, Kagen LJ. Clinical presentation of the idiopathic inflammatory myopathies. *Rheum Dis Clin North Am.* 2002;28:823–832.

53 NEPHROLITHIASIS

General Discussion

The lifetime risk of passing a kidney stone is approximately 8% to 10% among North American males, with a peak incidence at age 30 years. Women have a risk of approximately one-half that of men. Among patients who have passed one kidney stone, the lifetime recurrence rate is 60% to 80%.

Approximately 80% of kidney stones contain calcium, and the majority of these stones are composed of calcium oxalate. A minority contain calcium phosphate or admixtures of oxalate and phosphate salts. Approximately 10% of stones are composed of uric acid. Another 10% are struvite stones that develop exclusively in patients with urinary tract infections (UTIs) caused by urease-producing organisms, such as the *Proteus* species. Cystine accounts for approximately 1% of all stones, but it only occurs in patients with cystinuria, an autosomal recessive disorder.

Some controversy exists about the extent of investigation required after the passage of a single stone. Because the rate of recurrence is high, many experts favor a thorough evaluation for anyone who has passed a stone. A comprehensive urinary evaluation or referral is required for patients in whom multiple stones are detected clinically or radiographically, patients with anatomic abnormalities of the urinary tract, patients with a strong family history of nephrolithiasis, and patients with cystine or uric acid stones.

Plain abdominal radiography, ultrasonography, intravenous pyelography (IVP), helical computed tomography (CT) scanning, and magnetic resonance image scanning can be used to demonstrate stones in the renal tract. Non-contrast helical CT scanning is the preferred imaging modality because it is faster and more sensitive than IVP and does not require the use of intravenous contrast material. In addition, CT scanning may identify other causes of abdominal pain masquerading as renal colic.

Medications Associated with Nephrolithiasis

Acetazolamide
Allopurinol
Amiodarone
Amoxicillin
Ampicillin
Ascorbic acid
Calcium supplementation
Carbonic anhydrase inhibitors
Ceftriaxone
Corticosteroids
Cytotoxic agents used for malignancies
Dalfampridine

Furan antibiotics
Highly active antiretroviral therapy (reverse transcriptase inhibitors and
    protease inhibitors)
Laxatives
Pyridine antibiotics
Quinolones
Silicate
Sotalol
Sulfonamides
Sulfonylureas
Topiramate
Triamterene

Causes of Nephrolithiasis

Hypercalciuria
Hyperoxaluria
Hyperuricosuria
Hypocitraturia
Idiopathic
Infection (*Proteus, Klebsiella, Serratia,* and *Mycoplasma* UTIs)
Renal tubular acidosis type I

Key Historical Features

✓ Patient age
✓ Frequency of stone formation
✓ Medical history
- Anatomic abnormalities of the renal system
- Crohn disease
- Cystinuria
- Gout
- Hypercalciuria
- Hyperoxaluria
- Hyperparathyroidism
- Hyperthyroidism
- Hypocitraturia
- Immobilization
- Immunocompromised status
- Lesch-Nyhan syndrome
- Malignancy
- Milk alkali syndrome
- Polycystic kidney disease
- Recurrent or chronic UTIs
- Renal tubular acidosis

- • Sarcoidosis
- • Skeletal disease
- • Solitary functioning kidney
✓ Surgical history
- • Renal transplantation
- • Small bowel resection
✓ Medications
✓ Family history
- • Stone disease
- • Parathyroid disease
- • Gout
- • Occupational history, especially significant sweating
✓ Alcohol use
✓ Dietary history
- • Fluid intake
- • Calcium intake
- • Excessive intake of protein-rich foods
- • Excessive intake of chocolate or nuts
- • Sodium intake

Key Physical Findings

✓ Vital signs
✓ General examination for diaphoresis or ill appearance
✓ Cardiac examination for tachycardia
✓ Pulmonary examination for tachypnea
✓ Abdominal examination for tenderness, bruits, pulsatile masses, and symmetry of femoral pulses. The bladder should be examined for tenderness and evidence of retention. There should be no peritoneal signs in a patient with nephrolithiasis.
✓ Back examination for flank or costovertebral angle tenderness
✓ Genitourinary and rectal examinations should be unremarkable in nephrolithiasis

Suggested Work-Up of a Patient with First Stone Episode

Serum electrolytes	Used to calculate the anion gap. Type I renal tubular acidosis presents with a nonanion gap acidosis with concomitant hypokalemia.
Blood urea nitrogen and creatinine	To evaluate renal function
Serum calcium	To evaluate for hypercalcemia and hyperparathyroidism
Serum phosphorus	To evaluate for hypophosphatemia

Serum uric acid	To evaluate for hyperuricemia
Pregnancy test	To rule out pregnancy
Urinalysis	Hematuria is present in 90% of patients with stones. Urinalysis may reveal the presence of a UTI. Hexagonal crystals suggest cystinuria. Low urinary pH is associated with uric acid stone formation. High urinary pH may suggest a struvite stone. High urinary pH accompanied by a low-serum bicarbonate concentration may occur with type I renal tubular acidosis.
Urine culture	If urinary infection is suspected
Complete blood count	If infection is suspected
Stone analysis	If the stone is available
Imaging study with helical CT, ultrasonography, or IVP (helical CT generally preferred)	To evaluate for additional stones, radiolucent stones, or anatomic abnormalities
Serum bicarbonate	If type I renal tubular acidosis is suspected

Suggested Work-Up of a Patient with Recurrent Stone Formation

24-hour urine collection for volume, pH, calcium, phosphate, sodium, uric acid, oxalate, citrate, creatinine	Used for initial management and to guide therapy. May need to be repeated to monitor effectiveness of treatment.

Further Reading

Bushinsky DA. Nephrolithiasis. *J Am Soc Nephrol.* 1998;9:917–924.

Frassetto L, Kohlstadt I. Treatment and prevention of kidney stones: an update. *Am Fam Physician.* 2011;84:1234–1242.

Goldfarb DS, Coe FL. Prevention of recurrent nephrolithiasis. *Am Fam Physician.* 1999;60:2269–2276.

Manthey DE, Teichman J. Nephrolithiasis. *Emerg Med Clin North Am.* 2001;19:633–654.

Morton AR, Iliescu EA, Wilson JWL. Nephrology: investigation and treatment of recurrent kidney stones. *Can Med Assoc J.* 2002;166:213–218.

Tiselius HG. Medical evaluation of nephrolithiasis. *Endocrinol Metab Clin North Am.* 2002;31:1031–1050.

General Discussion

Definitions of night sweats vary and may include unusual sweating that occurs only or mainly at night, sweating at night even when it is not hot in the bedroom, or drenching sweats that require the patient to change bedclothes.

Sweating helps to reduce core body temperature when it rises above a certain threshold, which is called the thermoneutral zone (TNZ). Sweating can happen because of environmental heat exposure, decreased heat dissipation (e.g., excessive clothing or bed coverings), or increased heat production (e.g., excessive muscular activity). Release of inflammatory mediators during infections, autoimmune diseases, and malignancies can temporarily raise the TNZ, inducing chills and shivering that cause the core body temperature to rise. Sweating occurs when the levels of these mediators and the TNZ return to normal.

Some people who report night sweats may simply be more aware or concerned about nighttime sweating because they are awake for other reasons. Most patients who report night sweats to their physician probably do not have a serious disease causing the symptoms. Two studies of older primary care patients revealed that life expectancy did not differ between those with night sweats and those without. The differential diagnosis of night sweats is broad, but it can be narrowed with the history and physical examination.

If the history and physical examination do not reveal a suspected etiology of the patient's symptoms, an initial evaluation with complete blood count (CBC), purified protein derivative (PPD), chest x-ray, and thyroid-stimulating hormone (TSH) can be performed. An HIV test and erythrocyte sedimentation rate (ESR) may be added, if indicated. An elevated ESR and positive blood culture are present in more than 90% of cases of endocarditis. If these screening tests are normal, and nocturnal gastroesophageal reflux disease (GERD) is suspected, a trial of antireflux medications and measures may be considered. If night sweats continue, a diary of temperature variations may be useful to reveal febrile micropulses. Febrile pulses should prompt an evaluation for lymphoma or endocarditis.

Medications Associated with Night Sweats

Acetaminophen
Antidepressants
Antihypertensives
Aspirin
Cyclosporine
Daclizumab
Donepezil
Efavirenz

Indinavir
Interferon alfa-2a
Leuprolide
Niacin
Pegaspargase
Phenothiazines
Rituximab
Salicylates
Saquinavir
Tamoxifen
Zalcitabine

Causes of Night Sweats

Endocrine
- Diabetes mellitus (nocturnal hypoglycemia)
- Hyperthyroidism
- Ovarian failure

Infections
- Coccidioidomycosis
- Cysticercosis
- Endocarditis
- Eosinophilic pneumonia
- Histoplasmosis
- HIV
- Lung abscess
- Mononucleosis
- *Mycobacterium avium* complex
- Pneumonia

Malignancy
- Carcinoid tumor
- Essential thrombocythemia
- Leukemia
- Lymphoma
- Mesothelioma
- Myelofibrosis
- Other neoplasms
- Pancreatic cancer
- Pheochromocytoma

Other
- Anxiety and panic disorder
- Autonomic overactivity
- Chronic fatigue syndrome
- Diabetes insipidus
- GERD
- Granulomatous disease

- Lymph node hyperplasia
- Night terrors
- Obesity
- Obstructive sleep apnea
- Over-bundling
- Pregnancy
- Prinzmetal angina
- Sports overtraining

Rheumatologic/autoimmune
- POEMS syndrome
- Rheumatoid arthritis
- Takayasu arteritis
- Temporal arteritis

Substance abuse
- Alcohol
- Heroin

Key Historical Features

- ✓ Fever
- ✓ Cough
- ✓ Fatigue
- ✓ Malaise
- ✓ Weight loss
- ✓ Nervousness
- ✓ Palpitations
- ✓ Menstrual irregularities
- ✓ Symptoms suggestive of myocardial ischemia
- ✓ Symptoms suggestive of anxiety or depression
- ✓ Sleep habits, including snoring, apneic episodes, and daytime sleepiness
- ✓ Recent upper respiratory infection
- ✓ Risk factors for tuberculosis
- ✓ Risk factors for HIV infection
- ✓ Risk factors for endocarditis
- ✓ Symptoms suggestive of rheumatologic disease
- ✓ Travel history
- ✓ Symptoms of menopause in women
- ✓ Gastroesophageal reflux symptoms
- ✓ Medical history
- ✓ Medications

Key Physical Findings

- ✓ Vital signs, especially temperature and blood pressure
- ✓ General assessment of well-being and body habitus
- ✓ Head examination for oral candidiasis or redundant tissue in the oropharynx

- ✓ Eye examination for exophthalmos
- ✓ Neck examination for thyroid abnormalities
- ✓ Cardiovascular examination for murmurs
- ✓ Pulmonary examination
- ✓ Lymphatic examination for lymphadenopathy
- ✓ Abdominal examination for splenomegaly
- ✓ Neurologic examination for tremor or hyperreflexia
- ✓ Signs of endocarditis, such as splinter hemorrhages, Janeway lesions, or Osler nodes

Suggested Work-Up

CBC	To evaluate for underlying infection
PPD	To evaluate for tuberculosis
Chest x-ray	To evaluate for tuberculosis, other lung infections, malignancy, and lymphadenopathy
TSH	To evaluate for hyperthyroidism

Additional Work-Up

HIV test	To evaluate for HIV infection
ESR	To help rule out inflammatory disorders
Diary of nocturnal temperature	To evaluate for febrile pulses
Blood cultures, including HACEK group organisms	If endocarditis is suspected
Echocardiogram	If endocarditis is suspected
Computed tomography scan of chest, abdomen, and pelvis	If silent neoplastic or granulomatous disease is suspected
Lymph node biopsy	If firm lymphadenopathy is found in the absence of current or recent infection
Bone marrow biopsy	To evaluate for neoplastic or granulomatous disease
Sleep study	If obstructive sleep apnea is suspected
24-hour urinary catecholamines or metanephrines	If pheochromocytoma is suspected
Urinary 5-hydroxyindoleacetic acid	If carcinoid tumor is suspected (cyanotic flushing, watery diarrhea, wheezing, hypotension, or edema)

Further Reading

Fred HL. Night sweats. *Hosp Pract.* 1993;28:88.

Holtzclaw BJ. Circadian rhythmicity and homeostatic stability in thermoregulation. *Biol Res Nurs.* 2001;2:221–235.

Mold JW, Holtzclaw BJ, McCarthy L. Night sweats: a systematic review of the literature. *J Am Board Fam Med.* 2012;25:878–893.

Mold JW, Lawler F. The prognostic implications of night sweats in two cohorts of older patients. *J Am Board Fam Med.* 2010;23:97–103.

Viera AJ, Bond MM, Yates SW. Diagnosing night sweats. *Am Fam Physician.* 2003;67:1019–1024.

General Discussion

Osteoporosis is characterized by low bone mass and structural deterioration of bone, leading to an increased risk of fractures. The World Health Organization (WHO) defines osteoporosis as a spinal or hip bone mineral density of 2.5 SDs or more below the mean for healthy, young women (T-score of -2.5 or below) as measured by dual energy x-ray absorptiometry.

Primary osteoporosis results from deterioration of bone mass that is related to aging and decreased gonadal function, but it is not associated with any chronic illness. Because primary osteoporosis results from decreased gonadal function, early menopause or premenopausal estrogen deficiency may hasten the development of osteoporosis. Other risk factors for primary osteoporosis include female gender, white or Asian ancestry, sedentary lifestyle, tobacco use, low calcium intake, and low body weight.

Secondary osteoporosis results from chronic conditions that contribute to accelerated bone density loss. Men are more likely than women to have a secondary cause of osteoporosis. Chronic conditions that may contribute to secondary osteoporosis are listed in the following. Long-term glucocorticoid therapy is a common cause of osteoporosis. Medications that may cause osteoporosis are listed in the following.

In the patient with osteoporosis, initial evaluation should begin with a risk factor assessment (see the risk factors listed below), and a history and physical examination focusing on signs of chronic disease. If the clinical evaluation does not raise suspicion of a secondary cause, there is little evidence to warrant additional testing in postmenopausal women. Approximately 50% of men and 50% of pre- and perimenopausal women with osteoporosis have an associated underlying cause. If secondary osteoporosis is suspected based on findings from the history and physical examination, a workup should be performed.

Recommendations about which persons with osteoporosis should receive treatment vary. The National Osteoporosis Foundation recommends treatment of postmenopausal women and men with a personal history of hip or vertebral fracture, a T-score of -2.5 or below, low bone mass (T-score between -1 and -2.5), and a 10-year probability of hip fracture of at least 3% or 10-year probability of any major fracture of at least 20%. The 10-year probability of fracture is calculated using the WHO fracture risk assessment tool (http://osteoed.org/tools.php).

Medications Associated with Osteoporosis

Cyclosporine
Glucocorticoids
Gonadotropin-releasing hormone agonists

Heparin (prolonged treatment)
Methotrexate
Phenobarbital
Phenothiazines
Phenytoin
Tacrolimus
Thyroid hormone excess

Risk Factors for Osteoporosis

Advancing age
Alcohol abuse
Caucasian or Asian race
Chronic kidney disease
Early menopause
Family history of osteoporosis
Female gender
High caffeine intake
Impaired calcium absorption
Late menarche
Low intake of calcium, phosphorus, or vitamin D
Nulliparity
Low body weight or petite body frame
Personal history of osteoporotic fracture
Sedentary lifestyle
Tobacco use

Causes of Secondary Osteoporosis

Acromegaly
Alcoholism
Amyloidosis
Ankylosing spondylitis
Athletic amenorrhea
Anorexia nervosa
Celiac disease
Chronic liver disease
Chronic obstructive pulmonary disease
Cushing syndrome
Diabetes mellitus type I
Glycogen storage diseases
Hemochromatosis
Homocystinuria
HIV

Hyperadrenocorticism
Hyperparathyroidism (primary)
Hyperprolactinemia
Hyperthyroidism
Hypogonadism (primary and secondary)
Hypophosphatemia
Inflammatory bowel diseases
Malabsorption syndromes and gastric operations
Marfan syndrome
Multiple myeloma
Osteogenesis imperfecta
Renal insufficiency or renal failure
Rheumatoid arthritis
Systemic lupus erythematosus
Vitamin D deficiency

Suggested Work-Up for Patients with Suspected Secondary Osteoporosis

Serum creatinine	To evaluate for renal disease
Alanine aminotransferase and aspartate aminotransferase	To evaluate for liver disease
Alkaline phosphatase	To evaluate for liver disease, Paget disease, or other bone pathology
Serum calcium	Decreased level may indicate malabsorption or vitamin D deficiency. Increased level may indicate primary hyperparathyroidism or malignancy.
Complete blood count (CBC)	To evaluate for bone marrow malignancy or malabsorption
Thyroid-stimulating hormone	To evaluate for hyperthyroidism
Testosterone (males)	To evaluate for hypogonadism
25-hydroxyvitamin D	To evaluate for vitamin D deficiency

Additional Work-Up

Albumin	If malnutrition is suspected
Serum iron and ferritin	Levels are increased with hemochromatosis
Serum phosphorus	Decreased level may indicate osteomalacia

Serum protein electrophoresis (SPEP), CBC, serum calcium, parathyroid hormone (PTH)	Abnormal SPEP/elevated urine protein electrophoresis, erythrocyte sedimentation rate, anemia, hypercalcemia, and depressed PTH suggest multiple myeloma
Estrogen (females)	Decreased levels in premenopausal women suggest hypogonadism
1,25 hydroxyvitamin D	Elevated levels occur with hyperparathyroidism
24-hour urine calcium measurement	Decreased urinary calcium excretion suggests malabsorption or vitamin D deficiency
Dexamethasone suppression test	May be indicated when Cushing syndrome is suspected
Stool for fat or xylose breath test	Used when there is a history of gastrectomy or diarrhea to rule out malabsorption

Further Reading

Harper KD, Weber TJ. Secondary osteoporosis. Diagnostic considerations. *Endocrinol Metab Clin North Am.* 1998;27:325–348.

Kenny AM, Prestwood KM. Osteoporosis: pathogenesis, diagnosis, and treatment in older adults. *Rheum Dis Clin North Am.* 2000;26:569–591.

Mauck KF, Clarke BL. Diagnosis, screening, prevention, and treatment of osteoporosis. *Mayo Clin Proc.* 2006;81:662–672.

National Osteoporosis Foundation. Physician's guide to prevention and treatment of osteoporosis. (http://www.nof.org/professionals/Clinicians_Guide.htm). Accessed 27.01.16.

Simon LS. Osteoporosis. *Clin Geriatr Med.* 2005;21:603–629.

South-Paul JE. Osteoporosis: part I: evaluation and assessment. *Am Fam Physician.* 2001;63:897–904.

Sweet MG, Sweet JM, Jeremiah MP, Galazka SS. Diagnosis and treatment of osteoporosis. *Am Fam Physician.* 2009;79:193–200.

Tresolini CP, Gold DT, Lee LS, eds. *Working with Patients to Prevent, Treat and Manage Osteoporosis: A Curriculum Guide for Health Professions.* 2nd ed. San Francisco: National Fund for Medical Education; 1998.

56 PALPITATIONS

General Discussion

Palpitations are a common presenting problem in the outpatient setting and emergency department. Although usually benign, palpitations occasionally are a manifestation of potentially life-threatening conditions.

The etiology of palpitations can be divided into arrhythmias, nonarrhythmic cardiac causes, extracardiac causes, psychiatric causes, and drug or medication effects. Patient characteristics that increase the likelihood of an arrhythmic cause of palpitations include visible neck pulsations, palpitations affecting sleep, palpitations at work, known history of cardiac disease, male sex, and palpitations lasting more than 5 minutes. Patient age may be important, because supraventricular tachycardias, particularly ones that use a bypass tract, may be first experienced earlier in life.

Arrhythmias include any bradycardia and tachycardia, premature ventricular and atrial contractions, sick sinus syndrome, advanced arteriovenous block, or ventricular tachycardia. Palpitations associated with dizziness, near-syncope, or syncope suggest tachyarrhythmia and are potentially more serious. The challenge in evaluating palpitations is to capture a recording of the cardiac rhythm during symptoms.

Anxiety and panic disorders are the most common noncardiac causes of palpitations. Panic disorder is the cause of palpitations in 15% to 31% of patients. No specific cause of palpitations can be identified in 16% to 20% of patients. However, it is essential to rule out clinically significant arrhythmias before attributing palpitations to a psychiatric condition.

Patients should be asked to tap out the rhythm of their palpitations to help identify the regularity and speed of the palpitations. Single skipped beats or a sensation of the heart stopping and then starting with a pounding, jumping, or flipping sensation, especially while sitting quietly or lying in bed and lasting only for brief periods, have traditionally been attributed to premature atrial or ventricular extra systoles. An irregular heartbeat, both in rhythm and strength, that begins and terminates abruptly suggests atrial fibrillation.

Medications and Substances Associated with Palpitations

Alcohol
Amphetamines
Antiarrhythmics
- Amiodarone
- Disopyramide
- Procainamide

- Quinidine
- Sotalol

Anticholinergics
Beta agonists
Beta-blocker withdrawal
Caffeine
Cocaine
Decongestants
Digitalis
Diuretics
Fluoroquinolones
Macrolides
Nicotine
Phenothiazines
Protease inhibitors
Selective serotonin reuptake inhibitors
Theophylline
Tobacco
Tricyclic antidepressants
Vasodilators

Causes of Palpitations

Arrhythmias
- Atrial fibrillation/flutter
- Bradycardia due to advanced arteriovenous block or sinus node dysfunction
- Bradycardia-tachycardia syndrome (sick sinus syndrome)
- Long QT syndrome
- Multifocal atrial tachycardia
- Premature supraventricular contractions
- Premature ventricular contractions
- Sinus arrhythmia
- Sinus tachycardia
- Supraventricular tachycardia
- Ventricular tachycardia
- Wolff-Parkinson-White syndrome

Extracardiac causes
- Anemia
- Electrolyte imbalance
- Fever
- Food poisoning
- Hyperthyroidism

- Hypoglycemia
- Hypovolemia
- Mastocytosis
- Paget disease
- Pheochromocytoma
- Pulmonary disease
- Vasovagal syndrome

Nonarrhythmic cardiac causes

- Atrial myxoma
- Atrial or ventricular septal defect
- Cardiomyopathy
- Congenital heart disease
- Congestive heart failure
- Mitral valve prolapse
- Pacemaker-mediated tachycardia
- Pericarditis
- Valvular disease

Psychiatric causes

- Anxiety disorder
- Panic attacks
- Stress

Key Historical Features

✓ Description of the palpitations
✓ Occurrence at rest or with exercise
✓ Circumstances in which the palpitations occur
✓ Precipitating factors
✓ Associated symptoms (dizziness, near-syncope, syncope)
✓ Termination of the palpitations on their own or with maneuvers
✓ Nervousness
✓ Heat intolerance
✓ Medical history
✓ Family history of cardiac disease
✓ Medications, especially those that can prolong the QT interval

Key Physical Findings

✓ Vital signs for bradycardia, tachycardia, or blood pressure derangements
✓ Neck examination for thyroid abnormalities
✓ Cardiovascular examination for murmurs, extra sounds, or cardiac enlargement

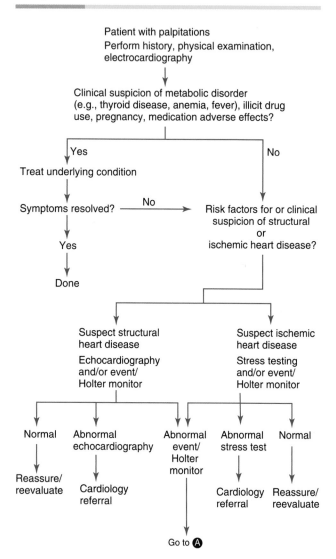

Figure 56-1. Algorithm for the evaluation and management of palpitations. (From Wexler RK, Pleister A, Raman S. Outpatient approach to palpitations. *American Family Physician* 2011;84:63–69; Figure 2.)

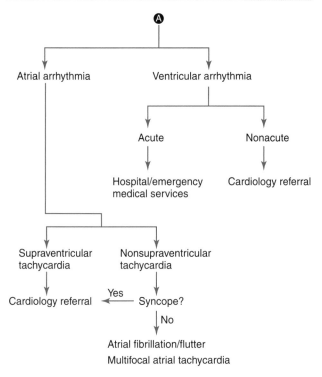

Figure 56-1—Cont'd

Suggested Work-Up

Electrocardiogram   Appropriate in all patients who complain
                                 of palpitations, to evaluate for arrhythmia,
                                 ventricular hypertrophy, previous
                                 myocardial infarction, atrioventricular
                                 block, short PR interval, delta waves (Wolff-
                                 Parkinson-White syndrome), or prolonged
                                 QT interval

Additional Work-Up

Further diagnostic testing is generally indicated for three groups of patients:
(1) those in whom the initial evaluation suggests an arrhythmic cause; (2) those
who are at high risk (those with organic heart disease or any myocardial

abnormality that can lead to serious arrhythmias) for an arrhythmia; and (3) those who remain anxious to have a specific explanation for their symptoms.

Complete blood count	If anemia or infection is suspected
Electrolytes	If arrhythmia secondary to electrolyte disturbance is suspected
Thyroid-stimulating hormone	If hyperthyroidism or hypothyroidism is suspected
Urine drug screen	If illicit drug use is suspected
Treadmill stress testing	Appropriate for patients who have palpitations with physical exertion or patients with suspected coronary artery disease or myocardial ischemia
Echocardiography	If structural abnormalities or abnormal ventricular function is suspected
Ambulatory cardiac monitoring (Holter or intermittent event recorder)	Allow for prolonged monitoring, typically 24 to 48 hours for Holter monitoring and weeks to months for intermittent event recorders
Implantable loop recorder	May be considered when palpitations occur infrequently or are associated with serious events, such as syncope, that cannot be identified using intermittent event recorders
Electrophysiology study	May be warranted in patients with palpitations preceded by syncope or near-syncope, and in those in whom there is a high index of suspicion of a cardiac origin not diagnosed with other studies

Further Reading

Abbott AV. Diagnostic approach to palpitations. *Am Fam Physician*. 2005;71:743–750.

Barsky AJ, Cleary PD, Coeytaux RR, Ruskin JN. Psychiatric disorders in medical outpatients complaining of palpitations. *J Gen Intern Med*. 1994;9:306–313.

Thavendiranathan P, Bagai A, Khoo C, et al. Does this patient with palpitations have a cardiac arrhythmia? *JAMA*. 2009;302:2135–2143.

Weber BE, Kapoor WN. Evaluation and outcomes of patients with palpitations. *Am J Med*. 1996;100:138–148.

Wexler RK, Pleister A, Raman S. Outpatient approach to palpitations. *Am Fam Physician*. 2011;84:63–69.

Zimetbaum P, Josephson ME. Evaluation of patients with palpitations. *N Engl J Med*. 1998;338:1369–1373.

General Discussion

Peripheral neuropathy represents one of the most common neurologic disorders encountered by primary care physicians. The term *peripheral neuropathy* is usually used to describe symmetric and universal damage to adjacent nerves. The damage and clinical manifestations usually are located distally with a proximal progression. Peripheral neuropathy may be the result of hereditary, toxic, infectious, inflammatory, metabolic, ischemic, or paraneoplastic causes. Diabetes and alcoholism are the most common etiologies of peripheral neuropathy in adults living in developed countries. It is important to differentiate a true neuropathy from other disorders that can have a similar clinical presentation (Figure 57-1). Despite extensive evaluation, an etiology is not found in 13% to 22% of cases.

The first step in the evaluation is to determine whether the symptoms are the result of a peripheral neuropathy or a lesion in the central nervous system, as well as whether a single nerve root, multiple nerve roots, or a peripheral nerve plexus is involved. Central nervous system lesions may be associated with additional features, such as diplopia, cranial nerve involvement, speech difficulty, or ataxia. Deep tendon reflexes are usually brisk, and muscle tone is spastic. Lesions of the peripheral nerve roots typically are asymmetric, follow a dermatomal pattern of sensory symptoms, and may be associated with neck or low back pain. Lesions of a peripheral nerve plexus are asymmetric with sensorimotor involvement of multiple nerves in one extremity.

Most patients can be diagnosed, classified, and managed based on the history and physical examination. Classifying the patient's neuropathy clinically based upon time course (acute, subacute, chronic, or lifelong), functional modalities affected (motor or sensory), and the distribution (distal, proximal, or patchy) can assist in diagnosis. Other important information includes medication use, medical history, age of onset, and family history.

Medications Associated with Neuropathy

Alfa interferon
Amiodarone
Amitriptyline
Chloramphenicol
Chloroquine
Cimetidine
Cisplatin
Colchicine
Dapsone
Didanosine

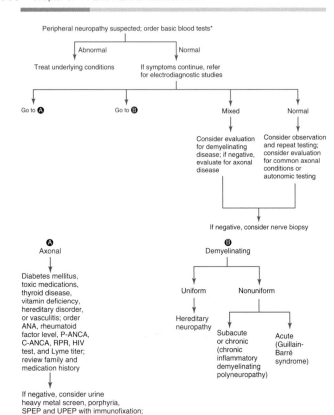

Figure 57-1 Diagnosis of suspected peripheral neuropathy. (From Azhary H, Farooq MU, Bhanushali M, Majid A, Kassab MY. Peripheral neuropathy: differential diagnosis and management. *American Family Physician* 2010;81:887–892; Figure 1.)

Dideoxycytidine
Dideoxyinosine
Digoxin
Disulfiram
Docetaxel
Ethambutol
Gold

Hydralazine
Isoniazid
Lithium
Metronidazole
Nitrofurantoin
Nitrous oxide
Paclitaxel
Phenytoin
Procainamide
Pyridoxine (vitamin B_6) excess
Statins
Suramin
Thalidomide
Vincristine

Causes of Peripheral Neuropathy

Acute pandysautonomia
Alcoholism
Amyloidosis
Carcinomatous axonal sensorimotor polyneuropathy
Charcot-Marie-Tooth disease
Chronic gluten enteropathy
Chronic inflammatory demyelinating polyradiculopathy
Chronic liver disease
Crohn disease
Churg-Strauss vasculitis
Compressive neuropathies
Critical illness neuropathy
Cryoglobulinemia
Diabetes mellitus
Diphtheria toxin
End-stage renal disease
Entrapment
- Acromegaly
- Amyloidosis
- Myxedema
- Rheumatoid arthritis

Folate deficiency
Friedreich ataxia
Gastric restriction surgery for obesity
Gouty neuropathy
Guillain-Barré syndrome
Hereditary motor sensory neuropathy
Heroin
HIV/AIDS

Hypophosphatemia
Hypothyroidism
Idiopathic sensory neuronopathy
Ischemic lesions
Leprosy
Lyme disease
Lymphoma
Lymphomatous axonal sensorimotor polyneuropathy
Metachromatic leukodystrophy
Metal neuropathy
- Acute arsenic polyneuropathy
- Chronic arsenic intoxication
- Lead neuropathy
- Mercury
- Gold
- Thallium

Monoclonal gammopathy
Monoclonal gammopathy of undetermined significance
Multiple myeloma
Neoplastic infiltration or compression
Organophosphates
Osteosclerotic myeloma
Paraneoplastic neuropathy
Paraproteinemias
Plasmacytoma
Polyarteritis nodosa
Porphyria
Postgastrectomy syndrome
Primary biliary cirrhosis
Refsum disease
Rheumatoid arthritis
Sarcoidosis
Sjögren syndrome
Styrene-induced peripheral neuropathy
Syphilis
Systemic lupus erythematosus
Tetanus
Thiamine deficiency
Tic paralysis
Toxic neuropathy
- Acrylamide
- Carbon disulfide
- Carbon monoxide
- Dichlorophenoxyacetic acid
- Ethylene oxide

- • Glue sniffing
- • Hexacarbons
- • Organophosphorus esters

Trauma
Vasculitis
Vitamin B_6 deficiency
Vitamin B_{12} deficiency
Vitamin E deficiency
Waldenström macroglobulinemia
Whipple disease

Suggested Work-Up

Fasting serum glucose and glycosylated hemoglobin	To evaluate for diabetes mellitus
Alanine aminotransferase and aspartate aminotransferase	To evaluate for occult alcoholism
Comprehensive metabolic panel	To evaluate for metabolic derangement or renal disease
Complete blood count	To evaluate for evidence of infection
Erythrocyte sedimentation rate, antinuclear antibody (ANA), rheumatoid factor	To evaluate for inflammatory and rheumatologic disorders
Urinalysis	To evaluate renal function
Vitamin B_{12} level	To evaluate for pernicious anemia
Thyroid-stimulating hormone level	To evaluate for thyroid abnormalities
Electromyography (EMG) and nerve conduction studies (NCS)	Indicated if the diagnosis remains unclear after initial diagnostic testing. Used to confirm the presence of a neuropathy and provide information regarding the types of fibers involved, the pathophysiology, and a symmetric versus asymmetric or multifocal pattern.

Neurologic consultation should be obtained early for any acute progressive neuropathy. EMG and/or NCS, electrocardiogram, lumbar puncture, chest radiograph, and pulmonary function tests are often performed in patients with acute progressive neuropathy.

Additional Selected Work-Up

Serum and urine protein electrophoresis	To evaluate for paraproteinemic and/or demyelinating neuropathies or multiple myeloma
HIV antibodies	If HIV infection is suspected
Cerebrospinal fluid analysis	Useful in the evaluation of myelinopathies and polyradiculopathies
Angiotensin-converting enzyme level	If sarcoidosis is suspected
Cryoglobulins	If cryoglobulinemia is suspected
Lyme polymerase chain reaction	If Lyme disease is suspected
Rapid plasma reagin (RPR); venereal disease research laboratory (VDRL)	If syphilis is suspected
Urinalysis, including 24-hour collection	If heavy metal toxicity or porphyria is suspected
Antinuclear antibody (ANA); perinuclear anti-neutrophil cytoplasmic antibody (P-ANCA); cytoplasmic anti-nuclear cytoplasmic antibody (C-ANCA)	If vasculitis is suspected
Cytology	If lymphoma is suspected
Nerve biopsy	Used in specific cases to diagnose vasculitis, leprosy, amyloid neuropathy, leukodystrophies, and sarcoidosis
Paraneoplastic panel	If underlying malignancy is suspected
Antisulfatide antibodies	If autoimmune polyneuropathy is suspected
Genetic testing	If hereditary neuropathy is suspected
Salivary flow rate, Shirmer test, rose bengal test	If Sjögren syndrome is suspected

Further Reading

Azhary H, Farooq MU, Bhanushali M, Majid A, Kassab MY. Peripheral neuropathy: differential diagnosis and management. *Am Fam Physician.* 2010;81:887–892.

Chalk CH. Acquired neuromuscular diseases; acquired peripheral neuropathy. *Neurol Clin.* 1997;15:501–528.

Dyck PJ, Oviatt KF, Lambert EH. Intensive evaluation of referred unclassified neuropathies yields improved diagnosis. *Ann Neurol.* 1981;10:222–226.

Griffin JW, Hsieh ST, McArthur JC, Cornblath DR. Diagnostic testing in neurology: laboratory testing in peripheral nerve disease. *Neurol Clin.* 1996;14:119–133.

McLeod JG, Tuck RR, Pollard JD, Cameron J, Walsh JC. Chronic polyneuropathy of undetermined cause. *J Neurol Neurosurg Psychiatry.* 1984;47:530–535.

Poncelet AN. An algorithm for the evaluation of peripheral neuropathy. *Am Fam Physician.* 1998;57:755–764.

Sabin TD, Swift TR, Jacobson RR. Leprosy. In: Dyck PJ, Thomas PK, eds. *Peripheral Neuropathy.* Philadelphia: Saunders; 1993:1354–1379.

General Discussion

Pituitary adenomas present clinically in three ways: (1) syndromes of hormone hypersecretion or deficiency; (2) neurologic manifestations from a mass effect of an expanding gland; or (3) an incidental finding on an imaging study performed for an unrelated indication.

Many of the so-called pituitary incidentalomas are associated with partial hypopituitarism, and some are associated with compression of the optic chiasm; therefore, further workup of these asymptomatic tumors is indicated.

Pituitary adenomas are categorized based on the type of hormone secreted, primary cell type, and size. Tumors that secrete hormones are called functioning adenomas, whereas those that do not secrete hormones are called nonfunctioning adenomas. Prolactinomas are the most common cell type (40%–57% of all adenomas), followed by nonfunctioning adenomas (28%–37%), growth hormone–secreting adenomas (11%–13%), and adrenocorticotropic hormone (ACTH)–secreting adenomas (1%–2%). If the tumor is 10 mm or larger, it is considered a macroadenoma; a tumor less than 10 mm is considered a microadenoma.

The most common syndromes of hormone hypersecretion are hyperprolactinemia, acromegaly, and Cushing disease. Partial or complete hypopituitarism (most often hypogonadism) may develop as a result of interference with normal hormone secretion. This occurs either from direct compression of the pituitary gland or inhibition of the pulsatile secretion of luteinizing hormone (LH). The goals of investigation are to identify a known or suspected pituitary adenoma and assess pituitary function to identify hormonal excess or deficiency with a basic endocrinological workup as outlined in the following.

The clinical presentation of pituitary lesions often depends on the patient's sex. Prolactinomas tend to be diagnosed later in men than women, partly because men delay seeking professional help for reduced libido or erectile dysfunction. Women of childbearing age with hyperprolactinemia develop menstrual irregularities or infertility, often prompting medical evaluation earlier. The most common neurologic symptoms in patients with pituitary adenomas are headaches and visual changes. Neurologic symptoms are more common in nonfunctioning adenomas or gonadotroph (LH and/or follicle-stimulating hormone [FSH]–secreting) adenomas.

Key Historical Features

✓ Fatigue
✓ Menstrual changes
✓ Decreased libido
✓ Erectile dysfunction

✓ Galactorrhea
✓ Hirsutism
✓ Headache
✓ Visual problems
✓ Muscle weakness
✓ Depression
✓ Weight gain
✓ Medical history, especially osteoporosis, seizures, diabetes, or cardiac disease

Key Physical Findings

✓ Vital signs for hypertension
✓ General examination for suggestions of acromegaly (change in facial features, large mandible)
✓ Thyroid examination for goiter
✓ Cardiac examination for evidence of cardiomyopathy
✓ Neurologic examination for cranial nerve defects
✓ Skin examination for acne, thin skin, striae, and bruising
✓ Genitourinary examination for testicular atrophy

Suggested Work-Up

Serum prolactin	To evaluate for prolactin excess
Early morning (9 am) basal insulin-like growth factor I level	To evaluate for growth hormone excess
LH and FSH	To evaluate for gonadotropin-secreting tumor (levels elevated) or hypogonadism (levels decreased)
Thyroid-stimulating hormone (TSH) and free T_4	To evaluate thyroid function. Low T_4 with normal or low TSH indicates secondary hypothyroidism.
24-hour urine free cortisol or late night salivary cortisol or low-dose dexamethasone suppression test	To evaluate for cortisol excess
Testosterone (men)	To evaluate for hormone deficiency in men
Estradiol (women)	To evaluate for hormone deficiency in females. Not accurate in women taking oral contraceptives or on hormone therapy.

| Magnetic resonance imaging of the pituitary sella with and without gadolinium enhancement symptoms | To establish the presence and size of pituitary adenoma and to rule out other causes of symptoms |
| Formal assessment of visual acuity and visual field | Should be undertaken at time of diagnosis of pituitary adenoma |

Additional Work-Up

Serum cortisol	If cortisol deficiency is suspected
ACTH	To evaluate for cortisol excess. Elevated with pituitary or ectopic source of excess cortisol.
Oral glucose suppression	To confirm growth hormone excess
Serum α-subunit	Useful if LH/FSH levels are elevated, but the etiology of the elevation is unknown. May be produced in some pituitary adenomas.

Further Reading

Freda PU, Beckers AM, Katznelson L, et al. Endocrine Society. Pituitary incidentaloma: an Endocrine Society clinical practice guideline. *J Clin Endocrinol Metab*. 2008;93:1526–1540.

Lake MG, Krook LS, Cruz SV. Pituitary adenomas: an overview. *Am Fam Physician*. 2013;88:319–327.

Rogers A, Karavitaki N, Wass JAH. Diagnosis and management of prolactinomas and non-functioning pituitary adenomas. *BMJ*. 2014;349:G5390.

Sivakumar W, Chamoun R, Nguyen V, Couldwell WT. Incidental pituitary adenomas. *Neurosurg Focus*. 2011;31:E18.

59 PLEURAL EFFUSION

General Discussion

Patients with pleural effusion can be asymptomatic or may present with dyspnea, cough, or pleuritic chest pain. When pleural effusion is suspected, chest radiography should be performed to confirm the diagnosis. Lateral decubitus films may be considered to help determine the size of the effusion and whether it is free-flowing or loculated. Computed tomography or ultrasound may be useful if chest radiography is inconclusive.

Potential mechanisms of pleural fluid accumulation include increased interstitial fluid in the lungs, secondary to increased pulmonary capillary pressure or permeability, decreased intrapleural pressure, decreased plasma oncotic pressure, increased pleural membrane permeability, obstructed lymphatic flow, diaphragmatic defects, and thoracic duct rupture. The most common causes in adults are heart failure, malignancy, pneumonia, tuberculosis, and pulmonary embolism. Heart failure is the most common cause of bilateral pleural effusion. However, if cardiomegaly is not seen with bilateral pleural effusion, other causes such as malignancy should be pursued.

The first step in identifying the underlying cause of a pleural effusion is determining whether the effusion is exudative or transudative. Thoracentesis should be performed in all patients with more than a minimal pleural effusion, unless heart failure is the clear diagnosis. If heart failure is present, thoracentesis may be indicated if atypical circumstances are present, such as fever, pleuritic chest pain, unilateral effusion, effusions of markedly disparate size, or absence of cardiomegaly, or if the effusion does not respond to treatment for heart failure.

Exudative effusions can be differentiated from transudative effusions using Light's criteria. Light's criteria are nearly 100% sensitive for diagnosing exudative effusion. An effusion is an exudate if one or more of the following criteria are present:

- Pleural fluid lactate dehydrogenase (LDH) is more than two-thirds the upper limit of normal for serum LDH;
- The pleural fluid-to-serum LDH ratio is more than 0.6; and
- The pleural fluid-to-serum protein ratio is more than 0.5.

A patient with heart failure who has received diuretics may fulfill criteria for an exudative effusion. In this case, if the difference between protein levels in the serum and the pleural fluid is greater than 3.1 g/dL, the patient actually has a transudative effusion.

Additional tests used to identify an exudative pleural effusion include the following:

- Pleural fluid-serum albumin gradient more than 1.2 g/dL;
- Pleural fluid-to-serum cholesterol ratio of more than 0.3;
- Pleural cholesterol level more than 55 mg/dL; and
- Pleural LDH more than 200 U/L.

Any drug should be considered as a potential cause for an undiagnosed exudative effusion before pursuing an extensive diagnostic evaluation. The presentation of drug-induced pleural disease may vary from an asymptomatic pleural effusion to acute pleuritis to symptomatic pleural thickening. Pleural disease due to medications may occur as a result of hypersensitivity or allergic reaction, direct toxic effect, increased oxygen free radical production, suppression of antioxidant defenses, or chemical-induced inflammation. Pleural fluid eosinophilia, defined as more than 10% of nucleated cells, may provide evidence for the presence of drug-induced pleural disease. However, the presence or absence of eosinophilia in the pleural fluid is a nonspecific finding. Other causes of pleural fluid eosinophilia include pneumothorax, fungal disease, parasitic infection, hemothorax, Hodgkin lymphoma, benign asbestos pleural effusion, and pulmonary emboli with pulmonary infarction.

Medications Associated with Pleural Effusion

Absolute alcohol
Acyclovir
Amiodarone
Beta blockers
Bleomycin
Bromocriptine
Clozapine
Cyclophosphamide
Dantrolene
Hihydroergotamine
Docetaxel
D-penicillamine
Ergotamine
Gliclazide
Granulocyte colony-stimulating factor
Interleukin-2
Intravenous immunoglobulin
Isotretinoin
Itraconazole
L-tryptophan
Mesalamine
Methotrexate
Methysergide
Minoxidil
Mitomycin
Nitrofurantoin
Oxyprenolol
Phenytoin
Practolol

Procarbazine
Propylthiouracil
Simvastatin
Sodium morrhuate
Troglitazone
Valproic acid

Causes of Pleural Effusion

Abdominal abscess
Atelectasis
Benign asbestos pleural effusion
Chylothorax
Cirrhosis
Dressler syndrome
Duropleural fistula
Empyema
Endometriosis
Esophageal perforation
Heart failure
Hemothorax
Hepatic hydrothorax
Hypoalbuminemia
Kaposi sarcoma
Lupus pleuritis
Lymphoma
Malignancy
Medications
Meigs syndrome
Mesothelioma
Nephrotic syndrome
Ovarian cancer
Ovarian hyperstimulation syndrome
Pancreatitis
Pericarditis
Pleural infection
Pleural malignancy
Pneumonia (bacterial or viral)
Postoperative pleural effusion (especially after coronary artery bypass graft
    surgery; also can occur after abdominal surgery)
Postpartum pleural effusion
Pseudochylothorax
Pulmonary embolism
Pulmonary vein stenosis

Rheumatoid arthritis/pleuritis
Subphrenic abscess
Superior vena cava obstruction
Trapped lung
Tuberculosis
Uremia
Urinothorax
Viral disease
Yellow nail syndrome

Key Historical Features

- ✓ Cough
- ✓ Dyspnea, orthopnea
- ✓ Pleuritic chest pain
- ✓ Fever
- ✓ Weight loss
- ✓ Hemoptysis
- ✓ Medical history
- ✓ Surgical history
- ✓ Medications
- ✓ Family history
- ✓ Social history

Key Physical Findings

- ✓ Vital signs
- ✓ General appearance
- ✓ Cardiac examination for evidence of heart failure
- ✓ Pulmonary examination for dullness to percussion, decreased or absent tactile fremitus, or decreased breath sounds
- ✓ Abdominal examination for hepatosplenomegaly, ascites, or masses
- ✓ Pelvic examination if ovarian malignancy is a potential diagnosis

Suggested Work-Up

Chest x-ray	To confirm the presence of a pleural effusion
Thoracentesis with pleural fluid sent for cell count and differential, gram stain, culture, cytology, pH, glucose, LDH, and protein	Routine tests on pleural fluid
Serum LDH and protein	Used to derive pleural fluid-to-serum ratios (Light's criteria)

Additional Work-Up

Ultrasound or computed tomography (CT)	If doubt exists about the pleural effusion, to detect small effusions, and to differentiate pleural fluid from pleural thickening. CT may be used in a patient suspected of having pulmonary embolism.
Polymerase chain reaction or culture for *Mycobacterium tuberculosis*	If tuberculosis is suspected
Brain natriuretic peptide	If heart failure is suspected
Liver transaminase levels	If cirrhosis is suspected
Thyroid-stimulating hormone level	If hypothyroidism is suspected
Urine protein level	If nephrotic syndrome is suspected
Pleural fluid amylase	If esophageal rupture or pancreatic disease is suspected
Pleural fluid adenosine deaminase	If tuberculosis is suspected
Pleural fluid cholesterol	If chylothorax or pseudochylothorax is suspected. May also be used to differentiate exudate from transudate.
Hematocrit fluid-to-blood ratio	If pleural fluid is bloody, to evaluate for hemothorax
Bronchoscopy	Useful when an endobronchial malignancy is suspected
Pleural biopsy	Useful when an exudative effusion remains undiagnosed or when tuberculosis or malignancy is suspected
Thoracoscopy	Useful in cytology-negative pleural effusion when pleural malignancy is suspected

Further Reading

Burgess L, Maritz FJ, Taljaard JF. Comparative analysis of the biochemical parameters used to distinguish between pleural transudates and exudates. *Chest.* 1995;107:1604–1609.

Heffner JE. Evaluating diagnostic tests in the pleural space: differentiating transudates from exudates as a model. *Clin Chest Med.* 1998;19:277–293.

Huggins JT, Sahn SA. Drug-induced pleural disease. *Clin Chest Med.* 2004;25:141–153.

Light RW. Pleural effusion. *N Engl J Med.* 2002;346:1971–1976.

Morelock SY, Sahn SA. Drugs and the pleura. *Chest.* 1999;116:212–221.

Porcel JM, Light RW. Diagnostic approach to pleural effusion in adults. *Am Fam Physician.* 2006;73:1211–1220.

Saguil A, Wyrick K, Hallgren J. Diagnostic approach to pleural effusion. *Am Fam Physician.* 2014;90:99–104.

General Discussion

The effective preoperative evaluation seeks to perform several tasks that include: (1) decreasing surgical morbidity; (2) minimizing expensive delays and cancellations on the day of surgery; (3) evaluating and optimizing patient health status; (4) facilitating the planning of anesthesia and perioperative care; and (5) reducing patient anxiety through education. The complete consultation should include recommendations for evaluation and treatment, including prophylactic therapies to minimize the perioperative risk.

Surgical complications occur frequently and generally include cardiac, respiratory, and infectious complications. The overall risk for surgical complications depends on individual factors and the type of surgical procedure being considered. Diseases associated with an increased risk for surgical complications include respiratory disease, cardiac disease, diabetes mellitus, and malnutrition. Cardiac complications are the most common cause of morbidity and mortality in the surgical patient.

Ideally, the patient should be evaluated several weeks before the planned surgical procedure. Emergency surgery requires expedited preoperative cardiac assessment and management. Patients undergoing elective or semi-elective procedures can proceed with preoperative cardiac testing, if indicated.

The patient's medical history usually is the most important component of the preoperative evaluation. The value of routine medical testing before elective surgery is unclear, because most abnormalities in laboratory values can be predicted from the patient's history and findings on the physical examination. Current recommendations call for fewer routine tests and instead recommend selective ordering of laboratory tests based on the specific indication in a given patient.

Aspirin and nonsteroidal anti-inflammatory drugs (NSAIDs) should be discontinued 1 week before surgery to minimize the risk of excessive bleeding. If the patient smokes, the patient should quit smoking at least 8 weeks before surgery to minimize the surgical risks associated with smoking.

Cardiac Assessment

Patients with active cardiovascular signs or symptoms should undergo electrocardiography (ECG). The decision to perform ECG in asymptomatic patients depends on whether the planned surgery is low, intermediate, or high risk (Table 60-1). ECG is not needed in patients undergoing low-risk procedures. ECG is recommended before intermediate-risk procedures in patients with at least one clinical risk factor identified by the Revised Cardiac Risk Index. Those with two or more clinical risk factors are at significantly higher risk of a major cardiac event. Patients should have preoperative ECG before undergoing a high-risk procedure.

Risk of Procedure	Examples
High (>5%)	Aortic and major vascular surgery, peripheral vascular surgery
Intermediate (1%–5%)	Intraperitoneal or intrathoracic surgery, carotid endarterectomy, head and neck surgery, orthopedic surgery, prostate surgery
Low (<1%)	Ambulatory surgery, breast surgery, endoscopic procedures, superficial procedures, cataract surgery

(From Fleisher LA, Beckman JA, Brown KA, et al.; American College of Cardiology; American Heart Association Task Force on Practice Guidelines (Writing Committee to Revise the 2002 Guidelines on Perioperative Cardiovascular Evaluation for Noncardiac Surgery); American Society of Echocardiography; American Society of Nuclear Cardiology; Heart Rhythm Society; Society of Cardiovascular Anesthesiologists; Society for Cardiovascular Angiography and Interventions; Society for Vascular Medicine and Biology; Society for Vascular Surgery. ACC/AHA 2007 guidelines on perioperative cardiovascular evaluation and care for noncardiac surgery. *J Am Coll Cardiol* 2007;50:e170 [published corrections appear in *J Am Coll Cardiol* 2007;50:e242 and *J Am Coll Cardiol*. 2008;52:793–794]).

Table 60-1 Risk of Cardiac Death and Nonfatal Myocardial Infarction for Noncardiac Surgical Procedures

Risk Factor	Points
Cerebrovascular disease	1
Congestive heart failure	1
Creatinine level >2.0 mg/dL (176.80 μmol/L)	1
Diabetes mellitus requiring insulin	1
Ischemic cardiac disease	1
Suprainguinal vascular surgery, intrathoracic surgery, or intra-abdominal surgery	1
Total points:	

Risk of Major Cardiac Event	
Points	Risk (%) (95% confidence interval)
0	0.4 (0.05–1.5)
1	0.9 (0.3–2.1)
2	6.6 (3.9–10.3)
≥3	≥11 (5.8–18.4)

(From American Heart Association. ACC/AHA Guideline Update for Perioperative Cardiovascular Evaluation for Noncardiac Surgery—Executive Summary A Report of the American College of Cardiology/American Heart Association Task Force on Practice Guidelines (Committee to Update the 1996 Guidelines on Perioperative Cardiovascular Evaluation for Noncardiac Surgery). *Circulation* 2002;105:1257–1267.)

Table 60-2 Revised Cardiac Risk Index

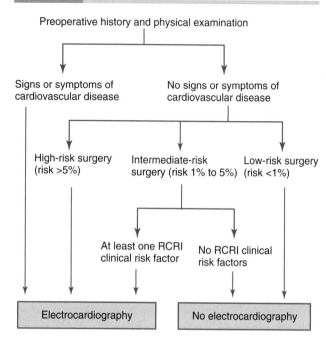

Figure 60-1 Determining the need for preoperative electrocardiography.
RCRI, Revised Cardiac Risk Index.
(From Feely MA, Collins CS, Daniels PR, Kebede EB, Jatoi A, Mauck KF. Preoperative testing before noncardiac surgery: guidelines and recommendations. *American Family Physician* 2013;87:414–418.)

Chest Radiography

Guidelines concur that routine preoperative chest radiography in asymptomatic, otherwise healthy patients is not indicated. However, if a patient has new or unstable cardiopulmonary signs or symptoms on examination, chest radiography is clearly indicated, regardless of the procedure. Risk factors for perioperative pulmonary complications include chronic obstructive pulmonary disease, age older than 60 years, American Society of Anesthesiologists score of 2 or greater, function dependence, hypoalbuminemia, congestive heart failure, emergency procedure, prolonged procedures, and certain surgical sites (e.g., head, neck, upper abdomen). Chest radiography may be considered for these patients if the results will alter perioperative management.

Routine Laboratory Tests

No guidelines recommend indiscriminate preoperative complete blood count (CBC) or hemoglobin testing. Testing is recommended for select patients who have conditions that increase the pretest probability of diagnosing anemia. These include chronic kidney disease, chronic liver disease, chronic inflammatory conditions, and clinical signs or symptoms of anemia. Testing is also recommended for procedures in which significant blood loss is anticipated.

Indiscriminate preoperative coagulation testing with prothrombin time, activated partial thromboplastin time, and platelet count is not warranted. Coagulation testing should be reserved for patients with medical conditions associated with impaired hemostasis (e.g., liver disease, diseases of hematopoiesis), patients taking anticoagulants, and those in whom an underlying coagulation disorder is suspected on the basis of history and physical examination findings.

Routine urinalysis is not recommended in asymptomatic patients, except in those undergoing invasive urologic procedures or surgical implantation of foreign material, such as a heart valve or a prosthetic joint.

The decision to perform preoperative electrolyte and creatinine testing should be made on the basis of compelling historical findings, such as hypertension, heart failure, chronic kidney disease, complicated diabetes, or liver disease. Likewise, testing may be appropriate for patients taking certain medications, such as diuretics, angiotensin-converting enzyme inhibitors, angiotensin receptor blockers, digoxin, or NSAIDs.

There is no clear consensus on preoperative glucose testing, and guidelines reflect the opinion that preoperative glucose assessment should be undertaken when the results could alter perioperative management. Guidelines suggest that preoperative random glucose measurement could be considered in patients at high risk of undiagnosed diabetes on the basis of history, examination, or use of certain medications (e.g., glucocorticoids) and in patients with signs or symptoms of undiagnosed diabetes.

Key Historical Features

✓ Surgical procedure being considered
✓ Medical history, especially heart and lung disease
  • Coronary artery disease
  • Previous cardiovascular procedural interventions or testing
  • Symptoms suggestive of angina or congestive heart failure
✓ Surgical history
✓ Anesthetic history
✓ Medications, including over-the-counter medications and herbal supplements
✓ Recent use of anticoagulants, aspirin, or NSAIDs
✓ Allergies to medications

- ✓ Smoking history
- ✓ Alcohol or drug use
- ✓ Complete review of systems, especially cough, dyspnea, and chest pain
- ✓ Functional status
- ✓ Self-reported exercise tolerance
- ✓ Risk factors for malnutrition, such as social isolation, limited financial resources, poor dentition, and weight loss

Key Physical Findings

- ✓ Vital signs
- ✓ Cardiac examination for evidence of heart murmurs, signs of congestive heart failure, or cardiovascular disease
- ✓ Pulmonary examination for evidence of pulmonary disease
- ✓ Evidence of malnutrition

Suggested Work-Up

Please see the preceding discussion and Figure 60-2.

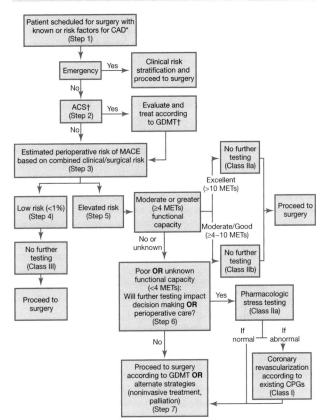

*See Sections 2.2, 2.4, and 2.5 in the full-text clinical practice guidelines (CPGs) for recommendations for patients with symptomatic HF, VHD, or arrhythmias.
†See UA/NSTEMI and STEMI CPGs (Table 2).
ACS, acute coronary syndrome; MACE, major adverse cardiovascular event; METs, metabolic equivalents.

Figure 60-2 Stepwise approach to perioperative cardiac assessment for coronary artery disease (CAD).
(From ACC/AHA Guideline Update for Perioperative Cardiovascular Evaluation for Noncardiac Surgery—Executive Summary A Report of the American College of Cardiology/American Heart Association Task Force on Practice Guidelines (Committee to Update the 1996 Guidelines on Perioperative Cardiovascular Evaluation for Noncardiac Surgery). *Circulation* 2002;105:1257–1267.)

Further Reading

American Society of Anesthesiologists Task Force on Preanesthesia Evaluation. Practice advisory for preanesthesia evaluation. *Anesthesiology.* 2002;96:485–496.

Chee YL, Crawford JC, Watson HG, Greaves M. British Committee for Standards in Haematology. Guidelines on the assessment of bleeding risk prior to surgery or invasive procedures. *Br J Haematol.* 2008;140:496–504.

Feely MA, Collins CS, Daniels PR, Kebede EB, Jatoi A, Mauck KF. Preoperative testing before noncardiac surgery: guidelines and recommendations. *Am Fam Physician.* 2013;87:414–418.

Fischer SP. Cost-effective preoperative evaluation and testing. *Chest.* 1999;115:96–100.

Fleisher LA, Fleischmann KE, Auerbach AD, et al. 2014 ACC/AHA guideline on perioperative cardiovascular evaluation and management of patients undergoing noncardiac surgery: a report of the American College of Cardiology/American Heart Association Task Force on Practice Guidelines. *J Am Coll Cardiol.* 2014;64:e77–e137.

Institute for Clinical Systems Improvement. *Health Care Guideline: Preoperative Evaluation.* 10th ed. Bloomington, MN: Institute for Clinical Systems Improvement; 2012.

King MS. Preoperative evaluation. *Am Fam Physician.* 2000;62:387–396.

Lee TH, Marcantonio ER, Mangione CM, et al. Derivation and prospective validation of a simple index for prediction of cardiac risk of major noncardiac surgery. *Circulation.* 1999;100:1043–1049.

Michota FA, Frost SD. Perioperative management of the hospitalized patient. *Med Clin North Am.* 2002;86:731–748.

National Institute for Clinical Excellence. *Preoperative Tests: The Use of Routine Preoperative Tests for Elective Surgery.* Available at: http://www.nice.org.uk/nicemedia/pdf/ CG3NICEguideline.pdf. Accessed 13.01.15.

Qaseem A, Snow V, Fitterman N, et al. Clinical Efficacy Assessment Subcommittee of the American College of Physicians. Risk assessment for and strategies to reduce perioperative pulmonary complications for patients undergoing noncardiothoracic surgery. *Ann Intern Med.* 2006;144:575–580.

General Discussion

Proteinuria is a frequent finding on dipstick testing of urine specimens; however, less than 2% of these represent serious and treatable urinary tract disorders. Proteinuria is defined as urinary protein excretion of more than 150 mg/day and can be classified pathophysiologically as glomerular, tubular, or overflow.

Causes of false-positive results include prolonged immersion of the dipstick, highly concentrated urine, alkaline urine, gross hematuria, the use of penicillin, sulfonamides, or tolbutamide, or the presence of semen, vaginal secretions, or pus.

If proteinuria is found on a dipstick urinalysis, the urinary sediment should be examined microscopically. Findings on the microscopic urinalysis are outlined in the following. If the dipstick urinalysis shows trace to 2+ protein, and the results of the microscopic urinalysis are inconclusive, the dipstick test should be repeated on a morning specimen at least twice during the next month. If a subsequent dipstick test is negative, the patient has transient proteinuria, which is associated with high fevers, vigorous exercise, and congestive heart failure. Transient proteinuria does not require follow-up.

If the dipstick urinalysis shows persistent proteinuria or if proteinuria of 3+ or 4+ is found, the evaluation should proceed to a quantitative evaluation of a specimen. Quantitative measurement of protein excretion can be performed with either a spot urine protein-to-creatinine ratio in a random urine specimen or a 24-hour urine specimen.

Individuals aged younger than 30 years who excrete less than 2 g of protein per day and who have a normal creatinine clearance should be tested for orthostatic (postural) proteinuria. This is a benign condition associated with prolonged standing that is confirmed with a negative urinalysis result after 8 hours of recumbency.

The diagnosis of isolated proteinuria can be made in a patient who has proteinuria of less than 2 g/day with normal renal function, no evidence of systemic disease that affects renal function, a normal urine sediment, and normal blood pressure. These patients should be observed with blood pressure measurement, urinalysis, and creatinine clearance every 6 months.

An adult with proteinuria greater than 2 g per 24 hours or with proteinuria and decreased creatinine clearance requires aggressive workup in consultation with a nephrologist. If the creatinine clearance is normal and the patient has a medical diagnosis such as congestive heart failure or diabetes mellitus, the underlying disease can be treated with close monitoring of the proteinuria and renal function. Consultation with a nephrologist should be considered if the renal function or amount of proteinuria changes.

Causes of Proteinuria

Overflow proteinuria
- Amyloidosis
- Hemoglobinuria
- Multiple myeloma
- Myoglobinuria

Primary glomerular causes
- Focal segmental glomerulonephritis
- Idiopathic membranous glomerulonephritis
- Immunoglobulin (Ig)-A nephropathy
- IgM nephropathy
- Membranoproliferative glomerulonephritis
- Membranous nephropathy
- Minimal change disease

Secondary glomerular causes
- Alport syndrome
- Amyloidosis
- Diabetes mellitus
- Drugs
  - Angiotensin-converting enzyme inhibitors
  - Gold
  - Heavy metals
  - Heroin
  - Lithium
  - Nonsteroidal anti-inflammatory drugs (NSAIDs)
  - Penicillamine
- Fabry disease
- Infection
  - Endocarditis
  - Hepatitis B
  - Hepatitis C
  - HIV
  - Leprosy
  - Malaria
  - Parasitic diseases
  - Poststreptococcal infection
  - Shunt nephritis
  - Syphilis
- Malignancy (lymphoma, solid tumors)
- Preeclampsia
- Sarcoidosis

- Sickle cell disease
- Systemic lupus erythematosus and other collagen vascular diseases

Transient proteinuria
- Congestive heart failure
- Dehydration
- Emotional distress
- Exercise
- Fever
- Orthostatic (postural proteinuria)
- Seizures

Tubular causes
- Aminoaciduria
- Drugs
  - Antibiotics
  - NSAIDs
- Fanconi syndrome
- Heavy metal ingestion
- Hypertensive nephrosclerosis
- Interstitial nephritis
- Sickle cell disease
- Uric acid nephropathy

Key Historical Features

✓ Recent illness or fever
✓ Facial or extremity swelling
✓ Medical history, especially those listed previously that are causes of proteinuria
✓ Medications
✓ Exercise habits
✓ Risk factors for sexually transmitted diseases
✓ Heavy metal exposure

Key Physical Findings

✓ Vital signs, especially evidence of hypertension
✓ Signs of systemic disease
✓ Funduscopic examination
✓ Cardiovascular examination
✓ Pulmonary examination
✓ Abdominal examination, including bruits
✓ Edema (periorbital or peripheral)
✓ Rash

Suggested Work-Up

Microscopic examination of urine sediment	Fatty casts or oval fat bodies suggest nephrotic syndrome. Leukocytes or leukocyte casts with bacteria suggest urinary tract infection. Leukocytes or leukocyte casts without bacteria suggest renal interstitial disease. Normal red cells suggest a lower urinary tract lesion. Dysmorphic red cells suggest an upper urinary tract lesion. Red cell casts suggest glomerular disease. Waxy, granular, or cellular casts suggest advanced chronic renal disease. Eosinophils suggest drug-induced acute interstitial nephritis. Hyaline casts are not suggestive of renal disease but are present with dehydration and diuretic therapy.
24-hour urine specimen or spot measurement of protein-to-creatinine ratio	To quantify urinary protein excretion
If proteinuria is confirmed: Antinuclear antibody	Elevated in systemic lupus erythematosus
Antistreptolysin O titer	Elevated levels indicate poststreptococcal glomerulonephritis
Complement C3 and C4	Levels decreased in glomerulonephritides
Erythrocyte sedimentation rate	Elevation may indicate inflammatory or infectious causes
Fasting serum glucose	To evaluate for diabetes mellitus
Complete blood count	Anemia may indicate chronic renal failure
HIV, venereal disease research laboratory test, hepatitis B and hepatitis C serologies	HIV, syphilis, hepatitis B, and hepatitis C are associated with glomerular proteinuria

Serum albumin and lipids	Albumin is decreased and cholesterol level is increased in nephrotic syndrome
Serum electrolytes, calcium, and phosphorus	To screen for derangements following renal disease
Serum and urine protein electrophoresis	To evaluate for multiple myeloma
Serum urate	Elevated urate can cause tubulointerstitial disease
Renal ultrasound	To evaluate for structural renal disease
Chest x-ray	To examine for systemic disease, such as sarcoidosis

Additional Work-Up

Renal biopsy	Usually recommended for nephrotic range proteinuria (>3.5 g in 24 hours)

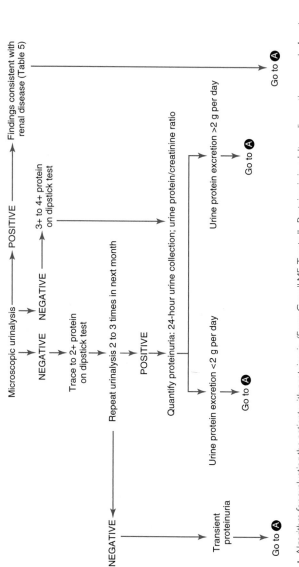

Figure 61-1 Algorithm for evaluating the patient with proteinuria. (From Carroll MF, Temte JL. Proteinuria in adults: a diagnostic approach. *American Family Physician* 2000;62:1333–1340; Figure 1.)

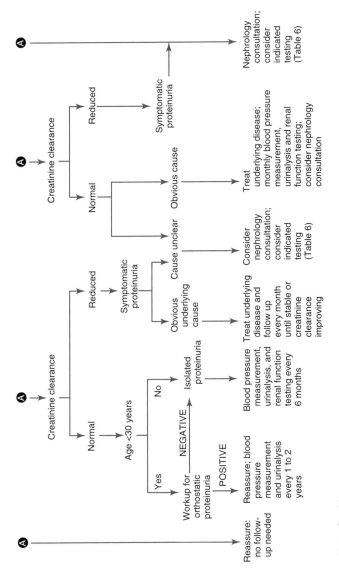

Figure 61-1—Cont'd

Microscopic Finding	Pathologic Process
Fatty casts, free fat, or oval fat bodies	Nephrotic range proteinuria (>3.5 g per 24 h)
Leukocytes, leukocyte casts with bacteria	Urinary tract infection
Leukocytes, leukocyte casts without bacteria	Renal interstitial disease
Normal-shaped erythrocytes	Suggestive of lower urinary tract lesion
Dysmorphic erythrocytes	Suggestive of upper urinary tract lesion
Erythrocyte casts	Glomerular disease
Waxy, granular, or cellular casts	Advanced chronic renal disease
Eosinophiluria*	Suggestive of drug-induced acute interstitial nephritis
Hyaline casts	No renal disease; present with dehydration and with diuretic therapy

*A Wright stain of the urine specimen is necessary to detect eosinophiluria.

(From Carroll MF, Temte JL. Proteinuria in adults: a diagnostic approach. *American Family Physician* 2000;62:1333–1340; Table 5).

Table 61-1 Interpretation of Findings on Microscopic Examination of Urine

Further Reading

Ahmed Z, Lee J. Asymptomatic urinary abnormalities: hematuria and proteinuria. *Med Clin North Am.* 1997;81:641–652.

Carroll MF, Temte JL. Proteinuria in adults: a diagnostic approach. *Am Fam Physician.* 2000;62:1333–1340.

Glassrock RJ. Proteinuria. In: Massry SJ, Glassrock RJ, eds. *Textbook of Nephrology.* 3rd ed. Baltimore: Williams & Wilkins; 1995:602.

Simerville JA, Maxted WC, Pahira JJ. Urinalysis: a comprehensive review. *Am Fam Physician.* 2005;71:1153–1162.

Woolhandler S, Pels RJ, Bor DH, Himmelstein DU, Lawrence RS. Dipstick urinalysis screening of asymptomatic adults for urinary tract disorders: hematuria and proteinuria. *JAMA.* 1989;262:1214–1219.

62 PRURITUS

General Discussion

The sensation of itching, or pruritus, is the most common symptom of dermatologic conditions, but it may also be associated with systemic disease, even in the absence of primary cutaneous findings. Pruritus can be broadly categorized into four major groups: dermatologic causes, systemic causes (e.g., cholestasis, chronic kidney disease, hyperthyroidism, myeloproliferative disorders), neuropathic causes (e.g., notalgia paresthetica, brachioradial pruritus), and psychogenic causes.

The mechanisms underlying the various types of pruritus are complex. Histamine is the main mediator of itching, but other mediators may be involved, including serotonin, neuropeptides, and prostaglandins. Patients with chronic itch often have peripheral and central neural hypersensitization in which sensitized itch fibers overreact to noxious stimuli that usually inhibit itch, such as heat and scratching. Misinterpretation of non-noxious stimuli also occurs, such as touch being perceived as itch.

Pruritus is frequently encountered as a symptom of common dermatologic conditions, such as atopic dermatitis, contact dermatitis, psoriasis, scabies, lichen planus, and urticaria. Additional dermatologic causes of itching are outlined in the following. When primary skin findings are absent, the approach shifts to attempting to detect an underlying systemic disorder. In patients with pruritus, the prevalence of underlying systemic disease ranges from 10% to 50%.

Pruritus is commonly listed as a medication side effect. Pruritus that is attributable to systemic medications can be classified into three categories: (1) pruritus with a transient eruption or with no rash; (2) pruritus caused by drug-induced cholestasis; and (3) pruritus with a skin eruption or rash. If no specific dermatologic disorder is identified after a thorough history and physical examination, laboratory and radiologic tests should be ordered to try to identify the presence of systemic disease.

Medications That Cause Cholestasis or Cholestatic Hepatitis

Angiotensin-converting enzyme inhibitors
Allopurinol
Ampicillin
Anabolic steroids
Antibiotics
- Amoxicillin/clavulanic acid
- Azithromycin
- Clarithromycin
- Dapsone
- Erythromycin

- Flucloxacillin
- Nitrofurantoin
- Trimethoprim/sulfamethoxazole

Arsenic
Azathioprine
Barbiturates
Benzodiazepines
Captopril
Carbamazepine
Chlorpromazine
Chlorpropamide
Cimetidine
Clindamycin
Co-trimoxazole
Cyclohexyl propionate
Cyclosporin A
Cyproheptadine
Cytosine-arabinoside
Danazol
Erythromycin
Fosinopril
Gold
Haloperidol
Infliximab
Loracarbef
Mesalamine
Methimazole
Nifedipine
Nonsteroidal anti-inflammatory drugs

- Diclofenac
- Ibuprofen
- Nimesulide
- Sulindac

Phenytoin
Pizotyline
Prochlorperazine
Propoxyphene
Risperidone
Sex steroids
Tamoxifen
Terbinafine
Terfenadine
Tetracyclines
Thiabendazole
Tricyclic antidepressants
Troglitazone

Conditions Associated with Pruritus

Advanced age
Anorexia nervosa
Chronic kidney disease
Cutaneous mastocytosis
Dermatologic conditions
- Atopic dermatitis
- Bullous pemphigoid
- Contact dermatitis
- Dermatitis herpetiformis
- Miliaria
- Parasitic infestations
- Pruritus ani/scroti/vulvae
- Psoriasis
- Urticaria
- Xerosis

Endocrine disorders
- Carcinoid syndrome
- Diabetes mellitus
- Hyperthyroidism
- Hypothyroidism
- Multiple endocrine neoplasia type 2

Hematopoietic diseases
- Hodgkin disease
- Iron-deficiency anemia
- Leukemia
- Lymphoma
- Mastocytosis
- Mycosis fungoides
- Plasma cell dyscrasias
- Polycythemia vera

HIV infection/AIDS
Linear immunoglobulin-A dermatosis
Liver and biliary disease
- Drug-induced cholestasis
- Extrahepatic biliary obstruction
- Infectious hepatitis
- Primary biliary cirrhosis
- Pruritus gravidarum
- Sclerosing cholangitis

Malignancy
Medications
Neurologic/neuropathic disorders
- Brachioradial pruritus
- Cerebral abscess

- Cerebral tumor
- Multiple sclerosis
- Notalgia paresthetica
- Post-herpetic itch
- Stroke

Psychiatric illness
- Delusions of parasitosis
- Obsessive-compulsive disorder

Renal disease
- Chronic renal failure

Substance use

Key Historical Features

✓ Duration and quality of the itching
✓ Distribution of itching
✓ Exacerbating and ameliorating factors
✓ Medical history
✓ Medications
✓ Illicit drug use
✓ Personal or family history of atopy or skin disease
✓ Occupation and hobbies
✓ Environmental exposures
✓ Animal exposure
✓ Travel history
✓ Sexual history
✓ Bathing habits
✓ Thorough review of systems

Key Physical Findings

✓ Thorough skin examination for rash, excoriations, dyspigmentation, or lichenification
✓ Palpation of lymph nodes for lymphadenopathy
✓ Palpation of liver and spleen for organomegaly
✓ Inspection of fingers, axillae, and genitals to evaluate for scabies

Suggested Work-Up

Complete blood count with differential	To evaluate for hematopoietic disorders
Alanine aminotransferase, aspartate aminotransferase, bilirubin, gamma-glutamyl transpeptidase (GGT), albumin	To evaluate for hepatobiliary disease
Blood urea nitrogen and creatinine	To evaluate for renal disease

Thyroid-stimulating hormone	To evaluate for hypo- or hyperthyroidism
Plasma glucose	To evaluate for diabetes mellitus
Erythrocyte sedimentation rate	To evaluate for inflammation/infection
Urinalysis	To evaluate for renal disease
Chest x-ray	To evaluate for pulmonary parasitic infestation
Stool for occult blood and parasites	To evaluate for intestinal parasitic infestation
HIV antibody	If risk factors for HIV infection are present

Additional Work-Up

| Punch biopsy of the skin | May be considered if the cause of the itching cannot be determined from history, physical examination, and laboratory/radiologic evaluation |
| Drug screening | If substance use is suspected |

Further Reading

Berger TG, Shive M, Harper GM. Pruritus in the older patient: a clinical review. *JAMA.* 2013;310:2443–2450.

Charlesworth EN, Beltrani VS. Pruritus dermatoses: overview of etiology and therapy. *Am J Med.* 2002;113(Suppl 9A):255–335.

Etter L, Myers SA. Pruritus in systemic disease: mechanisms and management. *Dermatology Clinics.* 2002;20:459–472.

Kantor G, Lookingbill D. Generalized pruritis and systemic disease. *J Am Acad Dermatol.* 1983;9:375–382.

Krajnik M, Zylicz Z. Pruritus in advanced internal diseases: pathogenesis and treatment. *Neth J Med.* 2001;58:27–40.

Levy C, Lindor KD. Drug-induced cholestasis. *Clin Liver Dis.* 2003;7:7311–7330.

Yosipovitch G, Bernhard JD. Chronic pruritus. *N Engl J Med.* 2013;368:1625–1634.

Yosipovitch G, David M. The diagnostic and therapeutic approach to idiopathic generalized pruritus. *Int J Dermatol.* 1999;38:881–887.

63 RECURRENT URINARY TRACT INFECTION

General Discussion

In the general population, urinary tract infection (UTI) is primarily an infection in sexually active women, with the prevalence of UTI in women outnumbering men by a ratio of 30:1. However, the prevalence of UTI increases in both sexes with advancing age, reducing the ratio to 2:1 in older adults. Recurrent UTIs are symptomatic UTIs that occur after resolution of an appropriately treated earlier episode. Recurrent UTIs include relapses (symptomatic recurrent UTIs with the same organism following adequate therapy) and reinfection (recurrent UTIs with previously isolated bacteria after treatment and with a negative intervening urine culture, or a recurrent UTI caused by a second bacterial isolate). Most recurrent UTIs are believed to represent reinfection with the same organism.

Recurrent UTIs are common among otherwise healthy young women with anatomically and physiologically normal urinary tracts, and are usually related to sexual intercourse. In older adults, recurrence is primarily a lower tract disease as a result of different risk or contributing factors, which may include incomplete bladder emptying or age-related diseases (e.g., diabetes mellitus).

The decision to evaluate recurrent UTI radiologically, endoscopically, urodynamically, or otherwise should be based on the patient's clinical presentation, history, findings, response to antimicrobial therapy, and pattern of recurrent UTIs. A patient with a severe UTI warrants further evaluation. Severe UTI is defined as sepsis, fever, history of UTI lasting more than 7 days, gross hematuria, signs or symptoms of obstruction, or history of stones. Risk factors such as diabetes mellitus, immunosuppression, debilitating disease, or pregnancy may also warrant further evaluation.

If a patient has a history of recurrent UTI, urine culture should be used to document the infection, identify the pathogen, and determine the frequency of infection. Urine culture is also used to distinguish between unresolved and recurrent infection. If the same pathogen is documented repeatedly and at close intervals, an underlying abnormality should be suspected, and an evaluation should be initiated. If the same pathogen is not found or UTIs do not occur in a close temporal relationship, the likelihood of the infections being associated with functional, metabolic, or anatomic abnormalities is low, and the patient may be treated with low-dose antimicrobial prophylaxis. Men with recurrent infections should be evaluated further because the infections usually are associated with an anatomic or functional urinary tract abnormality.

Conditions Associated with Recurrent Urinary Tract Infection

Advancing age
Bacterial resistance
Bladder outlet obstruction
Chronic bacterial prostatitis
Chronic renal insufficiency
Cystocele
Diabetes mellitus
Genitourinary anatomic abnormalities
- Bladder polyp
- Fistula
- Medullary sponge kidney
- Polycystic kidney disease
- Urethral diverticula

Genitourinary calculi
Immunosuppression
Incomplete bladder emptying
- Advancing age
- Multiple sclerosis
- Neurogenic bladder
- Spinal cord injury

Indwelling urinary catheter
Intermittent urinary catheterization
Medication noncompliance
Nephrostomy tube
Perinephric abscess
Pregnancy
Pyelonephritis
Poor hygiene
Renal abscess
Renal transplant
Sexual intercourse
Ureteral stent
Urethral valves
Urinary diversion procedure
Urolithiasis
Urologic instrumentation
Vesicoureteral reflux

Key Historical Features

✓ Age
✓ Previous response to therapy and culture results
✓ Presence of fever, nausea, or malaise
✓ Frequency of infection and temporal relationship to intercourse
✓ Contraceptive practices

- ✓ Dysuria
- ✓ Urinary frequency
- ✓ Urgency
- ✓ Hematuria
- ✓ Vaginal discharge
- ✓ Odor
- ✓ Dyspareunia
- ✓ Pruritus
- ✓ History of childhood infections
- ✓ Medical history, especially urolithiasis, known urinary tract abnormality, immunosuppression, or diabetes mellitus
- ✓ Previous urologic surgery or instrumentation
- ✓ Medications

Key Physical Findings

- ✓ Vital signs
- ✓ General examination to evaluate patient's overall health
- ✓ Abdominal examination
- ✓ Back examination to evaluate for costovertebral angle tenderness
- ✓ Genitourinary examination to distinguish evaluate for urethritis or vaginitis
- ✓ Gynecologic examination to rule out vaginal pathology
- ✓ Prostate examination

Suggested Work-Up

Urinalysis	To determine whether the urine is infected
Urine culture	To document infection, identify the pathogen, and determine the frequency of infection
Blood urea nitrogen and creatinine	To evaluate renal function
Quantification of post-void residual bladder volume	To evaluate bladder emptying
Renal ultrasound	To evaluate upper urinary tract architecture and establish the presence of hydronephrosis or abscess
Computed tomography scan	To evaluate anatomic detail and to diagnose the presence of urinary stones
Intravenous pyelogram	To evaluate for filling defects or diagnose obstructive uropathy

Additional Work-Up

Voiding cystogram	If an anatomic abnormality is suspected
Cystoscopy	If tumor or mass is suspected
Prostatic secretion wet mount or gram stain	If chronic bacterial prostatitis is suspected in a male
Urology consult	For obstructive uropathy, calculi, abscess, or genitourinary abnormalities

Further Reading

Engel JD, Schaeffer AJ. Evaluation of and antimicrobial therapy for recurrent urinary tract infections in women. *Urol Clin North Am.* 1998;25:685–701.

Kodner CM, Gupton EK. Recurrent urinary tract infections in women: diagnosis and management. *Am Fam Physician.* 2010;82:638–643.

McLaughlin SP, Carson CC. Urinary tract infections in women. *Med Clin North Am.* 2004;88:417–429.

Pewitt EB, Schaeffer AJ. Urinary tract infection in urology, including acute and chronic prostatitis. *Infect Dis Clin North Am.* 1997;11:623–646.

Yoshikawa TT, Nicolle LE, Norman DC. Management of complicated urinary tract infection in older patients. *J Am Geriatr Soc.* 1996;44:1235–1241.

General Discussion

Renal masses are common, with approximately 40% of patients having at least one renal cyst incidentally discovered on abdominal computed tomography (CT). Renal masses can be categorized into cysts, tumors, and inflammatory lesions. Simple cysts are usually asymptomatic but may cause flank pain, abdominal pain, hematuria, or a palpable mass. Malignant lesions may produce the same symptoms and may be associated with paraneoplastic syndromes. Inflammatory lesions are almost always associated with a history of fever, chills, or urinary tract infection.

Ultrasound is good for differentiating between cystic and solid lesions. Simple renal cysts must be distinguished from complex cysts and solid masses. The ultrasound criteria for the diagnosis of a simple renal cyst (Bosniak category I; see the following) include:

1. Spherical or ovoid shape;
2. Absence of internal echoes;
3. Presence of a thin, smooth wall that is separate from the surrounding parenchyma; and
4. Enhancement of the posterior wall, indicating ultrasound transmission through the water-filled cyst.

When these ultrasound criteria are met, the likelihood of malignancy is extremely small. Asymptomatic patients with incidental renal cysts that meet these criteria require no additional evaluation.

When visualization of the mass is inadequate on ultrasonography or when the ultrasound shows evidence of calcifications, septa, or multiple cysts that may obscure a potential malignancy, renal CT scanning with contrast should be performed.

Classification of Renal Masses

The Bosniak system is the most widely used categorization system for cystic renal masses. The system uses the thickness of the cyst wall, the presence or absence of calcifications, and the measurement of Hounsfield units to categorize lesions in order of increasing probability of malignancy.

Category I masses are simple benign cysts. These lesions are round or oval in shape with no perceptible wall, have the same density as water, and exhibit no enhancement on radiographs after contrast medium is administered. No further evaluation or follow-up is required. If the patient becomes symptomatic, as rarely occurs with large cysts, urologic consultation should be obtained.

Category II masses are minimally complicated cysts that can be reliably considered as benign. These lesions include septated cysts, minimally calcified cysts, infected cysts, or cysts with higher density due to the presence of blood, protein, or colloid. These lesions should not enhance with contrast medium. Bosniak category II cysts can be considered benign and do not require follow-up.

Category IIF masses (F for follow-up) have more features than those defined in the category II masses. Category IIF lesions are likely benign, but these lesions require follow-up imaging to demonstrate stability. These masses may contain multiple thin septa and thick or nodular calcification. A suggested follow-up regimen is CT (or magnetic resonance imaging [MRI] if that was the original imaging modality) imaging at 6, 12, 24, and 36 months. At 36 months, a decision can be made regarding further annual follow-up. Some authors recommend 5-year follow-up, and if the cyst has not significantly changed in a period of 5 years, it is likely benign.

Class III lesions are more complicated cystic lesions with thick, irregular calcifications, multilocular form, thick irregular borders, thickened or enhancing septa, small nonenhancing nodules, or irregular calcifications. Urologic referral is indicated for these lesions. MRI may help to better characterize the lesions. Most category III masses are treated by surgical resection to ensure that a malignancy is not missed.

Class IV lesions are clearly malignant cystic masses, until proved otherwise. The lesions are heterogeneous with a shaggy appearance, thickened walls, or enhancing nodules resulting from necrosis and liquefaction of a solid tumor or a tumor growing in the wall. Surgical excision is indicated.

Further Reading

Bosniak MA. The current radiologic approach to renal cysts. *Radiology*. 1986;158:1–10.

Bradley AJ, Lim YY, Singh FM. Imaging features, follow-up, and management of incidentally detected renal lesions. *Clin Radiol*. 2011;66:1129–1139.

Curry NS, Bissada NK. Radiologic evaluation of small and indeterminant renal masses. *Urol Clin North Am*. 1997;24:493–505.

Higgins JC, Fitzgerald JM. Evaluation of incidental renal and adrenal masses. *Am Fam Physician*. 2001;63:288–291.

Israel GM, Silverman SG. The incidental renal mass. *Radiol Clin N Am*. 2011;49:369–383.

Kissane JM. Congenital malformations. In: Jennette JC, et al., eds. *Heptinstall's pathology of the kidney*. 5th ed. Philadelphia: Lippincott-Raven; 1998.

Wolf JS. Evaluation and management of solid and cystic renal masses. *J Urol*. 1998;159:1120–1233.

65 RHINITIS

General Discussion

Rhinitis can be practically viewed as a heterogeneous group of nasal disorders characterized by symptoms such as rhinorrhea, nasal congestion, nasal itching, and sneezing. These classic symptoms of rhinitis overlap significantly with allergic rhinitis and other forms of rhinitis, as well as with various anatomic abnormalities of the upper airway. Rhinitis may be caused by allergic, nonallergic, hormonal, infectious, occupational, and other factors. Allergic rhinitis is the most common type of chronic rhinitis, although 30% to 50% of patients with rhinitis have nonallergic causes.

Allergic rhinitis can be categorized as seasonal, perennial, or occupational. Characteristics of allergic rhinitis include onset of symptoms early in life, a positive family history of allergic rhinitis, seasonal variability, itching in the nose, throat, or eyes, and the presence of identifiable suspected allergens. Physical examination often reveals moist and slightly blue nasal turbinates.

The diagnosis of nonallergic rhinitis is made after allergic or immunoglobulin-E (IgE)–mediated causes have been eliminated. Characteristics that suggest nonallergic rhinitis include onset of symptoms after age 30 years, a negative family history of allergic rhinitis, perennial symptoms, the absence of nasal or throat itching, symptoms that are precipitated by irritants or weather changes, and the presence of viral- or flu-like symptoms. Physical examination often reveals nasal mucosa that is dry, erythematous, or irritated.

Nonallergic rhinitis may be classified as vasomotor rhinitis, gustatory rhinitis, nonallergic rhinitis with eosinophil syndrome (NARES), rhinitis medicamentosa, occupational rhinitis, hormonal rhinitis, drug-induced rhinitis, atrophic rhinitis, cold air–induced rhinitis, and anatomic rhinitis.

Several expert panels have published reviews of rhinitis. None of the three reports on rhinitis provides specific recommendations on when to perform allergy testing for patients with rhinitis. Empiric treatment is appropriate in patients with classic symptoms. In general, diagnostic tests may be appropriate if they change outcomes or change treatment plans, if the symptoms are severe, if the diagnosis is unclear, or if the patient is a potential candidate for allergen avoidance treatment or immunotherapy.

The most common diagnostic tests for allergic rhinitis are the percutaneous skin test and the allergen-specific IgE antibody test, which are also known as radioallergosorbent testing (RAST). Other diagnostic tools include nasal cytology and nasolaryngoscopy. Skin testing involves introducing allergen and control substances into the skin. The primary goal of skin testing is to detect the immediate allergic response caused by the release of mast cell or basophil IgE-specific mediators. RAST is highly specific, but it is not as sensitive as skin testing. RAST is useful for identifying common allergens, such as pet dander, dust mites, pollen, and common molds, but it is less useful for identifying food, venom, and drug allergies. Generally speaking, skin testing or RAST should be used to confirm suspicions, but these should not be relied on to make a diagnosis.

Medications Associated with Rhinitis

Angiotensin-converting enzyme inhibitors
Alpha antagonists
Antihypertensives
Aspirin
Beta-blockers
Chlorpromazine
Nonsteroidal anti-inflammatory drugs
Oral contraceptives
Phentolamine
Phosphodiesterase-5 selective inhibitors

Causes of Rhinitis

Allergic rhinitis
- Occupational rhinitis
- Perennial rhinitis
- Seasonal rhinitis

Anatomic abnormalities
- Adenoidal hypertrophy
- Choanal atresia
- Deviated septum
- Foreign body in the nose
- Hypertrophic turbinates
- Nasal polyps
- Nasal and sinus tumors

Atrophic rhinitis
Cerebrospinal fluid leak
Ciliary dyskinesia syndrome
Cocaine abuse
Cold air–induced rhinitis
Diabetes mellitus
Emotional rhinitis
Ethanol ingestion
Exercise-induced rhinitis
Gustatory
Hormonal
- Hypothyroidism
- Menstrual cycle

- Oral contraceptives
- Pregnancy

Infectious rhinitis
- Bacterial infection
- Coronavirus
- Rhinovirus

Inflammatory or immunologic conditions
- Midline granuloma
- Nasal polyposis
- Sarcoidosis
- Sjögren syndrome
- Systemic lupus erythematosus
- Wegener granulomatosis

Medication-induced rhinitis

NARES

Postural reflexes

Primary ciliary dyskinesia

Reflux-induced rhinitis (gastroesophageal reflux disease)

Relapsing polychondritis

Rhinitis medicamentosa

Vasomotor rhinitis

Key Historical Features

✓ Specific symptoms, such as nasal congestion, rhinorrhea, sneezing, or pruritus
✓ Duration and chronicity
✓ Magnitude of reaction
✓ Eye itching and lacrimation
✓ Pattern of symptoms (intermittent, seasonal, perennial)
✓ Precipitating factors/triggers
✓ Response to treatment
✓ Coexisting conditions
✓ Environmental history (home and occupational exposures)
✓ Medical history, including trauma
✓ Medications
✓ Family history

Key Physical Findings

✓ Presence of fever
✓ Nasal examination for nasal discharge, swollen turbinates, bluish or pale mucosa, nasal polyps, septal deviation, and masses
✓ Ocular examination for conjunctivitis
✓ Evidence of infraorbital darkening or transverse nasal crease

- ✓ Ear examination for air-fluid levels
- ✓ Examination of the oropharynx for enlarged tonsils or pharyngeal postnasal discharge
- ✓ Neck examination for lymphadenopathy
- ✓ Pulmonary examination for evidence of asthma
- ✓ Skin examination for evidence of eczema

Suggested Work-Up

Empiric treatment is appropriate in patients with classic symptoms. In general, diagnostic tests may be appropriate if they will change outcomes, change treatment plans, if the symptoms are severe, if an unclear diagnosis is present, or if the patient is a potential candidate for allergen avoidance treatment or immunotherapy.

Skin testing	To identify specific allergens when avoidance measures or allergen immunotherapy is being considered
RAST	Highly specific, but not as sensitive as skin testing. RAST is useful for identifying common allergens, such as pet dander, dust mites, pollen, and common molds, but is less useful for identifying food, venom, and drug allergies.

Additional Work-Up

Nasal smear	Staining the nasal secretions for eosinophils with Hansel's stain can help suggest an allergic cause, but it is not specific. Irritant and infectious rhinitis produce a neutrophil predominance.
Fiberoptic nasal endoscopy	Typically reserved for patients with atypical symptoms or those with inadequate response to treatment
Computed tomography scan or magnetic resonance imaging	May be helpful if anatomic abnormality is suspected

Further Reading

Beard S. Rhinitis. *Prim Care Clin Office Pract.* 2014;41:33–46.

Dykewicz MS. Allergic disorders. *J Allergy Clin Immunol.* 2003;111:S520–S529.

Dykewicz MS, Fineman S, Skoner DP, et al. Diagnosis and management of rhinitis: complete guidelines of the Joint Task Force on Practice Parameters in Allergy, Asthma, and Immunology. American Academy of Allergy, Asthma, and Immunology. *Ann Allergy Asthma Immunol.* 1998;81(pt 2):478–518.

Knight A. Anticholinergic therapy for allergic and nonallergic rhinitis and the common cold. *J Allergy Clin Immunol.* 1995;95:1080–1083.

Quillen DM, Feller DB. Diagnosing rhinitis: allergic vs. nonallergic. *Am Fam Physician.* 2006;73:1583–1590.

Wallace D, Dykewicz M. The diagnosis and management of rhinitis: an updated practice parameter. *J Allergy Clin Immunol.* 2008;122:S1–S84.

Weldon D. Diagnosis and management of rhinitis. *Primary Care: Clinics in Office Practice.* 1998;25:831–848.

Wheeler PW, Wheeler SF. Vasomotor rhinitis. *Am Fam Physician.* 2005;72:1057–1062.

General Discussion

When evaluating a scrotal mass, it should be determined whether the mass is extra-testicular or intra-testicular, solid or cystic, and painless or painful. Painless masses may either be benign or malignant, but painful masses are much more likely to require urgent intervention. Masses that arise from the testicle are more likely to represent malignancies, whereas extra-testicular masses are more likely to be benign. Likewise, solid masses are much more likely to represent neoplastic conditions, especially when painless. Transillumination using a hand-held light source may help differentiate between solid and cystic structures. Extra-testicular tumors are uncommon but do occur in the form of para-testicular rhabdomyosarcoma or adenomatoid tumors of the epididymis.

Painful scrotal masses include testicular torsion, epididymitis and/or orchitis, torsion of the testicular appendage, hematocele, and testicular rupture. Testicular cancer and inguinal hernias may present with or without pain. Painless scrotal masses include hydrocele, varicocele, spermatocele, and epididymal cysts.

Although a careful history and physical examination may be diagnostic, confirmation using scrotal ultrasonography is recommended to confirm the location of the mass and to differentiate between solid and cystic lesions.

Cystic lesions of the scrotum are much more common than solid lesions. A cystic mass within the epididymis is usually a spermatocele. A cyst within the spermatic cord usually represents a hydrocele. A cystic mass that surrounds the entire testicle usually represents a hydrocele.

A testicular tumor usually presents as a painless mass, although the patient may complain of scrotal heaviness or a dull ache. If testicular cancer is suspected, the patient should also be examined for lymphadenopathy, gynecomastia, and abdominal masses.

A hydrocele is a collection of peritoneal fluid between the layers of the tunica vaginalis surrounding the testicle. A hydrocele usually presents as a painless scrotal swelling that can be transilluminated. The swelling often worsens during the course of the day, and the patient may complain of weight and bulk as a result of the hydrocele. A new hydrocele or one that hemorrhages as a result of minor trauma may indicate an underlying testicular cancer.

A spermatocele usually presents as a painless cystic mass superior and posterior to the testis. This mass is separate from the testis, is freely mobile, and transilluminates easily.

A varicocele is present in up to 20% of all males and is a tortuous and dilated pampiniform venous plexus and internal spermatic vein. Varicoceles are often described as a "bag of worms" superior to and distinct from the testicle. Varicoceles usually first appear near midpuberty. Most varicoceles occur on the left side and are often asymptomatic, although they may cause male infertility. The dilatation and tortuosity are most noticeable when the patient is upright and may be accentuated if the patient performs a Valsalva maneuver.

Causes of Testicular Masses

Acute orchitis
Epididymal cyst
Epididymitis
Hematocele or testicular rupture
Hydrocele
Inguinal hernia
Orchitis
Skin cancer
Spermatocele
Testicular cancer
Testicular torsion with associated swelling
Torsion of the testicular appendage
Varicocele

Key Historical Features

✓ Duration of the mass
✓ How the mass was discovered
✓ Presence of pain and character of the pain, if present
✓ Associated trauma
✓ History of scrotal issues, such as an undescended testicle
✓ Constitutional symptoms, such as weight loss, fever, chest pain, cough, headache
✓ Recent infection
✓ Medical history
✓ Surgical history
✓ Family history

Key Physical Findings

✓ Careful palpation and identification of the intrascrotal contents
✓ Testicular examination for volume, masses, or tenderness
✓ Transillumination of the testicular mass
✓ Palpation of the epididymis
✓ Assessment of the spermatic cord
✓ Cremasteric reflex
✓ Examination of the inguinal canals for a hernia or cord tenderness
✓ Valsalva maneuver to evaluate for hernia or varicocele
✓ Abdominal examination for masses

✓   Breast examination for gynecomastia
✓   Lymph node examination

Suggested Work-Up

Scrotal ultrasound	To help define suspected lesions and differentiate between intra-testicular and extra-testicular lesions

Additional Work-Up

C-reactive protein	May be helpful in diagnosing epididymitis and/or orchitis if the level is greater than 24 mg/L
Serum-α fetoprotein (AFP)	If testicular cancer is suspected. Elevated AFP level implies non-seminomatous germ cell tumor or mixed tumor.
Serum human chorionic gonadotropin (HCG)	If testicular cancer is suspected. HCG is secreted by one-half of non-seminomatous germ cell tumors and mixed tumors, as well as 10% of pure seminomas.
Lactate dehydrogenase	If testicular cancer is suspected. Lactate dehydrogenase is elevated in 60% of non-seminomatous germ cell tumors.
Computed tomography (CT) scan of the abdomen and pelvis, chest x-ray	Performed for staging purposes if a testicular malignancy is identified
CT scan of the chest	If abdominal or pelvic metastases are seen on initial staging workup

Further Reading

Crawford P, Crop JA. Evaluation of scrotal masses. *Am Fam Physician*. 2014;89:723–727.

Haynes JH. Inguinal and scrotal disorders. *Surg Clin North Am*. 2006;86:371–381.

Jayanthi VR. Adolescent urology. *Adolesc Med Clin*. 2004;15:521–534.

Junnila J, Lassen P. Testicular masses. *Am Fam Physician*. 1998;57:685–692.

Montgomery JS, Bloom DA. The diagnosis and management of scrotal masses. *Med Clin N Am*. 2011;95:235–244.

General Discussion

Seizures may be classified as localized (partial or focal) or generalized based on clinical and electroencephalographic changes. A generalized seizure involves the cerebral hemispheres bilaterally and symmetrically at the time of onset. In contrast, a partial seizure originates in a specific region of the cerebral cortex. These seizures may be associated with signs or symptoms related to the cerebral region of origin, and they may occur with or without mental status changes or loss of consciousness.

A first seizure can range from a fleeting subjective experience, such as déjà vu, or a myoclonic jerk (a twitch) to a tonic-clonic convulsion. A single seizure may be provoked (with an acute precipitant) or unprovoked (idiopathic or of unknown cause). Epilepsy is defined as more than one seizure.

Seizures have a bimodal frequency, declining in frequency from childhood until the age of 60 years, and then increasing again. In adults younger than 60 years of age, anticonvulsant discontinuation and/or withdrawal, and low antiepileptic drug levels are the most common causes of seizures. Alcohol is the cause of most seizures for people between the ages of 30 and 60 years, and is the second most common cause in all adults. Other common causes of seizures are drug overdose, metabolic disorders, central nervous system (CNS) infections, and trauma. Hypoglycemia and hyponatremia are the most common metabolic disorders.

The first step in the evaluation of a seizure is to determine if the event is truly a seizure. The physician should attempt to obtain a moment-by-moment description of the event from the patient or a witness. Clarifying whether the seizure occurred with or without loss of consciousness is useful. The differentiation of tonic-clonic seizure from syncope is important but may be difficult to assess if no eyewitness account is possible. Postictal confusion, lateral tongue biting, cyanosis, confirmed unresponsiveness, preceding déjà vu, head or eye turning to one side, rhythmic limb shaking, and dystonic posturing are strong seizure markers. When unable to obtain a reliable history, the examining physician should assume that the seizure is a first-time event and proceed with a new-onset seizure workup.

Special consideration should be given to the possibility of toxic exposure or underlying complicating medical conditions, such as alcoholism, diabetes, and renal failure. The second step is to identify possible acute precipitants for seizures. Seizures may be the manifestation of an underlying medical illness that requires specific treatment.

Medications and Substances Associated with Seizure

Amantadine
Amphetamines

Bupropion
Caffeine
Camphor
Carbamazepine
Citalopram
Cocaine
Cyclic antidepressants
Diphenhydramine
Disopyramide
Fluoride
Gamma-hydroxybutyric acid
Hydroxychloroquine
Iron
Isoniazid
Lidocaine
Lithium
Meperidine
N-methyl-D-aspartate
Nicotine
Olanzapine
Phencyclidine
Phenytoin
Procainamide
Propoxyphene
Quinidine
Quinine
Salicylates
Selective serotonin reuptake inhibitors
Theophylline
Thioridazine
Thujone
Tramadol
Venlafaxine
Water hemlock

Causes of Seizure

Boric acid ingestion
Brain tumor
- Brain metastases
- CNS lymphoma
- Malignant glioma
- Meningiomas

Carbamates
Carbon monoxide exposure
Cerebrovascular accident or transient ischemic attack

CNS infection
- Abscess
- AIDS dementia
- Bacterial meningitis
- Cryptococcal meningitis
- Cysticercosis
- Encephalitis, especially herpes
- Tuberculous meningitis

Cyanide ingestion

Degenerative disorders
- Alzheimer dementia
- Amyloid angiopathy

Dialysis disequilibrium

Dialysis encephalopathy

Elapid envenomation

Encephalopathy

Ephedra

Granulomatous angiitis of the CNS

Gyromitra esculenta mushroom

Head trauma

Heavy metal poisoning
- Arsenic
- Lead
- Thallium

Hydrogen sulfide

Hypertensive encephalopathy

Medications and substances (listed previously)

Metabolic causes
- Hyperglycemia
- Hypoglycemia
- Hyponatremia
- Hypoxia
- Uremia

Multiple sclerosis

Organochlorine pesticides
- Dichlorodiphenyltrichloroethane
- Lindane

Organophosphates

Polyarteritis nodosa

Porphyria

Rodenticides
- Bromethalin
- Zinc phosphide

Scorpion envenomation

Sickle cell anemia

Subdural hematoma

Systemic lupus erythematosus
Thrombotic thrombocytopenia purpura
Wegener granulomatosis
Withdrawal syndromes
- Alcohol
- Baclofen
- Sedative-hypnotic

Conditions That May Mimic Seizures

Breath-holding spells
Cardiac arrhythmia
Conversion disorders
Dementia
Disassociation
Episodic dyscontrol syndrome
Fugue state
Hyperventilation
Malingering
Migraine
Movement disorders, such as tics or Tourette syndrome
Panic attacks
Paroxysmal ataxia
Paroxysmal kinesigenic choreoathetosis
Paroxysmal vertigo
Periodic paralysis
Pseudoseizure
Psychosis
Sleep disorders (narcolepsy, sleep paralysis)
Somatization
Startle syndrome
Syncope
Transient global amnesia

Key Historical Features

✓ Detailed description of the event
✓ Pain or injury from the seizure
✓ Risk factors for seizure (head trauma, cerebrovascular disease)
✓ Fever
✓ Infectious symptoms
✓ Headache
✓ Complaints of focal neurologic deficits
✓ Seizure history

✓ Medical history, especially diabetes, cancer, cardiac and vascular diseases, renal failure, hepatic failure, and bleeding disorders or coagulopathies
✓ Pregnancy
✓ Medications, including over-the-counter agents
✓ Alcohol and substance abuse
✓ Toxin exposure
✓ HIV risk factors
✓ Thorough review of systems
✓ Evidence of sleep disorders

Key Physical Findings

✓ Vital signs, including presence of fever
✓ Evaluation of level of consciousness and mental status
✓ Evaluation for injuries preceding or experienced during the seizure
✓ Funduscopic examination
✓ Neck examination for nuchal rigidity
✓ Thorough neurologic examination
✓ Cardiovascular examination
✓ Thorough examination for evidence of underlying systemic disease, infection, or toxic exposure

Suggested Work-Up

Glucose level	To evaluate for hypoglycemia or hyperglycemia
Complete blood count	To evaluate for anemia or evidence of infection or platelet disorder
Electrolytes	To evaluate for hyponatremia or hypernatremia
Blood urea nitrogen and creatinine	To evaluate for uremia
Calcium	To evaluate for hypocalcemia or hypercalcemia
Magnesium	To evaluate for magnesium disturbance
Phosphorus	To evaluate for phosphorus disturbance
Erythrocyte sedimentation rate	To evaluate for inflammatory disorder or vasculitis
Liver function tests	To evaluate for liver disease
Thyroid-stimulating hormone	To evaluate for hypothyroidism

Pregnancy test	For women of reproductive age
Electrocardiogram	May be helpful in diagnosing long QT syndrome presenting as a seizure. A seizure with a widened QRS interval on electrocardiogram may be a clue to cyclic antidepressants, propoxyphene, venlafaxine, diphenhydramine, or other agents.
Chest x-ray	Rarely adds to the discovery of seizure etiology but can indicate a need for further workup (such as malignancy)
Electroencephalogram	To help establish the diagnosis of epilepsy and classify the seizure type. Yield is highest in the first 24 hours after the seizure.
Head computed tomography (CT) or magnetic resonance imaging (MRI)	Many guidelines advocate for MRI in all first seizure patients. It is superior in resolution to CT scanning. CT scanning is useful for first seizure patients with acute head injury or patients with reduced level of consciousness.

Additional Work-Up

Serum drug levels	If the patient is taking anticonvulsant medications
Toxicology screen and alcohol level	If substance abuse is suspected or the patient's mental status is not returning to normal after a seizure
Blood alcohol level and prothrombin time	For the evaluation of an alcoholic patient
Prothrombin time and activated partial thromboplastin time	For patients taking anticoagulants or with known coagulopathies or platelet disorders
HIV testing	If HIV infection is suspected
Blood cultures	If bacterial meningitis is suspected
Lumbar puncture	Indicated if the patient is febrile or recently febrile, if the patient is immunocompromised, or if

	meningitis is suspected. Also indicated in patients in whom subarachnoid hemorrhage is suspected after a negative CT is obtained. May also be indicated if a clear precipitant is not found on initial evaluation.
Echocardiogram, carotid Doppler ultrasonography, Holter monitoring	Often indicated in the patient with suspected cardiogenic syncope, transient ischemic attack, or stroke
Cerebrospinal fluid for herpes simplex polymerase chain reaction	If encephalitis is suspected
Creatine kinase and troponin	In patients with known or suspected heart disease to help rule out a myocardial ischemia-induced arrhythmia
In-patient monitoring	May be indicated if the diagnosis is uncertain

Further Reading

Angus-Leppan H. First seizures in adults. *BMJ.* 2014;348:g2470.

Bradford JC, Kyriakedes CG. Evaluation of the patient with seizures: an evidence based approach. *Emerg Med Clin North Am.* 1999;17:203–220.

Roth HL, Drislane FW. Seizures. *Neurol Clin.* 1998;16:257–284.

Schachter SC. Seizure disorders. *Primary Care: Clinics in Office Practice.* 2004;31:85–94.

Velez L, Selwa LM. Seizure disorders in the elderly. *Am Fam Physician.* 2003;67:325–332.

Willmore LJ. Epilepsy emergencies: the first seizure and status epilepticus. *J Neurol.* 1998;51:S034–38.

Wills B, Erickson T. Drug- and toxin-associated seizures. *Med Clin North Am.* 2005;89:1297–1321.

68 SOLITARY PULMONARY NODULE

General Discussion

A solitary pulmonary nodule is radiologically defined as an intraparenchymal lung lesion that is less than 3 cm in diameter and is not associated with atelectasis or adenopathy. Lung lesions greater than 3 cm in diameter are defined as lung masses. Approximately 1 in 500 chest radiographs demonstrates a lung nodule, most of which are incidental findings. The incidence of cancer in patients with solitary nodules ranges from 10% to 70%. Infectious granulomas cause approximately 80% of the benign lesions, and hamartomas cause approximately 10% of these lesions. Factors that increase the probability that a solitary pulmonary nodule is malignant include older age, a history of cigarette smoking, and a history of malignancy.

Certain radiologic characteristics also influence the probability of malignancy. The size of a lung nodule is correlated with the likelihood of malignancy. Most lung nodules greater than 2 cm in size are malignant, whereas 50% of nodules less than 2 cm are malignant. Two patterns of the margins of a nodule suggest cancer. The first is the corona radiata sign, consisting of very fine linear strands that extend 4 to 5 mm outward from the nodule. These have a spiculated appearance on plain radiographs. The second potentially concerning pattern is a scalloped border, which is associated with an intermediate probability of cancer. A smooth border is more suggestive of a benign diagnosis. Likewise, if benign-appearing central calcifications are seen within the solitary pulmonary nodule, further diagnostic testing usually is not indicated. Calcification patterns that are stippled or eccentric may be suggestive of malignancy and warrant further evaluation.

If a solitary pulmonary nodule is found on a chest x-ray, all previous chest x-rays should be reviewed. Rate of growth can aid in determining the likelihood of malignancy. Malignant lesions typically have a doubling time between 1 month and 1 year. Thus, a solitary pulmonary nodule that is unchanged on chest x-ray for at least 2 years is more likely to be benign. The growth rate of a nodule can be estimated if previous images are available. A 30% increase in diameter represents a doubling of volume. If a lesion doubles in less than 1 month or if a nodule was not present on a radiograph obtained less than 2 months before the current image, it is not likely to be malignant.

All patients with unclearly characterized solitary pulmonary nodules on chest radiography should be evaluated with chest computed tomography (CT). CT is the imaging modality of choice to reevaluate pulmonary nodules seen on chest radiographs and to follow nodules on subsequent studies for change in size. In addition to characterizing the nodule, CT can also be used to identify other lung lesions, metastatic disease, or lymphadenopathy.

Fluorodeoxyglucose-positron emission tomography (FDG-PET) has a high sensitivity and specificity for evaluating nodules greater than 8 to 10 mm in diameter. Increased activity is demonstrated in cells with high metabolic rates, as is seen in tumors and areas of inflammation. FDG-PET may also provide staging information. FDG-PET is likely most cost-effective for patients with discordant pretest probability and CT results.

In a patient with a new finding of a solitary pulmonary nodule and a recent history of pneumonia or pulmonary symptoms, the patients may be followed for 4 to 6 weeks to rule out an infectious etiology. If the nodule persists, further diagnostic evaluation is indicated.

Any patient who has evidence of a nodule with notable growth during follow-up or with a positive FDG-PET result should undergo further evaluation, typically with biopsy by excision, needle biopsy, or bronchoscopy. For operable patients with a solitary pulmonary nodule who decline surgical intervention, transthoracic needle aspiration or transbronchial needle biopsy is the preferred procedure for establishing a diagnosis. For patients with a solitary pulmonary nodule who are not operable candidates or are at high risk, transthoracic needle aspiration may be helpful to establish tissue diagnosis. Bronchoscopy is often a good approach for obtaining a tissue diagnosis for a large central lung mass or in those with endobronchial encroachment. There is little role for bronchoscopy in patients with a peripheral lung nodule.

If a solitary pulmonary nodule is new and does not have benign-appearing calcifications, it should be considered to be a malignancy until proven otherwise. Surgical resection is the ideal approach, because it is both diagnostic and therapeutic.

Fleischner Society Recommendations for Follow-up and Management of Nodules Smaller Than 8 mm Detected Incidentally at Nonscreening CT		
Nodule Size (mm)*	Low-Risk Patient†	High-Risk Patient‡
≤4	No follow-up needed§	Follow-up CT at 12 mo; if unchanged, no further follow-up‖
>4–6	Follow-up CT at 12 mo; if unchanged, no further follow-up‖	Initial follow-up CT at 6–12 mo then at 18–24 mo if no change‖
>6–8	Initial follow-up CT at 6–12 mo then at 18–24 mo if no change	Initial follow-up CT at 3–6 mo then at 9–12 and 24 mo if no change
>8	Follow-up CT at around 3, 9, and 24 mo, dynamic contrast-enhanced CT, PET, and/or biopsy	Same as for low-risk patient

Note.—Newly detected indeterminate nodule in persons 35 years of age or older.
* Average of length and width.
† Minimal or absent history of smoking and of other known risk factors.
‡ History of smoking or of other known risk factors.
§ The risk of malignancy in this category (<1%) is substantially less than that in a baseline CT scan of an asymptomatic smoker.
‖ Nonsolid (ground-glass) or partly solid nodules may require longer follow-up to exclude indolent adenocarcinoma.

Figure 68-1. *CT,* Computed tomography; *PET,* positron emission tomography. (From MacMahon H, Austin JH, Gamsu G, et al. Guidelines for management of small pulmonary nodules detected on CT scans: a statement from the Fleischner Society. *Radiology* 2005;237:395–400, Table 1.)

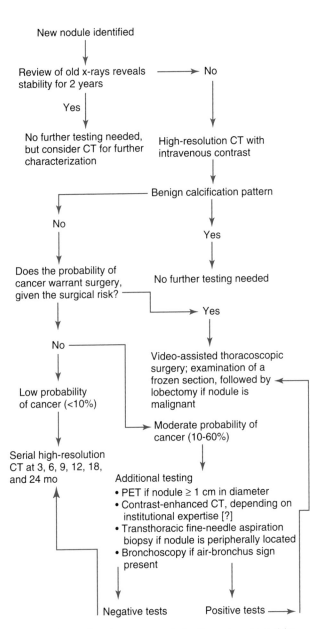

Figure 68-2. Approach to the management of solitary pulmonary nodules. *CT*, Computed tomography; *PET*, positron emission tomography. (From Ost D, Fein AM, Feinsilver SH. The solitary pulmonary nodule. *New England Journal of Medicine* 2003;348:2535–2542; Figure 2.)

Further Reading

Albert RH, Russell JJ. Evaluation of the solitary pulmonary nodule. *Am Fam Physician.* 2009;80:827–831.

Hodnett PA, Ko JP. Evaluation and management of intermediate pulmonary nodules. *Radiol Clin N Am.* 2012;50:895–914.

Lederlin M, Revel MP, Khalil A, et al. Management strategy of pulmonary nodule in 2013. *Diagnostic and Interventional Imaging.* 2013;94:1081–1094.

Lippy DM, Smith JP, Altorki NK, et al. Managing the small pulmonary nodule discovered by CT. *Chest.* 2004;125:1522–1529.

MacMahon H, Austin JH, Gamsu G, et al. Guidelines for management of small pulmonary nodules detected on CT scans: a statement from the Fleischner Society. *J Radiol.* 2005;237:395–400.

Ost D, Fein AM, Feinsilver SH. The solitary pulmonary nodule. *N Engl J Med.* 2003; 348:2535–2542.

Skouras VS, Tanner NT, Silvestri GA. Diagnostic approach to the solitary pulmonary nodule. *Semin Repir Crit Care Med.* 2013;34:762–769.

Tan BB, Flaherty KR, Kazerooni EA, Iannettoni MD. The solitary pulmonary nodule. *Chest.* 2003;123:89–96.

Yankelevitz DF, Henschke CI. Small solitary pulmonary nodules. *Radiol Clin North Am.* 2000;38:471–478.

69 SYNCOPE

General Discussion

Syncope is a sudden, unexpected loss of consciousness associated with a loss of postural tone with spontaneous recovery. A syncopal event is one of the more dramatic and anxiety-provoking symptoms encountered by patients and often produces a diagnostic dilemma for the clinician. However, syncope is a common manifestation of numerous disorders, with a final common pathway of insufficient cerebral blood flow to maintain consciousness. Syncope must be differentiated from other disorders of altered consciousness, including seizures, sleep disorders, metabolic disorders, vertigo, presyncope, and psychiatric disorders.

In the evaluation of syncope, proving a specific diagnosis is often difficult because of a lack of residual abnormalities on examination or on initial diagnostic studies. The clinician must remember that syncope is a symptom, and not a disease. By possessing an understanding of the common etiologies that cause syncope, the clinician can focus on the history, physical examination, and diagnostic evaluation in each specific case. An understanding of the available diagnostic tests and their indications is imperative.

The differential diagnosis of syncope is broad, and prevalence varies depending on the research methods used in each study. The most common causes are vasovagal syncope, arrhythmias, and orthostatic hypotension. As many as one-half of patients have syncope of an unknown cause after a standard diagnostic evaluation.

Many algorithms exist for the evaluation of syncope, and most emphasize the importance of the history and physical examination in making an accurate diagnosis. A position paper published by the American College of Physicians presents the following important features in guiding diagnosis:

- Separate patients into diagnostic, suggestive, and unexplained categories on the basis of the history, physical examination, and electrocardiographic (ECG) findings.
- Separate patients with unexplained syncope further on the basis of age and the presence of organic heart disease or an abnormal ECG.
- Use echocardiography and treadmill stress testing to evaluate and quantify the degree of heart disease.
- Reserve Holter monitoring and electrophysiology studies for patients with confirmed heart disease.
- Employ tilt table testing, loop recorders, and psychiatric evaluation in patients with recurrent unexplained syncope and no suspected heart disease, or a negative cardiac evaluation.
- Although algorithms may provide a guide for the evaluation of syncope, the various available algorithms each contain

controversial elements. In addition, algorithms do not consider every clinical situation and are not designed to replace individual clinician judgment. The physician should understand the approach to the patient with syncope first, and then consult algorithms to focus the diagnostic evaluation.

Medications Associated with Syncope

Alpha-agonists
Antiarrhythmics
Anticholinergic agents
Antiemetics
Antihypertensives
Antiparkinsonian agents
Antipsychotics
Beta-adrenergic blockers
Diuretics
Macrolides
Narcotics
Tricyclic antidepressants
Vasodilators

Causes of Syncope

Reflex-mediated
- Vasovagal
- Situational (cough, defecation, micturition, swallow)
- Carotid sinus hypersensitivity

Cardiac
- Arrhythmia
  - Atrial fibrillation
  - Atrioventricular conduction system disease
  - Implanted device malfunction
  - Sinus node dysfunction
  - Supraventricular tachycardias
  - Ventricular tachycardias
- Structural heart disease
  - Acute aortic dissection
  - Acute myocardial infarction/ischemia
  - Cardiac masses (e.g., atrial myxoma)
  - Congenital coronary artery anomaly
  - Hypertrophic cardiomyopathy
  - Pericardial disease/tamponade
  - Prosthetic valve dysfunction

- Tamponade
- Valvular disease

Intoxication (drugs or alcohol)

Medication effects

Metabolic disorders
- Adrenal failure
- Hypercapnia
- Hypernatremia
- Hypoglycemia
- Hyponatremia
- Hypoxia

Neurologic causes
- Cataplexy
- Drop attack
- Migraine headache
- Transient ischemic attack (especially vertebrobasilar)

Orthostatic hypotension
- Guillain-Barré syndrome
- HIV infection
- Medication effects
- Paraneoplastic neuropathies
- Primary autonomic failure
  - Lewy body dementia
  - Multiple system atrophy
  - Parkinson disease with autonomic failure
  - Pure autonomic failure
- Secondary autonomic failure
  - Amyloidosis
  - Chronic inflammatory polyneuropathy
  - Connective tissue diseases
  - Diabetes
  - Spinal cord injury
  - Uremia
- Shy-Drager syndrome
- Volume depletion

Pulmonary embolism

Psychiatric causes
- Major depression
- Panic disorder
- Pseudoseizure

Other causes
- Hyperventilation
- Seizure (not a true case of syncope)
- Subclavian steal syndrome

Unknown

Key Historical Features

✓ Situation in which syncope occurred (upon standing, in a fearful situation, during micturition, with coughing, with exertion)
✓ Prodromal symptoms (lightheadedness, warmth, nausea, sweating)
✓ Associated cardiac symptoms (chest pain, palpitations, shortness of breath)
✓ Associated neurologic symptoms (focal neurologic symptoms, headache, diplopia)
✓ Witnessed events (tonic/clonic movements, tongue biting, urinary incontinence)
✓ History of syncope
✓ Recent dehydration
✓ Postevent symptoms
  • Confusion may indicate seizure activity
  • Injuries related to a fall
  • Duration of recovery
✓ Medical history, particularly:
  • History of cardiac disease, including coronary artery disease, arrhythmia, or cardiomyopathy
  • History of cerebrovascular ischemia
  • History of pulmonary embolism or pulmonary hypertension
  • History of gastrointestinal bleeding
✓ Family history of syncope or sudden death
✓ Medications
  • Especially antihypertensive agents, antidepressants, vasodilators, narcotic analgesics, Q-T prolonging agents (tricyclic antidepressants), and hypoglycemic agents
✓ Social history
  • Alcohol or marijuana use
  • Smoking history, which places the patient at risk for cardiopulmonary disease

Key Physical Findings

✓ Vitals signs
✓ Evaluation for orthostatic hypotension (defined as at least a 20 mm Hg systolic or 10 mm Hg diastolic blood pressure within 3 minutes of standing)
✓ Cardiovascular examination
  • Carotid bruit
  • Murmur
  • Jugular venous distention
  • Loud S2
  • Presence of an S3

- • Pericardial friction rub
- • Blood pressures in both the arms
✓ Neurologic evaluation
  - • Mental status
  - • Pupil symmetry
  - • Evaluation for nystagmus
  - • Gait
  - • Balance

Suggested Work-Up

Complete blood count, electrolytes, blood urea nitrogen, creatinine, and glucose	Indicated when an underlying disorder is suspected as a potential cause of syncope.
Pregnancy test	Should be considered in women of childbearing age
ECG	To identify abnormalities that may suggest an underlying cardiac cause for syncope. Important findings include evidence of conduction disorders, signs of coronary artery disease, or left ventricular hypertrophy that may be associated with ventricular tachycardia.
Holter monitoring or telemetry monitoring	Recommended for patients with known or suspected cardiac disease or a suspected arrhythmic cause of syncope.

Additional Work-Up

Tilt table testing	May be useful in patients with recurrent unexplained syncope with a suspected neurocardiogenic cause. May also be useful in patients without cardiac disease or in whom cardiac testing has been negative.
Echocardiography	To rule out a cardiac cause of syncope in patients with suspected cardiac disease. In patients with exertional syncope, echocardiography can help exclude hypertrophic cardiomyopathy and aortic stenosis.

Exercise tolerance testing	To confirm and quantify coronary artery disease in patients with syncope in whom coronary artery disease is suspected. Exercise tolerance testing may also be used to rule out coronary artery disease and exercise-induced arrhythmias in patients with exertional syncope.
Electrophysiology study	To diagnose conduction disease or susceptibility for developing tachyarrhythmias in patients with a suspected arrhythmic cause for their syncope and a history of known heart disease, especially previous myocardial infarction or congestive heart failure. May also be used for patients with pre-excitation syndromes such as Wolff-Parkinson-White syndrome and in patients with a suspected bradyarrhythmic cause for syncope, particularly older patients.
Transtelephonic ECG monitoring	Most useful in patients with frequent syncope and either no suspected cardiac disease or a negative cardiac evaluation.
Insertable loop recorder	May be useful in patients without evidence of neurocardiogenic syncope or organic heart disease and with infrequent episodes of syncope that make the use of an external loop recorder impractical.
Electroencephalogram (EEG)	The diagnostic yield of EEG is very low and is indicated only when seizure is suspected.
Computed tomography (CT)	CT scanning of the head has a relatively low yield in patients with syncope and is not routinely indicated. It is recommended in patients with focal neurologic symptoms and signs. It may be performed in patients with seizure activity and head trauma to rule out intracranial hemorrhage.

Vascular studies	Carotid ultrasonography and transcranial Doppler add little in the evaluation of syncope. Carotid disease or vertebrobasilar disease significant enough to cause a loss of consciousness would be unlikely in the absence of other neurologic signs such as diplopia, dysarthria, or vertigo.
Carotid sinus massage	May be considered in selected patients 40 years or older with an otherwise nondiagnostic evaluation for syncope.
Psychiatric evaluation	Recommended for patients with recurrent unexplained syncope if there is no cardiac disease or if the cardiac evaluation is negative. Young patients and patients with many prodromal symptoms are at higher risk of having an underlying psychiatric disease associated with their episodes of syncope.

Further Reading

Abboud FM. Neurocardiogenic syncope. *N Engl J Med.* 1993;328:1117–1120.

Atkins D, Hanusa B, Sefcik T, et al. Syncope and orthostatic hypotension. *Am J Med.* 1991;91:179–185.

Benditt DG, Adkisson WO. Approach to the patient with syncope: venues, presentations, diagnoses. *Cardiol Clin.* 2013;31:9–25.

Calkins H. Pharmacologic approaches to therapy for vasovagal syncope. *Am J Cardiol.* 1999;84:20Q–25Q.

Cunningham R, Mikhail MG. Management of patients with syncope and cardiac arrhythmias in an emergency department observation unit. *Emerg Med Clin North Am.* 2001;19:105–121.

Davis TL, Freemon FR. Electroencephalography should not be routine in the evaluation of syncope in adults. *Arch Intern Med.* 1990;150:2027–2029.

Di Girolamo E, Di Iorio C, Sabatini P, et al. Effects of paroxetine hydrochloride, a selective serotonin reuptake inhibitor, on refractory vasovagal syncope: a randomized, double-blind, placebo-controlled study. *J Am Coll Cardiol.* 1999;33:1227–1230.

Gauer RL. Evaluation of syncope. *Am Fam Physician.* 2011;84:640–650.

Kapoor WN. Syncope. *N Engl J Med.* 2000;343:1856–1862.

Kaufmann H. Neurally mediated syncope: pathogenesis, diagnosis, and treatment. *Neurology.* 1995;45(suppl 5):S12–S18.

Linzer M, Yang EH, Estes 3rd NA, et al. Diagnosing syncope: Part 1: value of history, physical examination and electrocardiography. Clinical efficacy assessment project of the American College of Physicians. *Ann Intern Med.* 1997;126:989–996.

Linzer M, Yang EH, Estes 3rd NA, et al. Diagnosing syncope: Part 2. Unexplained syncope. Clinical efficacy project of the American College of Physicians. *Ann Intern Med.* 1997;127:76–86.

Mahanonda N, Bhuripanyo K, Kangkagate C, et al. Randomized double-blind, placebo-controlled trial of oral atenolol in patients with unexplained syncope and positive upright tilt table test results. *Am Heart J.* 1995;130:1250–1253.

Munro NC, McIntosh S, Lawson J, et al. Incidence of complications after carotid sinus massage in older patients with syncope. *J Am Geriatr Soc.* 1994;42:1248–1251.

Puppala VK, Dickinson O, Benditt DG. Syncope: classification and risk stratification. *J Cardiol.* 2014;63:171–177.

Saklani P, Krahn A, Klein G. Syncope. *Circulation.* 2013;127:1330–1339.

Schnipper JL, Kapoor WN. Diagnostic evaluation and management of patients with syncope. *Med Clin North Am.* 2001;85:423–456.

Sutton R, Brignole M, Menozzi C, et al. Dual chamber pacing in the treatment of neurally mediated positive cardioinhibitory syncope: pacemaker versus no therapy—a multicenter randomized study. The Vasovagal Syncope International Study (VASIS) Investigators. *Circulation.* 2000;102:294–299.

Sutton R, Petersen M, Brignole M, et al. Proposed classification for tilt induced vasovagal syncope. *Eur J Pacing Electrophysiol.* 1992;3:180–183.

Ward CR, Gray JC, Gilroy JJ, et al. Midodrine: a role in the management of neurocardiogenic syncope. *Heart.* 1998;79:45–49.

Weimer LH. Syncope and orthostatic intolerance for the primary care physician. *Prim Care Clin Office Pract.* 2004;31:175–199.

Zeng C, Zhu Z, Liu G, et al. Randomized, double-blind, placebo-controlled trial of oral enalapril in patients with neurally mediated syncope. *Am Heart J.* 1998;136:852–858.

Zimetbaum P, Kim KY, Ho KK, et al. Utility of patient-activated cardiac event recorders in general clinical practice. *Am J Cardiol.* 1997;79:371–372.

General Discussion

Analysis of synovial fluid plays a major role in the diagnosis of joint disease. Several classification schemes have been used to help classify joint diseases. When using classification schemes, it is important to realize that considerable overlap may occur in synovial fluid findings among different groups. In addition, more than one diagnosis may be present, such as a septic joint in a patient with rheumatoid arthritis (RA). Findings on synovial fluid analysis may be classified as normal, noninflammatory, inflammatory, infectious, crystal-associated, and hemorrhagic.

Routine examination of synovial fluid should include: (1) gross examination of color and clarity; (2) total leukocyte and differential counts; (3) gram stain and bacterial culture (both aerobic and anaerobic); and (4) crystal examination with polarizing microscopy.

Additional studies may be indicated under certain circumstances and should be guided by clinical suspicion. These studies include fungal and acid-fast stains and cultures, countercurrent immunoelectrophoresis for bacterial antigens, lactate levels, complement levels, and the presence of certain enzymes, such as lactate dehydrogenase.

Suggested Work-Up

Physical characteristics of the fluid
- Color
- Clarity
- Viscosity

Microscopic appearance
- White blood count and differential
- Crystals (polarized light)

Microbiology
- Gram stain
- Bacterial culture (aerobic and anaerobic)

See Table 70-1 for the interpretation of findings.

Additional Work-Up

Fungal culture	If fungal arthritis is suspected
Culture for *Mycobacterium tuberculosis*	If tuberculous arthritis is suspected
Serum and synovial fluid glucose levels	A serum-synovia differential is less than 10 mg/dL in normal fluid and many noninflammatory conditions. In septic arthritis, the differential ranges

from 20 to 60 mg/dL but overlaps with other inflammatory conditions.

Serum and synovial fluid complement levels

Complement levels in synovial fluid normally are approximately 10% of serum levels. Inflammatory conditions increases this to 40% to 70% of serum levels.

Classification	Appearance	WBCs/μL	PMNs (%)	Crystals	Culture
Normal	Clear to straw-colored	<150	<25	No	Negative

Noninflammatory

Classification	Appearance	WBCs/μL	PMNs (%)	Crystals	Culture
Osteoarthritis Traumatic arthritis Neuroarthropathy Early RA Paget disease Acromegaly Hyperparathyroidism	Yellow, transparent	<3000	<30	No	Negative

Inflammatory

Classification	Appearance	WBCs/μL	PMNs (%)	Crystals	Culture
RA Lupus erythematosus Scleroderma Reactive arthritis Ankylosing spondylitis Rheumatic fever Ulcerative colitis Sarcoidosis Polymyalgia rheumatica	Yellow, cloudy, or bloody	3000–75,000	>50	No	Negative

Infectious

Classification	Appearance	WBCs/μL	PMNs (%)	Crystals	Culture
Bacterial Mycobacterial Fungal Viral Spirochetal	Yellow, purulent	50,000–200,000	>90	No	Often positive

Crystal-induced

Classification	Appearance	WBCs/μL	PMNs (%)	Crystals	Culture
Gout CPPD	Cloudy, turbid	500–200,000	<90	Yes	Negative

Hemorrhagic

Classification	Appearance	WBCs/μL	PMNs (%)	Crystals	Culture
Traumatic arthritis Hemophiliac arthropathy Anticoagulation Thrombocytopenia	Red-brown	50-10,000	<50	No	Negative

CPPD, Calcium pyrophosphate dihydrate; PMN, polymorphonuclear leukocyte; RA, rheumatoid arthritis; WBC, white blood cell.

Table 70-1 Classification of Synovial Fluid

Further Reading

Henry JB. Cerebrospinal, synovial, and serous body fluids. In: *Clinical Diagnosis and Management by Laboratory Methods*. Philadelphia: Saunders; 1996:467–472.

Kjeldsberg CR, Knight JA. Body fluids: laboratory examinations of amniotic, cerebrospinal, seminal, serous and synovial fluids. 3rd ed. Chicago: American Society of Clinical Pathologists.

O'Connell TX. Interpreting tests from joint aspirates. *Atlas Office Procedures*. 2000;5:423–431.

Schmerling RH, et al. Synovial fluid tests—what should be ordered? *JAMA*. 1990;260:1009.

Schumacher HR. Synovial fluid analysis and synovial biopsy. In: *Textbook of Rheumatology*. 4th ed. Philadelphia: Saunders; 1993:562–570.

Tierney LM, McPhee SJ, Papadakis MA. Arthritis and musculoskeletal disorders. In: *Current Medical Diagnosis and Treatment*. New York: Lange; 2000:807–808.

General Discussion

Thrombocytopenia is defined as a platelet count of less than 150,000 μL. Healthy women may experience mild to moderate thrombocytopenia in the range of 75,000 to 150,000/μL during pregnancy and do not require any investigation.

Thrombocytopenia arises from three main causes: ineffective production of platelets by bone marrow (e.g., aplastic anemia, myelodysplastic syndrome, lymphoma, leukemia, multiple myeloma); accelerated destruction of platelets (e.g., disseminated intravascular coagulation, immune thrombocytopenia); or sequestration of platelets in the spleen (e.g., secondary to portal hypertension).

The diagnostic evaluation of thrombocytopenia begins by excluding artifactual thrombocytopenia, or pseudothrombocytopenia, as the etiology. This is caused by platelet clumping when ethylenediaminetetra-acetic acid is used as an anticoagulant in the blood sample. The presence of platelet clumps on examination of the peripheral smear and a normal repeat platelet count using citrated blood confirms pseudothrombocytopenia as the cause.

After pseudothrombocytopenia has been excluded, the possibility of thrombotic thrombocytopenic purpura/hemolytic uremic syndrome (TTP/HUS) should be considered. A peripheral blood smear with schistocytes, increased serum levels of lactate dehydrogenase (LDH), and decreased serum haptoglobin suggest TTP/HUS or disseminated intravascular coagulation (DIC). Coagulation studies are usually normal in TTP/HUS, but they are prolonged in DIC.

Once TTP/HUS and DIC have been excluded, drug-related thrombocytopenia and hypersplenism should be considered as possible causes. There are two types of drug-induced thrombocytopenia caused by different mechanisms. The first is by the direct myelosuppressive effect, and the second is by immune-mediated destruction of platelets caused by a drug-induced immune response. If heparin-induced thrombocytopenia is considered, the diagnosis may be confirmed by in vitro testing to detect heparin-dependent platelet antibodies. Typically, thrombocytopenia will occur between 5 and 14 days of the first heparin dose.

Idiopathic thrombocytopenic purpura (ITP) is a diagnosis of exclusion. Other causes of immune-mediated thrombocytopenia should be considered. These include connective tissue disease, lymphoproliferative disorders, and HIV infection.

Medications Associated with Thrombocytopenia

Abciximab
Acetaminophen

Aminoglutethimide
Aminosalicylic acid
Amiodarone
Amphotericin B
Ampicillin
Amrinone
Captopril
Carbamazepine
Chlorothiazide
Chlorpromazine
Chlorpropamide
Cimetidine
Cisplatin
Clopidogrel
Cyclosporine A
Danazol
Deferoxamine
Diatrizoate meglumine
Diazepam
Diazoxide
Diclofenac
Diethylstilbestrol
Digoxin
Eptifibatide
Furosemide
Gold
Haloperidol
Heparin
Hydrochlorothiazide
Ibuprofen
Interferon-α
Isoniazid
Levamisole
Lithium
Meclofenamate
Methicillin
Methyldopa
Minoxidil
Mitomycin A
Nalidixic acid
Naphazoline
Oxyphenbutazone
Oxytetracycline
Phenytoin
Piperacillin

Procainamide
Quinidine
Quinine
Ranitidine
Rifampin
Sulfasalazine
Sulfisoxazole
Sulindac
Tamoxifen
Thiothixene
Ticlopidine
Tirofiban
Trimethoprim/sulfamethoxazole
Valproic acid
Vancomycin

Causes of Thrombocytopenia

Amegakaryocytic thrombocytopenia
Antiphospholipid syndrome
Aplastic anemia
Bernard-Soulier syndrome
Bone marrow transplantation
Cardiac bypass
Cardiac valves
Common variable hypogammaglobulinemia
Congenital thrombocytopenia
Connective tissue diseases
DIC
Escherichia coli O157:H7 infection
Epstein-Barr virus
Gray platelet syndrome
Hemolysis, Elevated Liver enzymes, Low Platelet count
    (HELLP) syndrome
Hematologic malignancies
HUS
Heparin-induced thrombocytopenia
Hepatitis C infection
Hereditary thrombocytopenias
HIV infection
Hypersplenism
ITP
Immunoglobulin-A deficiency
Kasabach Merrit syndrome
May-Hegglin anomaly
Medications

Metastatic cancer to bone marrow
Myelodysplastic syndrome
Paroxysmal nocturnal hemoglobinuria
Post-transfusion purpura
Pregnancy
Primary bone marrow disorder
Radiation
Rheumatoid arthritis
Sepsis
Systemic lupus erythematosus
TTP
Vitamin D deficiency
X-linked Wiskott-Aldrich syndrome

Key Historical Features

✓ Easy bruising
✓ Gingival bleeding
✓ Epistaxis
✓ Menorrhagia
✓ Gastrointestinal bleeding
✓ Recent viral or bacterial infection
✓ Medical history (especially a history of low platelet count, bleeding tendency, malignancy)
✓ Medications (especially those started 1–2 weeks before the development of thrombocytopenia)
✓ Use of over-the-counter products
✓ Dietary habits
✓ Family history of platelet disorders or bleeding tendency
✓ Recent travel (e.g., exposure to malaria, rickettsiosis, dengue fever)
✓ Recent transfusion
✓ Recent vaccination
✓ Alcohol consumption
✓ HIV risk factors

Key Physical Findings

✓ Vital signs
✓ Head and neck examination for evidence of bleeding in the mucous membranes
✓ Funduscopic examination for evidence of retinal hemorrhage
✓ Lymphadenopathy
✓ Evidence of bleeding in the skin
✓ Cardiac examination for tachycardia
✓ Abdominal examination for splenomegaly or hepatomegaly

✓ Rectal examination including stool occult blood testing to evaluate for gastrointestinal bleeding

✓ Neurologic examination to help evaluate for intracranial bleed

Suggested Work-Up

Complete blood count	Particular attention should be paid to whether anemia and/or leukopenia are also present
Peripheral blood smear	To evaluate for schistocytes (hemolysis), atypical lymphocytes (many viral infections), blasts (leukemia), giant platelets (hereditary thrombocytopenias)
Serum LDH	Increased in hemolysis
Indirect bilirubin	Increased in hemolysis
Serum haptoglobin	Decreased in hemolysis
Prothrombin time (PT), partial thrombin time, fibrin split products, fibrinogen, D-dimer	Prolonged PT, low fibrinogen, and elevated D-dimer suggest disseminated intravascular coagulation
Blood urea nitrogen and creatinine	Elevated LDH with impaired renal function may indicate TTP or HUS
Liver function tests	Abnormal in hepatic diseases such as viral hepatitis, drug-induced hepatitis, and cirrhosis

Additional Work-Up

Pregnancy test	If pregnancy is suspected
Antiplatelet antibodies	If immune thrombocytopenia is suspected
Coombs test	If hemolysis is suspected
HIV antinuclear antibodies, and serum protein electrophoresis	Should be ordered before ITP is diagnosed to evaluate for HIV infection, autoimmune disease, and lymphoproliferative disease
Vitamin B_{12} and folate levels	If nutritional causes of thrombocytopenia are suspected
Blood cultures	If bacteremia is suspected
Bone marrow examination	Indicated when a platelet production problem is suspected. In older adult patients, patients with abnormalities in red and/or white cells, and patients without a definitive cause after initial workup, a bone marrow biopsy may elucidate the presence of a primary marrow disorder.

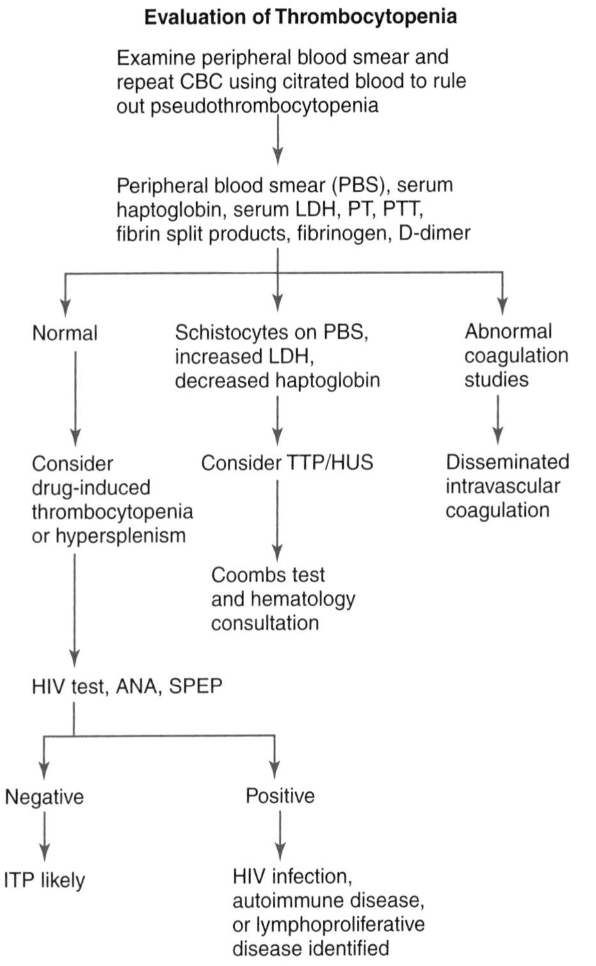

Evaluation of Thrombocytopenia

Examine peripheral blood smear and repeat CBC using citrated blood to rule out pseudothrombocytopenia

Peripheral blood smear (PBS), serum haptoglobin, serum LDH, PT, PTT, fibrin split products, fibrinogen, D-dimer

Normal

Schistocytes on PBS, increased LDH, decreased haptoglobin

Abnormal coagulation studies

Consider drug-induced thrombocytopenia or hypersplenism

Consider TTP/HUS

Disseminated intravascular coagulation

Coombs test and hematology consultation

HIV test, ANA, SPEP

Negative

Positive

ITP likely

HIV infection, autoimmune disease, or lymphoproliferative disease identified

Figure 71-1. Evaluation of Thrombocytopenia. *CBC*, complete blood count; *LDH*, lactate dehydrogenase; *PT*, prothrombin time; *PTT*, partial thromboplastin time; *TTP*, thrombotic thrombocytopenic purpura; *HUS*, hemolytic uremic syndrome; *ANA*, antinuclear antibody; *ITP*, idiopathic thrombocytopenic purpura; *SPEP*, serum protein electrophoresis.

Further Reading

Cines DB, Blanchette VS. Immune thrombocytopenic purpura. *N Engl J Med.* 2002;346:995–1008.

Izak M, Bussel JB. Management of thrombocytopenia. *F1000Prime Reports.* 2014;6:45.

Sekhon SS, Roy V. Thrombocytopenia in adults: a practical approach to evaluation and management. *South Med J.* 2006;99:491–498.

Tefferi A, Hanson CA, Inwards DJ. How to interpret and pursue an abnormal complete blood cell count in adults. *Mayo Clin Proc.* 2005;80:923–936.

Vandendries ER, Drews RE. Drug-associated disease: hematologic dysfunction. *Crit Care Clin.* 2006;22:347–355.

General Discussion

The prevalence of palpable thyroid nodules is 4% to 7% in adults in North America, but they are found incidentally in up to 40% of patients who undergo ultrasonography of the neck. Some studies estimate that 20% to 76% of the population has at least one thyroid nodule. Thyroid nodules are more common in older adults, in women, in those with iodine deficiency, and in those with a history of radiation exposure. The clinical importance of thyroid nodules is primarily the need to exclude the presence of malignancy. The rate of malignancy is 5% in palpable thyroid nodules, regardless of the size of the nodule, and 1.5% to 17% in nodules detected incidentally during imaging performed for non-thyroid–related reasons.

Factors that may increase the risk of thyroid cancer include a history of head and neck irradiation (especially in childhood), a family history of medullary thyroid carcinoma or multiple endocrine neoplasia type 2, age younger than 20 years or older than 70 years, male gender, a growing nodule, a firm nodule, cervical lymphadenopathy, a fixed nodule, dysphonia, dysphagia, or cough.

The primary goal when evaluating a thyroid nodule is to determine whether it is malignant. Current guidelines recommend the same diagnostic strategy for both palpable nodules and nodules found incidentally during diagnostic imaging performed for other reasons.

Key Historical Features

✓ Age
✓ Gender
✓ Symptoms of hypo- or hyperthyroidism
✓ Rate of growth of the nodule
✓ Duration of the nodule
✓ Pain
✓ History of radiation to the head or neck
✓ Recent pregnancy
✓ Family history of autoimmune thyroid disease, thyroid carcinoma, multiple endocrine neoplasia, or familial polyposis
✓ Symptoms such as dysphagia, dysphonia, or hemoptysis
✓ Difficulty swallowing

Key Physical Findings

✓ Size of the nodule
✓ Fixation of the nodule to skin or soft tissue
✓ Movement of the nodule with swallowing
✓ Tenderness to palpation
✓ Presence of cervical lymphadenopathy

Suggested Work-Up

Thyroid-stimulating hormone (TSH)	To confirm a euthyroid state or detect the presence of hypo- or hyperthyroidism
Thyroid ultrasound	To detect features suggestive of malignant growth and select the lesions to be recommended for fine needle aspiration biopsy, to look for coincidental thyroid nodules, to measure the baseline volume of the lesion, and to help choose the size of the biopsy needle
Fine needle aspiration	Recommended in the following situations:

1. Nodules larger than 1 cm
2. Nodules of any size if ultrasonography suggests extracapsular invasion by the lesion or shows cervical lymphadenopathy
3. History of head and neck irradiation
4. History of thyroid cancer
5. History of multiple endocrine neoplasia (MEN) type 2 in a first-degree relative

More than one nodule should be biopsied if multiple nodules are found on ultrasonography. Nodules 1 cm or smaller may be followed with serial ultrasonography. Hyperfunctioning nodules do not need to be biopsied.

Radionuclide scintigraphy with technetium-99 m or iodine-123	Should be performed if TSH is suppressed to determine whether there are hyperfunctioning nodules or whether the entire thyroid gland is overactive as in toxic multinodular goiter

Additional Work-Up

Calcitonin level	Guidelines are unclear about the utility of routinely measuring the calcitonin level. Calcitonin levels are elevated in patients with medullary thyroid carcinoma, but this disease is rare. Recent guidelines recommend measuring calcitonin levels in patients with thyroid nodules and a family history or clinical suspicion of medullary thyroid carcinoma or MEN type 2.
Complete blood count and erythrocyte sedimentation rate	If inflammatory or infectious thyroiditis is suspected
Thyroperoxidase antibody, T4, and thyroglobulin test	May be helpful in the diagnosis of Graves disease or Hashimoto thyroiditis when the initial TSH is elevated

Further Reading

Cooper DS, Doherty GM, Haugen BR, et al. American Thyroid Association (ATA) guidelines taskforce on thyroid nodules and differentiated thyroid cancer. Revised American Thyroid Association management guidelines for patients with thyroid nodules and differentiated thyroid cancer. *Thyroid.* 2009;19:1167–1214. [published corrections appear in Thyroid. 2010;20:674–675, and Thyroid 2010;20:942].

Gharib H, Papini E, Paschke R, et al. AACE/AME/ETA Task Force on Thyroid Nodules. American Association of Clinical Endocrinologists, Associazone Medici Endocrinologi, and European Thyroid Association medical guidelines for clinical practice for the diagnosis and management of thyroid nodules: executive summary of recommendations. *J Endocrinol Invest.* 2010;33(5 suppl):51–56.

Kim N, Lavertu P. Evaluation of a thyroid nodule. *Otolaryngol Clin North Am.* 2003;26:17–33.

Knox MA. Thyroid nodules. *Am Fam Physician.* 2013;88:193–196.

Marsh DJ, Learoyd DL, Robinson BG. Medullary thyroid carcinoma: recent advances and management update. *Thyroid.* 1995;5:407–424.

Stang MT, Carty SE. Recent developments in predicting thyroid malignancy. *Curr Opin Oncol.* 2009;21:11–17.

Welker MJ, Orlov D. Thyroid nodules. *Am Fam Physician.* 2003;67:559–566.

Yeung MJ, Serpell JW. Management of the solitary thyroid nodule. *Oncologist.* 2008;13:105–112.

Yoon DY, Chang SK, Choi CS, et al. The prevalence and significance of incidental thyroid nodules identified on computed tomography. *J Comput Assist Tomogr.* 2008;32:810–815.

73 TINNITUS

General Discussion

Tinnitus is an unwanted auditory perception in the absence of sound input external to the patient. Tinnitus affects 10% to 15% of the U.S. population, with the prevalence increasing with age. Other factors that may affect the prevalence of tinnitus include gender, race, socioeconomic status, hearing loss, and noise exposure.

The most accepted theory of tinnitus pathophysiology is that of outer hair cell damage, which results in altered stiffness and thus in increased discharge rates. When the discharge rate rises above the background level, tinnitus becomes troublesome. The physician's role is to determine which factors may have led to the increase in the discharge rate and which factors diminish it.

Tinnitus is often classified as either subjective or objective. Subjective tinnitus is the most common and is audible only to the patient without internal or external sound input. Objective tinnitus accounts for less than 1% of cases and involves the perception of an internal sound, such as a bruit, as tinnitus. Subjective tinnitus is heard only by the patient, whereas objective tinnitus can be heard by both the patient and the examiner. Objective tinnitus usually has an identifiable acoustic source, whereas subjective tinnitus is more commonly idiopathic. Tinnitus can be further classified by whether it is pulsatile or nonpulsatile, and it can also be graded based upon volume or severity. Unilateral or pulsatile tinnitus is more likely to represent serious underlying disease and generally warrants an evaluation by an otolaryngologist.

Medications Associated with Tinnitus

Aminoglycosides
Amphotericin B
Antiarrhythmics
Anticonvulsants
Antihypertensives
Antiulcer medications
Aspirin
Atorvastatin
Bumetanide
Bupivacaine
Bupropion
Chemotherapy agents
- Bleomycin
- Cisplatin
- Etoposide

- - Mechlorethamine
  - Methotrexate
  - Vincristine
- Chloramphenicol
- Chloroquine
- Erythromycin
- Ethacrynic acid
- Fluoroquinolones
- Furosemide
- Ganciclovir
- Heterocyclic antidepressants
- Hormones
- Imipenem/cilastatin
- Lidocaine
- Linezolid
- Loop diuretics
- Macrolides
- Nonsteroidal anti-inflammatory drugs
- Psychotropic medications
- Quinine
- Ribavirin
- Risedronate
- Sulfasalazine
- Sulfonamides
- Tetracyclines
- Vancomycin
- Varenicline
- Voriconazole

Causes of Tinnitus

- Acoustic neuroma
- Arterial bruit
- Arteriovenous malformation
- Carotid atherosclerosis
- Chiari malformation (type 1)
- Cholesteatoma
- Dissection
- Head or neck injury
- Hearing loss
- Heavy metal exposure (mercury, lead)
- Hyperlipidemia
- Idiopathic stapedial muscle spasm
- Idiopathic tensor tympani muscle spasm

Infectious etiology
- Bacterial
- Fungal
- Viral

Lead
Medications
Meniere disease
Mercury
Multiple sclerosis
Paget disease
Palatal myoclonus
Patulous eustachian tube
Spontaneous intracranial hypotension
Substance use
Temporomandibular joint dysfunction
Thyroid disorder
Vascular tumors
Venous hum
Vestibular migraine
Vestibular schwannoma
Vitamin B_{12} deficiency
Psychogenic causes
- Anxiety
- Depression
- Fibromyalgia

Key Historical Features

✓ Onset (gradual or abrupt)
✓ Unilateral or bilateral
✓ Pattern (continuous, episodic, pulsatile)
✓ Pitch, quality, loudness
✓ Exacerbating and ameliorating factors
✓ Associated vertigo, hearing loss, aural fullness
✓ Presence of hearing loss
✓ Exposure to ototoxic medications
✓ Previous long-term noise exposure
✓ Acoustic trauma
✓ Head or neck trauma
✓ Headaches
✓ Medical history, especially thyroid disorders, hyperlipidemia, vitamin B_{12} deficiency, anemia
✓ Family history of tinnitus or hearing loss
✓ Medications

Key Physical Findings

✓ Inspection of the external canal and tympanic membrane
✓ Examination of the head, eyes, nose, throat, and neck
✓ Cranial nerve examination
✓ Auscultation over the neck, peri-auricular area, mastoid, and orbits
✓ Weber and Rinne tests

Suggested Work-Up

Audiography	Helps determine need for more advanced diagnostic testing and evaluates for hearing loss
Speech discrimination testing	May help detect pathology in the central nervous system
Tympanometry	To help identify middle ear effusions, changes in tympanic membrane stiffness, or myoclonus of the stapedial muscle

Additional Work-Up

Magnetic resonance imaging (MRI) of the internal auditory canals	For patients with unilateral tinnitus and sensorineural hearing loss and those with asymmetric hearing loss suspicious of an acoustic neuroma
Computed tomography (CT) of the temporal bones	For patients suspected of having hereditary hearing loss, otosclerosis, Paget disease, or trauma
Vestibular testing with electronystagmography	For patients with suspected Meniere disease
Doppler ultrasonography or neck CT, or neck MRI	For patients with an arterial bruit
Magnetic resonance venography	For patients with suspected venous pulsatile tinnitus
Lumbar puncture with measurement of cerebrospinal fluid pressure	For patients with suspected idiopathic intracranial hypertension
Referral to an otolaryngologist	For patients with unilateral or pulsatile tinnitus

Laboratory tests seldom reveal a treatable cause of tinnitus. However, the following tests may be considered if the history and physical examination suggest an underlying medical abnormality:

Thyroid-stimulating hormone	To evaluate for thyroid disorder
Hemoglobin and hematocrit	To evaluate for anemia
Serum glucose	To evaluate for diabetes
Electrolytes, blood urea nitrogen, creatinine	To evaluate for metabolic derangements
Lipid panel	To evaluate for hyperlipidemia
Rapid plasma reagin (RPR)	To evaluate for neurosyphilis
Consider erythrocyte sedimentation rate, antinuclear antibody (ANA), rheumatoid factor (RF)	If autoimmune disease is suspected

Further Reading

Cianfrone G, Pentangelo D, Cianfrone E, et al. Pharmacologic drugs inducing ototoxicity, vestibular symptoms and tinnitus: a reasoned and updated guide. *Eur Rev Med Pharmacol Sci.* 2011;15:601–636.

Crummer RW, Hassan GA. Diagnostic approach to tinnitus. *Am Fam Physician.* 2004;69:120–126.

Heller AJ. Classification and epidemiology of tinnitus. *Otolaryngol Clin North Am.* 2003;36:239–248.

Lockwood AH. Tinnitus. *Neurol Clin.* 2005;23:893–900.

Meyerhoff WL, Cooper JC. Tinnitus. In: Paparella MM, ed. *Otolaryngology.* 3rd ed. Philadelphia: Saunders; 1991:1169–1175.

Schwaber MK. Medical evaluation of tinnitus. *Otolaryngol Clin North Am.* 2003;36:287–292.

Seligman H, Podoshin L, Ben-David J, Fradis M, Goldsher M. Drug-induced tinnitus and other hearing disorders. *Drug Saf.* 1996;14:198–212.

Tyler RS. Does tinnitus originate from hyperactive nerve fibers in the cochlea? *J Neurophysiol.* 1984;44:76–96.

Yew KS. Diagnostic approach to patients with tinnitus. *Am Fam Physician.* 2014;89:106–113.

General Discussion

The following discussion applies to mild elevations of liver transaminase levels (up to 5 times normal) in asymptomatic patients. If there is any evidence of chronic liver disease or hepatic decompensation by laboratory tests or physical examination findings, an expedited workup should be pursued. Both alanine aminotransferase (ALT) and aspartate aminotransferase (AST) are released into the blood in increasing amounts when the liver cell membrane is damaged. However, necrosis of liver cells is not required for the release of the aminotransferases, and there is a poor correlation between the level of the aminotransferases and the degree of liver cell damage.

The National Health and Nutrition Examination Survey found elevated liver transaminase levels in up to 8.9% of the survey population. Not all people with a single, isolated, mildly elevated liver enzyme value have underlying liver disease, nor do they require an extensive evaluation. Mildly elevated liver enzymes are common and potentially important, yet very few well-designed prospective studies have addressed the issue of what should be done once they are identified.

The first step in the evaluation of the patient is to confirm the abnormality by repeating the blood test. If an enzyme elevation is confirmed, further investigation is warranted. A detailed history, review of medications, and a physical examination can provide crucial clues in the initial workup. The history should include an assessment of the patient's risk factors for liver disease, with attention directed toward family history, medications, vitamins, herbal supplements, alcohol consumption, drug use, history of blood product transfusions, and symptoms of liver disease. Signs of liver disease are outlined in the following.

If medication or alcohol is a suspected cause, aminotransferase levels should be repeated after 6 to 8 weeks of abstinence. A patient who is initially seen with elevated aminotransferase can be monitored if: (1) there is no clear risk factor for liver disease; (2) liver enzyme levels are less than three times normal; (3) liver function (as gauged by serum bilirubin, albumin, and prothrombin time) is preserved; and (4) the patient feels well.

Nonalcoholic fatty liver disease (NAFLD) is the leading cause of mild transaminase elevations and is becoming more prevalent as the obesity rate increases. NAFLD includes hepatic steatosis and nonalcoholic steatohepatitis. Hepatic steatosis is more common and generally does not progress to severe liver disease or cirrhosis. Nonalcoholic steatohepatitis increases the risk of progression to end-stage liver disease, cirrhosis, and hepatocellular carcinoma. NAFLD should be considered in patients who are obese or who have diabetes mellitus, hypertriglyceridemia, or metabolic syndrome.

Other common causes of elevated aminotransferase levels are alcohol-related liver injury, hepatitis B, hepatitis C, and hemochromatosis. Less common causes include autoimmune hepatitis, Wilson disease, α_1-antitrypsin deficiency, and celiac disease.

Medications Associated with Transaminase Elevation

Acarbose
Acetaminophen
Allopurinol
Amiodarone
Amoxicillin-clavulanic acid
Azathioprine
Baclofen
Buproprion
Carbamazepine
Ciprofloxacin
Corticosteroids
Fluconazole
Glipizide
Glyburide
Highly active antiretroviral therapy
Heparin
Hydralazine
Isoniazid
Ketoconazole
Labetalol
Lisinopril
Losartan
Methotrexate
Methyldopa
Nitrofurantoin
Nonsteroidal anti-inflammatory drugs
Omeprazole
Phenytoin
Protease inhibitors
Pyrazinamide
Quinidine
Risperidone
Selective serotonin reuptake inhibitors
Statins
Sulfonamides
Synthetic penicillins
Tetracyclines
Trazodone
Valproic acid

Causes of Transaminase Elevation

Acquired muscle disorders/myopathy

Acute fatty liver of pregnancy

Acute viral hepatitis

Adrenal insufficiency

Alcoholic liver disease

Alpha$_1$-antitrypsin deficiency

Amyloidosis

Anorexia nervosa

Autoimmune hepatitis

Cardiac disease

Celiac disease

Cirrhosis

Hemolysis, Elevated Liver enzymes, Low Platelet count (HELLP) syndrome

Hemochromatosis

Hemolysis

Hepatitis A, B, C, D, E

Hyperthyroidism

Inherited disorders of muscle metabolism

Macro AST

Medications

Neoplasm

NAFLD

Nonprescription medications and supplements

- Alchemilla
- Anabolic steroids
- Chaparral leaf
- Cocaine
- Ecstasy (3,4-methylenedioxymethamphetamine; MDMA)
- Ephedra (mahuang)
- Gentian
- Germander
- Glues containing toluene
- Jin bu huan
- Kava
- Phencyclidine
- Scutellaria (skullcap)
- Senna
- Shark cartilage
- Solvents
- Trichloroethylene
- Vitamin A

Primary biliary cirrhosis

Primary sclerosing cholangitis

Sarcoidosis

Secondary cholangitis
Steatosis/steatohepatitis
Strenuous exercise
Thyroid disorders
Vascular disease
- Budd-Chiari syndrome
- Ischemic hepatitis
- Sinusoidal obstruction syndrome

Viral illnesses
- Cytomegalovirus
- Epstein-Barr virus
- Herpes simplex virus
- Severe acute respiratory syndrome
- Varicella zoster virus

Wilson disease (in patients younger than 40 years old)

Key Historical Features

✓ Abdominal pain
✓ Medical history
✓ Surgical history
✓ Family history, especially a history of liver disease
✓ Medications
- Prescription
- Over-the-counter
- Herbal supplements

✓ Alcohol use
✓ Risk factors for viral hepatitis
- Intravenous drug use
- Intranasal cocaine use
- Unsafe sexual activity
- Blood product transfusion

✓ Native of an endemic area of the world

Key Physical Findings

✓ Ascites
✓ Bleeding problems
✓ Caput medusae
✓ Gynecomastia
✓ Hemorrhoids
✓ Impotence
✓ Jaundice
✓ Liver size
✓ Mental status changes
✓ Palmar erythema
✓ Spider angiomata

✓ Splenomegaly
✓ Testicular atrophy

Suggested Work-Up

ALT and AST	To confirm the elevation: AST:ALT ratio >2 suggests alcohol abuse; AST:ALT ratio <1 suggests NAFLD
Lipid profile	To screen for hyperlipidemia and metabolic syndrome
Glucose level	To screen for diabetes and metabolic syndrome
Hepatitis B surface antigen	To screen for hepatitis B
Hepatitis C antibody	To screen for hepatitis C
Serum iron, ferritin, and total iron-binding capacity	To screen for hemochromatosis. Confirm with HFE genotyping.
Ultrasonography	Should be considered to evaluate for fatty liver disease and other causes of transaminase elevation
Complete blood count, prothrombin time, and albumin	If there are concerns about the synthetic function of the liver

Additional Work-Up

Serum ceruloplasmin, 24-hour urine copper level, and ophthalmologic examination	If Wilson disease is suspected. Decreased ceruloplasmin level suggests Wilson disease.
Serum protein electrophoresis	Increase in polyclonal immunoglobulins suggests autoimmune hepatitis. Marked decrease in α-globulin bands suggests α_1-antitrypsin deficiency.
Antimitochondrial antibody	To evaluate for primary biliary cirrhosis
Antinuclear antibody, anti-smooth muscle antibody, and anti-liver/kidney microsomal antibody type I testing	To evaluate for autoimmune hepatitis
Alpha$_1$-antitrypsin phenotyping	To evaluate for α_1-antitrypsin deficiency
Tissue transglutaminase antibody	To evaluate for celiac disease
Serum thyroid-stimulating hormone	To evaluate for thyroid disorders
Creatine kinase and aldolase	If rhabdomyolysis or polymyositis is suspected
Liver biopsy	Used on a case-by-case basis

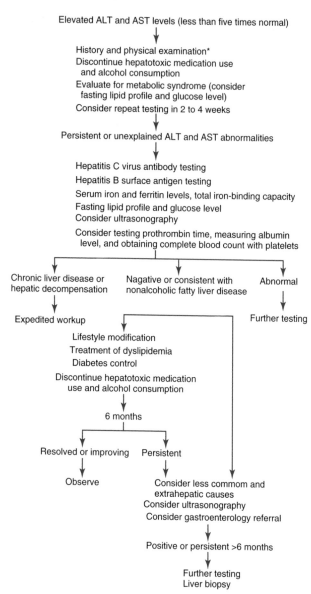

Elevated ALT and AST levels (less than five times normal)
↓
History and physical examination*
Discontinue hepatotoxic medication use
  and alcohol consumption
Evaluate for metabolic syndrome (consider
  fasting lipid profile and glucose level)
Consider repeat testing in 2 to 4 weeks
↓
Persistent or unexplained ALT and AST abnormalities
↓
Hepatitis C virus antibody testing
Hepatitis B surface antigen testing
Serum iron and ferritin levels, total iron-binding capacity
Fasting lipid profile and glucose level
Consider ultrasonography
Consider testing prothrombin time, measuring albumin
  level, and obtaining complete blood count with platelets

Chronic liver disease or   Nagative or consistent with   Abnormal
hepatic decompensation   nonalcoholic fatty liver disease
↓   ↓   ↓
Expedited workup   Further testing

Lifestyle modification
Treatment of dyslipidemia
Diabetes control
Discontinue hepatotoxic medication
  use and alcohol consumption
↓
6 months

Resolved or improving   Persistent
↓   ↓
Observe   Consider less commom and
                            extrahepatic causes
                          Consider ultrasonography
                          Consider gastroenterology referral
                          ↓
                          Positive or persistent >6 months
                          ↓
                          Further testing
                          Liver biopsy

*—If the history or physical examination suggests a diagnosis, targeted testing should
be pursued.

Figure 74-1 Management of mild liver transaminase abnormalities.
ALT, Alanine transaminase; *AST,* aspartate transaminase. (From Oh RC,
Hustead TR. Causes and evaluation of mildly elevated liver transaminase levels.
American Family Physician 2011;85:1003–1008; Fig. 1.)

Further Reading

American Gastroenterological Association. Medical position statement: evaluation of liver chemistry tests. *Gastroenterology*. 2002;123:1364–1366.

Aragon G, Younossi ZM. When and how to evaluate mildly elevated liver enzymes in apparently healthy patients. *Cleve Clin J Med*. 2010;77:195–204.

Clark JM, Brancati FL, Diehl AM. The prevalence and etiology of elevated aminotransferase levels in the United States. *Am J Gastroenterol*. 2003;98:960–967.

Giboney PT. Mildly elevated liver transaminase levels in the asymptomatic patient. *Am Fam Physician*. 2005;71:1105–1110.

Green RM, Flamm S. AGA technical review on the evaluation of liver chemistry tests. *Gastroenterology*. 2002;123:1367–1384.

Grover M, Rutkowski R, Nashelsky J. FPIN's Clinical Inquiries: evaluation of elevated serum transaminase levels. *Am Fam Physician*. 2012;86:1–2.

Ioannou GN, Boyko EJ, Lee SP. The prevalence and predictors of elevated serum aminotransferase activity in the United States in 1999-2002. *Am J Gastroenterol*. 2006;101:76–82.

Lee TH, Kim WR, Poterucha JJ. Evaluation of elevated liver enzymes. *Clin Liver Dis*. 2012;16:183–198.

Oh RC, Hustead TR. Causes and evaluation of mildly elevated liver transaminase levels. *Am Fam Physician*. 2011;85:1003–1008.

Pratt DS, Kaplan MM. Evaluation of abnormal liver enzyme results in asymptomatic patients. *N Engl J Med*. 2000;342:1266–1271.

Swartz MH. *Textbook of Physical Diagnosis*. 2nd ed. Philadelphia: Saunders; 1994;302–336.

75 TREMOR

General Discussion

Tremor is an involuntary, rhythmic, oscillatory movement of any body part. The first step in evaluating any patient with tremor is to characterize the tremor. All humans have physiologic tremor of the hands that may be enhanced under stressful circumstances. In addition to this normal form of tremor, there are several pathologic tremors that are generally categorized as resting tremor, action tremor, and intention tremor. Action tremor is the most prevalent of these types.

Resting tremor occurs while the limb is relaxed, stationary, and supported against gravity. The amplitude increases during mental stress, such as counting backward and with general movement (e.g., walking). Resting tremor diminishes with target-directed movement such as the finger-to-nose test.

Action tremor occurs during sustained extension of the arm or during voluntary motion such as writing or pouring. Action tremors can be subdivided into postural, isometric, and kinetic tremors. The differential diagnosis of an action tremor includes essential tremor, enhanced physiologic tremor, Parkinson disease, adult-onset idiopathic dystonia, and Wilson disease. Essential tremor is a visible tremor that occurs when the affected body part maintains position against gravity. It is the most common movement disorder worldwide and has a bimodal age distribution in the teenage years and in the 50s. Parkinson disease is 20 times less common than essential tremor, yet it affects approximately 1 million Americans. Initial symptoms include resting tremor beginning in one arm, typically as a flexion-extension elbow movement, a pronation-supination of the forearm, or a pill-rolling finger movement. This tremor worsens with stress and diminishes with voluntary movement. Other signs of Parkinson disease include rigidity, bradykinesia, impaired postural reflexes, and masked facies.

Intention tremor is a coarse terminal tremor that occurs during visually guided movements as the limb approaches a target. There is significant amplitude fluctuation as the target is approached.

Drug-induced tremor should be differentiated from other forms of tremor. First, other medical causes of tremor such as hyperthyroidism and hypoglycemia should be ruled out. Factors that suggest drug-induced tremor include a temporal relation to the start of therapy with the drug, a dose-response relation, and a lack of tremor progression. In addition, drug-induced tremor is symmetric for most drugs, except in the setting of drug-induced parkinsonism, in which patients commonly develop unilateral resting tremor. Older age places the patient at higher risk for drug-induced tremor.

Cerebellar tremor presents as unilateral or bilateral, low-frequency intention tremor caused by multiple sclerosis, stroke, or brainstem tumor. Finger-to-nose, finger-to-finger, and heel-to-shin testing results in worsening tremor as the extremity approaches its target. The patient may also have abnormalities of speech, gait, and ocular movements.

Psychogenic tremor is occasionally a consideration in the differential diagnosis of tremor. Psychogenic mimicking is usually diagnosed by distracting the patient with other motor or cognitive tasks. Psychogenic tremor decreases or stops with distraction while organic tremor stays the same or increases.

Medications and Substances Associated with Tremor

Amiodarone
Amitriptyline
Amphetamines
Amphotericin B
Beta-agonists
Caffeine
Calcitonin
Carbamazepine
Cimetidine
Corticosteroids
Co-trimoxazole
Cyclosporine
Cytarabine
Epinephrine
Fluoxetine
Haloperidol
Hypoglycemic agents
Ifosfamide
Interferon-alfa
Lithium
Medroxyprogesterone
Methyldopa
Methylphenidate
Metoclopramide
Mexiletine
Procainamide
Pseudoephedrine
Reserpine
Risperidone
Salbutamol
Salmeterol
Selective serotonin reuptake inhibitors

Tacrolimus
Tamoxifen
Terbutaline
Thalidomide
Theophylline
Thioridazine
Thyroxine
Tricyclic antidepressants
Valproic acid
Verapamil
Vidarabine

Causes of Tremor

Action tremor
- Adult-onset idiopathic dystonia
- Enhanced physiologic tremor
- Essential tremor
- Parkinson disease
- Wilson disease

Alcohol abuse
Caffeine
Cerebellar lesion
- Multiple sclerosis
- Stroke
- Traumatic brain injury

Cortical tremor
Drug withdrawal
Drugs of abuse
- Amphetamines
- Cocaine
- 3,4-methylenedioxymethamphetamine (MDMA)
- Nicotine

Intention tremor
Isolated chin tremor
Isolated voice tremor
Medications
Metabolic disorders
- Vitamin B_{12} deficiency
- Hyperparathyroidism
- Hyperthyroidism
- Hypocalcemia
- Hypoglycemia
- Hyponatremia

- Liver disease
- Renal disease
- Wilson disease

Movement disorders
Neuropathic tremor
Orthostatic tremor
Physiologic tremor
Psychogenic tremor
Resting tremor
Rubral or midbrain tremor
Withdrawal from alcohol, benzodiazepines, or cocaine

Key Historical Features

- ✓ Age at onset
- ✓ Exacerbating and relieving factors
- ✓ Functional limitations
- ✓ Type of tremor
- ✓ Rate of progression of the tremor
- ✓ Medical history
- ✓ Medications
- ✓ Family history
- ✓ Social history
    - Alcohol use
    - Caffeine
    - Illicit drug use
    - Tobacco use
- ✓ Review of systems
    - Diarrhea or weight loss to suggest hyperthyroidism
    - Sensation of muscles in the hand or neck being pulled or twisted to suggest dystonia
- ✓ Depressive symptoms, cognitive impairment, or other involuntary movements to suggest Wilson disease

Key Physical Findings

- ✓ Characteristics of the tremor
    - Amplitude
    - Frequency
    - Affected body part
    - Proximal or distal location
- ✓ Observation of the patient at rest, seated in a chair
- ✓ Observation of the patient performing maneuvers with the arms outstretched in front of the body to evaluate for postural tremor

✓ Observation of the patient performing the finger-to-nose movement to evaluate for an intention tremor

✓ Observation of the patient drinking from a glass, writing, or drawing a rhythmic pattern, such as a spiral

✓ Evaluation for rigidity and bradykinesia by flexing and extending the patient's arms

✓ Observation of the patient standing and walking to evaluate for difficulty initiating movement, decreased arm swing, or shuffling gait that may indicate Parkinson disease

✓ Evaluation for nystagmus

✓ General examination for signs of alcoholism, such as spider angiomata or an enlarged liver

✓ Head and neck examination for exophthalmos or thyroid enlargement

✓ Cardiac examination for tachycardia

✓ Neurologic examination for brisk reflexes that may suggest thyrotoxicosis or other abnormalities that may suggest multiple sclerosis

✓ Slit lamp examination for Kayser-Fleischer rings if Wilson disease is suspected

Suggested Work-Up

Serum glucose	To evaluate for hypoglycemia
Serum electrolytes	To evaluate for hyponatremia
Serum blood urea nitrogen and creatinine	To evaluate for renal disease
Thyroid function tests	To evaluate for hyperthyroidism
Liver function tests	To evaluate for liver disease
Serum ceruloplasmin level	In any patient with action tremor who is younger than 40 years of age to evaluate for Wilson disease. The level is <20 mg/dL in 95% of patients with Wilson disease.

Additional Work-Up

Computed tomography (CT) scan or magnetic resonance imaging (MRI)	If cerebellar tumor or stroke is suspected
MRI and cerebrospinal fluid examination of oligoclonal immunoglobulin-G bands	If multiple sclerosis is suspected
Single-photon emission CT	If Parkinson disease is suspected
Vitamin B_{12} level	If vitamin B_{12} deficiency is suspected

Serum calcium	If hypocalcemia is suspected
Serum parathyroid hormone (PTH)	If hyperparathyroidism is suspected
Lithium level	If lithium toxicity is suspected

Further Reading

Crawford P, Zimmerman E. Differentiation and diagnosis of tremor. *Am Fam Physician.* 2011;83:697–702.

Louis ED. Essential tremor. *N Engl J Med.* 2001;345:887–891.

Morgan JC, Sethi KD. Drug-induced tremors. *Lancet Neurol.* 2005;4:866–876.

Pahwa R, Lyons KE. Essential tremor: differential diagnosis and current therapy. *Am J Med.* 2003;115:134–142.

Smaga S. Tremor. *Am Fam Physician.* 2003;68:1545–1552.

Velickovic M, Gracies JM. Movement disorders: keys to identifying and treating tremor. *Geriatrics.* 2002;57:32–36.

General Discussion

Urinary incontinence is caused by a disturbance in the storage function, and occasionally in the emptying function, of the lower urinary tract. A continent sphincter mechanism requires proper angulation between the urethra and the bladder, as well as proper positioning of the urethra so that increases in intra-abdominal pressure are effectively transmitted to the urethra.

Women may undergo an anatomic or neuromuscular injury during childbirth, but they remain clinically asymptomatic as long as there is compensation by other components of the continence mechanism. Incontinence may not present in a woman until she loses a small percentage of muscle strength and innervation to the urethral sphincter due to aging or other injuries.

Stress incontinence is the involuntary loss of urine during an increase of intra-abdominal pressure. Stress urinary incontinence arises when bladder pressure exceeds urethral pressure during activities such as coughing, laughing, or exercising. The underlying abnormality is typically urethral hypermobility caused by a failure of the normal anatomic supports of the bladder neck. Intrinsic urethral sphincter deficiency, the lack of normal intrinsic pressure within the urethra, may also lead to stress incontinence.

Overactive bladder, also known as urge incontinence, is the involuntary loss of urine preceded by a strong urge to void whether or not the bladder is full. Urge incontinence results from bladder contractions that overwhelm the ability of the cerebral centers to inhibit them. This bladder oversensitivity may originate from the bladder epithelium or detrusor muscle as a result of altered neural activation in the voiding cycle.

Overflow incontinence is urine loss associated with overdistension of the bladder, typically caused by an underactive detrusor muscle and/or outlet obstruction. Patients may present with frequent or constant dribbling, overactive bladder, or stress incontinence. Causes of detrusor muscle underactivity are outlined in the following. Overflow incontinence is relatively uncommon, but it is more common in men because of the prevalence of obstructive prostate gland enlargement.

The first goal of the evaluation of urinary incontinence is to identify reversible causes of incontinence so that effective treatments may be instituted. The second goal is to identify conditions that may require specialty referral to urology or urogynecology. Once transient causes and indications for specialty evaluation or referral have been excluded, the third goal is to decide if the patient's symptoms are more suggestive of urge incontinence or stress incontinence. After this has been determined, treatment may be initiated accordingly. If the treatment is ineffective, specialty evaluation may be indicated.

Indications for special evaluation or referral detected by history include the following: recent onset within 2 months of urge incontinence or irritative bladder symptoms; previous surgery for incontinence; previous radical pelvic surgery; or incontinence associated with recurrent symptomatic urinary infections. Physical findings that usually require specialty referral include prostate nodules or asymmetry, gross pelvic prolapse, and neurologic abnormalities suggesting a systemic disorder or spinal cord lesion. Hematuria without infection or significant persistent proteinuria on urinalysis requires additional evaluation. Other situations that may require specialty referral are an abnormal post-void residual volume, treatment failure, consideration of surgical intervention, or an inability to arrive at a presumptive diagnosis and treatment plan.

Medications Associated with Urinary Incontinence

Alpha-adrenergic agonists
Angiotensin-converting enzyme inhibitors
Anticholinergic agents
Antidepressants
Antihistamines
Antiparkinsonian agents
Antipsychotics
Beta-blockers
Calcium channel blockers
Cyclo-oxygenase-2 selective nonsteroidal anti-inflammatory drugs
Diuretics
Lithium
Narcotics
Sedatives and hypnotics
Skeletal muscle relaxants
Thiazolidinediones

Causes of Urinary Incontinence

Overflow incontinence
- Diabetic neuropathy
- Fecal impaction
- Medications
- Prostatic enlargement
- Radiation
- Tumor
- Surgery
- Urethral stricture

Stress incontinence
- Intrinsic sphincter deficiency
- Medications

- Pelvic prolapse
- Radiation damage
- Surgical trauma
- Urethral hypermobility

Urge incontinence

- Alcohol
- Atrophic vaginitis
- Caffeine
- Calculi
- Dementia
- Encephalopathy
- Hypoxemia
- Impaired mobility
- Infection
- Malignancy
- Medications
- Parkinson disease
- Stroke

Key Historical Features

- ✓ Frequency of episodes
- ✓ Degree of bother and effect on quality of life
- ✓ Leakage of urine with coughing, laughing, lifting, or sneezing
- ✓ Leakage of urine associated with a strong urge to urinate
- ✓ Leakage of urine during sex
- ✓ Use of pad to protect from leaking urine
- ✓ Leakage of urine without the patient being aware of the leakage
- ✓ Time of day or night
- ✓ Relation to medication treatments
- ✓ Fluid intake
- ✓ Voiding habits
- ✓ How often sleep is interrupted by the need to urinate
- ✓ Presence of dysuria
- ✓ Presence of the sensation of incomplete bladder emptying
- ✓ Frequency of bowel movements
- ✓ Splinting of the vagina or perineum during defecation
- ✓ Presence of fecal incontinence
- ✓ Medical history
  - Chronic lung disease
  - Cognitive impairment
  - Diabetes
  - Fecal impaction
  - Lumbar disc disease
  - Stroke

✓   Obstetric and gynecologic history
  •   Gravity and parity
  •   Number of vaginal, instrument-assisted, and cesarean deliveries
  •   Estrogen status
  •   Time interval between deliveries
  •   Hysterectomy, vaginal surgery
  •   Bladder surgery
  •   Pelvic trauma
  •   Pelvic radiotherapy
✓   Surgical history
✓   Medications

Key Physical Findings

✓   General examination for mobility status
✓   Neurologic examination for cognitive status, upper motor neuron lesions (e.g., multiple sclerosis or Parkinson disease), and lower motor neuron lesions (e.g., sacral-nerve root lesions). The lumbosacral nerve roots should be assessed by checking deep tendon reflexes, lower extremity strength, and sharp and/or dull sensations.
✓   Cardiovascular and pulmonary examinations to assess for causes of cough
✓   Abdominal examination for masses, diastasis recti, ascites, or organomegaly
✓   Pelvic examination for pelvic masses, organ prolapse, or vaginal atrophy. The levator ani muscle function can be evaluated by asking the patient to tighten her vaginal muscles and hold the contraction as long as possible. The bulbocavernous and clitoral sacral reflexes should be evaluated. The examination should also include an evaluation for inflammation, infection, and atrophy.
✓   Rectal examination to evaluate for sphincter tone, fecal impaction, rectal lesions, prostate nodules, prostate asymmetry, or the presence of occult blood.
✓   Urine leakage should be assessed with coughing or Valsalva maneuver in both the supine and standing positions.
✓   Extremity examination for peripheral edema

Suggested Work-Up

Urinalysis	To evaluate for urinary tract infection, hematuria, proteinuria, or diabetes-induced glycosuria
Urine culture	Not routinely indicated but may be useful in identifying the causative organism of infections and in guiding antibiotic therapy.

Serum creatinine	May be elevated if there is urinary retention caused by bladder outlet obstruction or denervation of the detrusor
Assessment of post-void residual volume by catheterization or ultrasonography	To detect urinary retention. Less than 50 mL is normal, whereas more than 200 mL is abnormal.

If the cause of urinary incontinence is unclear after this assessment, referral to a urologist or urogynecologist should be considered.

Additional Work-Up

Cystometry	To measure bladder pressure during filling, which provides information about bladder capacity and the ability to inhibit detrusor contractions.
Cystoscopy	Indicated for the evaluation of patients with incontinence who also have any of the following: • hematuria or pyuria • irritative voiding symptoms, such as frequency, urgency, and urge incontinence in the absence of reversible causes • bladder pain • recurrent cystitis • suburethral mass • When urodynamic testing fails to duplicate symptoms of urinary incontinence
Cystometric testing	Indicated as part of the evaluation of more complex disorders of bladder filling and voiding, such as the presence of neurologic disease and other comorbid conditions. There are limited data suggesting its need in the routine evaluation of women with urinary incontinence.
Urodynamic testing	May be indicated when surgical treatment of stress incontinence is planned

| Pressure–flow voiding studies, uroflometry, and electromyography of the anal sphincter | May be indicated for the assessment of complex and neurogenic causes of urinary incontinence and voiding disorders |

Further Reading

Culligan PJ, Heit M. Urinary incontinence in women: evaluation and management. *Am Fam Physician.* 2000;62:2433–2444.

Khandelwal C, Kistler C. Diagnosis of urinary incontinence. *Am Fam Physician.* 2013;87:543–550.

Morantz CA. ACOG guidelines on urinary incontinence in women. *Am Fam Physician.* 2005;72:175.

Norton P, Brubaker L. Urinary incontinence in women. *Lancet.* 2006;367:57–67.

Wein AJ, Rackley RR. Overactive bladder: a better understanding of pathophysiology, diagnosis, and management. *J Urol.* 2006;175:S5–S10.

Weiss BD. Diagnostic evaluation of urinary incontinence in geriatric patients. *Am Fam Physician.* 1998;57:2675–2684.

General Discussion

Visual disturbances encompass a wide range of symptoms, including blurred vision, diplopia (double vision), visual field defects, and visual auras (such as flashes, halos, or scotomata). These may be a result of intraocular or extraocular pathology and can arise due to trauma, infection, inflammation, neoplasm, medication effect, or as a manifestation of systemic disease. One approach to categorizing visual disturbances is by anatomic location of injury. Affected structures may include the cornea, iris/pupil, lens, retina, optic nerve, extraocular muscles, vasculature, or cortex. A thorough history may help to identify which of these structures are damaged by characterizing the nature of the visual disturbance and determining the presence or absence of associated symptoms. Intraocular pathology is more likely to cause unilateral or asymmetric symptoms (e.g., with corneal injury or retinal detachment), whereas bilateral and symmetric visual disturbances are more likely to be the result of a cortical or systemic etiology. The physical examination should include a full ophthalmologic assessment, which may entail visual acuity, funduscopic examination, and slit lamp examination, as well as a complete neurologic evaluation.

Corneal causes of blurred vision include refractive errors due to irregular or abnormal corneal shape, as well as corneal abrasions, ulcers, or scarring (usually due to trauma, but these can be a result of infection). Corneal defects may be identified on slit lamp examination with fluorescein staining.

Abnormal and/or inappropriate pupillary dilation can result from medication effect or traumatic iris injury (rare); it may also reflect cranial nerve III palsy.

Cataract is an age-related disorder of the lens with high prevalence in the older adult population. Clouding of the lens is visible on inspection of the eye.

Paresis or entrapment of the extraocular muscles can result in diplopia. This can be caused by mass effect, trauma (e.g., orbital fractures), or cranial nerve deficit. Restricted extraocular movement is observed on examination.

Retinal disorders include diabetic or hypertensive retinopathy, retinal detachment, retinal toxicity, macular degeneration, and retinal tumors. Systemic vasculitides and other inflammatory vascular disorders, such as temporal arteritis and Takayasu arteritis, can cause visual loss due to retinal ischemia. Signs of retinal disease may be detected on funduscopic examination, which allows for visualization of the retina and macula.

The optic nerve or optic chiasm can be compressed due to mass effect, such as from a pituitary tumor. The characteristic visual field defect, bitemporal hemianopia, is pathognomonic for disruption of the optic chiasm. Optic neuritis (inflammation of the optic nerve) is commonly associated with multiple sclerosis, but can arise due to an infectious process or as an adverse medication effect. The optic nerve can also be damaged as a result of increased intraocular pressure (i.e., glaucoma); this can be a side effect of certain medications, particularly psychotropic agents.

Cortical and/or intracranial etiologies for visual disturbance can include trauma, intracranial mass, cerebrovascular accident, migraine, normal pressure hydrocephalus, and pseudotumor cerebri.

There are many other potential causes of visual disturbance. Rheumatologic disorders may have ocular manifestations; uveitis, keratoconjunctivitis sicca, scleritis, episcleritis, and iritis can cause decreased visual acuity or blurred vision and may be due to systemic autoimmune etiology. Proptosis, or protrusion of the globe, can cause blurred vision and may occur as a result of traumatic injury, orbital cellulitis or abscess, or Graves ophthalmopathy. Conjunctivitis can give the perception of blurred vision due to excessive ocular discharge, although visual acuity is usually normal if tested after the discharge has been removed by irrigation.

Medications Associated with Visual Disturbances

Amiodarone
Anticholinergics
- Antihistamines
- Antispasmodics (dicyclomine, hyoscyamine, oxybutynin)
- Chlorpromazine
- Thioridazine

Bisphosphonates
Deferoxamine
Ethambutol
Linezolid
Isoniazid
Isotretinoin
Sertraline
Tamoxifen
Topiramate
Tricyclic antidepressants

Causes of Visual Disturbances

Autoimmune disease/vasculitis
- Episcleritis
- Giant cell arteritis
- Graves disease
- Inflammatory bowel disease
- Iritis
- Myasthenia gravis
- Scleritis
- Systemic lupus erythematosus

- Takayasu arteritis
- Uveitis

Cataracts

Cerebrovascular accident (CVA)/transient ischemic attack (TIA)

Corneal abrasion/corneal ulcer

Cranial nerve palsy

Diabetic retinopathy

Dry eyes (keratoconjunctivitis sicca)

Excessive eye discharge (allergic reaction, conjunctivitis)

Extraocular muscle entrapment

Glaucoma

Hypertensive crisis

Intracranial tumor

Intraocular tumor

Macular degeneration/macular pucker

Migraine headache

Normal pressure hydrocephalus

Optic neuritis/multiple sclerosis

Pituitary tumor

Pseudotumor cerebri

Refractive error

Retinal detachment

Retinal toxicity

Key Historical Features

✓ Nature of symptom onset (sudden or gradual)
✓ Constant versus intermittent disturbance
✓ Unilateral or bilateral
✓ Eye pain
✓ Eye redness
✓ Headache
✓ Focal neurologic symptoms
✓ Recent head trauma
✓ Medical history
✓ Medications
✓ Family history

Key Physical Findings

✓ Blood pressure
✓ Visual acuity
✓ Visual fields
✓ Pupillary reactivity
✓ Extraocular movements

✓ Funduscopic examination
✓ Slit lamp examination
✓ Intraocular pressure
✓ Cranial nerve examination
✓ Tenderness over temporal artery

Suggested Work-Up

Erythrocyte sedimentation rate, C-reactive protein, Antinuclear antibody (ANA), antiphospholipid antibodies, complete blood count	If autoimmune process is suspected
Hemoglobin A$_{1c}$	If diabetic retinopathy is suspected
Thyroid-stimulating hormone, free T4	If Graves ophthalmology is suspected

Additional Work-Up

Orbital computed tomography	If extraocular muscle entrapment is suspected
Orbital or brain magnetic resonance imaging	If intraocular or intracranial mass, CVA, or demyelinating process is suspected
Carotid ultrasound	If CVA/TIA is suspected

Further Reading

Dafer RM, Jay WM. Headache and the eye. *Curr Opin Ophthalmol.* 2009;20:520–524.

Espinoza GM, Desai A, Akduman L. Ocular vasculitis. *Curr Rheumatol Rep.* 2013;15:355.

Friedman DI. The pseudotumor cerebri syndrome. *Neurol Clin.* 2014;32:363–396.

Hamideh F, et al. Ophthalmologic manifestations of rheumatic diseases. *Semin Arthritis Rheum.* 2001;30:217–241.

Li J, Tripathi RC, Tripathi BJ. Drug-induced ocular disorders. *Drug Saf.* 2008;31:127–141.

Pakdaman MN, Sepahdari AR, Elkhamary SM. Orbital inflammatory disease: pictorial review and differential diagnosis. *World J Radiol.* 2014;6:106–115.

Panda A, Sharma S, Jana M, Arora A, Sharma SK. Ophthalmic manifestations of systemic diseases—part 2: metabolic, infections, granulomatoses, demyelination, and skeletal dysplasias. *Curr Probl Diagn Radiol.* 2014;43:242–253.

Pelletier AL, Thomas J, Shaw FR. Vision loss in older persons. *Am Fam Physician.* 2009;79:963–970.

Richa S, Yazbek JC. Ocular adverse effects of common psychotropic agents: a review. *CNS Drugs.* 2010;24:501–526.

Sharma S, Panda A, Jana M, et al. Ophthalmic manifestations of systemic diseases—part 1: phakomatoses, hematologic malignancies, metastases, and histiocytosis. *Curr Probl Diagn Radiol.* 2014;43:175–185.

Uzelac A, Gean AD. Orbital and facial fractures. *Neuroimaging Clin N Am.* 2014;24:407–424. vii.

Ventura RE, Balcer LJ, Galetta SL. The neuro-ophthalmology of head trauma. *Lancet Neurol.* 2014;13:1006–1016.

Wipperman JL, Dorsch JN. Evaluation and management of corneal abrasions. *Am Fam Physician.* 2013;87:114–120.

General Discussion

Clinically significant weight loss can be defined as the loss of 10 pounds or more than 5% of the usual body weight over 6 to 12 months, especially when the weight loss is progressive. Weight loss greater than 10% represents protein–energy malnutrition, which is associated with impaired physiologic function such as impaired cell-mediated and humoral immunity. Weight loss greater than 20% represents severe protein–energy malnutrition and is associated with organ dysfunction.

Dieting and eating disorders, such as anorexia nervosa and bulimia nervosa, explain most cases of intentional weight loss. Unintentional weight loss can be divided into four problems: anorexia, dysphagia, weight loss despite normal intake, or socioeconomic problems.

Malignancies account for approximately one-third of all patients presenting with unintentional weight loss. Gastrointestinal disorders are the most common nonmalignant organic etiologies in patients with unintentional weight loss, accounting for approximately 15% of cases. Medications are a frequently overlooked potential etiology of unintentional weight loss, particularly in older adult patients. Polypharmacy can interfere with taste and cause anorexia. Adverse effects of medications, such as nausea, anorexia, diarrhea, dysphagia, and dysgeusia, may alter the intake, absorption, and use of nutrients.

Weight loss occurs commonly in older adult individuals. Among community-dwelling older adults, the most common causes of weight loss are depression, cancer, and benign gastrointestinal tract diseases. Among nursing home residents, psychiatric and neurologic illnesses account for the greatest proportion of weight loss.

In most patients, the etiology of unintentional weight loss may be identified through a detailed history and physical examination. The first step in evaluating a complaint of weight loss is quantifying the weight loss. The symptoms acquired from the history can guide the clinician to one of the four causal categories: anorexia, dysphagia, weight loss despite normal intake, and social factors. The suggested laboratory evaluation is outlined in the following. Additional testing should be directed by findings on history, physical examination, or initial laboratory evaluation. Patients with normal physical and laboratory findings are unlikely to have a serious physical illness.

Medications Associated with Weight Loss

Angiotensin-converting enzyme inhibitors
Alendronate
Allopurinol
Amantadine

Amphetamines
Antibiotics
- Atovaquone
- Ciprofloxacin
- Clarithromycin
- Doxycycline
- Ethambutol
- Griseofulvin
- Metronidazole
- Ofloxacin
- Pentamidine
- Rifabutin
- Tetracycline

Anticholinergics
Anticonvulsants
Antihistamines
Antipsychotics
Benzodiazepines
Bisphosphonates
Calcium-channel blockers
Carbamazepine
Chemotherapeutic agents
Clonidine
Corticosteroids
Decongestants
Digoxin
Dopamine agonists
Gold
Hormone replacement therapy
Hydralazine
Hydrochlorothiazide
Iron
Levodopa
Lithium
Loop diuretics
Metformin
Methimazole
Neuroleptics
Nicotine
Nitroglycerin
Nonsteroidal anti-inflammatory drugs
Opiates
Penicillamine
Pergolide

Phenytoin
Potassium
Propranolol
Quinidine
Selective serotonin reuptake inhibitors
Selegiline
Spironolactone
Statins
Theophylline
Tricyclic antidepressants

Causes of Weight Loss

Alcoholism
Cardiovascular disease
- Congestive heart failure
- Mesenteric ischemia
Cocaine use
Dietary factors (low-salt, low-cholesterol diets)
Endocrine disorders
- Adrenal insufficiency
- Diabetes mellitus
- Hyperparathyroidism
- Hyperthyroidism
- Hypothyroidism
- Panhypopituitarism
- Pheochromocytoma
Gastrointestinal disease
- Atrophic gastritis
- Celiac disease
- Cholelithiasis
- Chronic pancreatitis
- Constipation
- Diarrhea
- Dysphagia (oropharyngeal or esophageal)
- Gastroparesis
- Inflammatory bowel disease
- Malabsorption due to bacterial overgrowth, pancreatic exocrine deficiency, or celiac disease
- Peptic ulcer disease
- Pseudo-obstruction
- Reflux esophagitis
Inability to feed self
Infections

- Fungal disease
- HIV infection
- Parasites
- Subacute bacterial endocarditis
- Tuberculosis

Malignancies
- Breast
- Gastrointestinal
- Genitourinary
- Hepatobiliary
- Hematologic
- Lung
- Ovarian
- Prostate

Medications

Neurologic disease
- Cerebrovascular accident
- Delirium
- Dementia
- Multiple sclerosis
- Parkinson disease
- Quadriplegia
- Tardive dyskinesia

Nutritional disorders

Oral factors
- Periodontal disease
- Poor dentition
- Xerostomia

Pulmonary disease
- Chronic obstructive pulmonary disease

Psychiatric disorders
- Anorexia nervosa
- Anxiety disorders
- Depression
- Paranoia

Renal disease
- Hemodialysis
- Nephrotic syndrome
- Uremia

Rheumatologic disease
- Giant cell arteritis
- Scleroderma

Socioeconomic conditions

Swallowing disorders

Visual impairments

Key Historical Features

✓ Amount of weight loss
✓ Determine if the patient is predominantly not hungry, is feeling nauseated after meals, is having difficulty eating or swallowing, or is having functional or social problems that may be interfering with the ability to obtain or enjoy food
✓ Presence of indigestion or reflux symptoms
✓ Abdominal pain
✓ Changes in bowel habits
✓ Early satiety
✓ In geriatric patients, interview a knowledgeable caretaker
✓ Dietary history
   • Availability of food
   • Use of nutritional or herbal supplements
   • Amount of food consumed
   • Adequacy of the patient's diet
   • Daily caloric intake
✓ Discussion of functional and mental status
✓ Assessment for depression and dementia
✓ Medical history, especially previous gastrointestinal conditions
✓ Surgical history, especially previous gastrointestinal surgery
✓ Medications
✓ Social history
   • Financial situation
   • Lifestyle
   • Living arrangements/home environment
   • Occupation
   • Support network
   • Travel
   • Use of transportation
✓ Thorough review of systems
   • Fever
   • Fatigue
   • Dyspnea
   • Exertional fatigue

Key Physical Findings

✓ Vital signs
✓ Height, weight, and body mass index
✓ Examination of the oral cavity
✓ Cardiopulmonary examination
✓ Abdominal examination
✓ Rectal examination

✓ Mental status examination and formal cognitive testing with an instrument such as the Folstein Mini-Mental State Exam
✓ Evaluation for depression using an instrument such as the PHQ-9 or the Geriatric Depression Scale
✓ Examination of the nervous system
✓ Functional assessment, including evaluations of sight, hearing, gait, and self-care ability (tools include the Katz scale of activities of daily living and the Lawton scale of instrumental activities of daily living)

Suggested Work-Up

Complete blood count	To evaluate for infection, anemia, or lymphoproliferative disorder
Chemistry panel	To evaluate for diabetes mellitus, dehydration, or renal dysfunction
Thyroid-stimulating hormone	To evaluate for hypo- or hyperthyroidism
Liver function tests	To evaluate for liver pathology
Lactate dehydrogenase	To evaluate for malignancy
C-reactive protein and erythrocyte sedimentation rate	To evaluate for inflammatory/infectious processes
Urinalysis	To evaluate for infection, renal dysfunction, or dehydration
Fecal occult blood test	To screen for gastrointestinal malignancy
Chest x-ray	To evaluate for infection, malignancy, or cardiopulmonary disease

Additional Work-Up

Abdominal ultrasound	To evaluate for anatomic lesions
Upper endoscopy or upper gastrointestinal series	Should be considered in patients with anorexia, absence of other symptoms, and persistent weight loss because peptic ulcer disease and gastroesophageal reflux may be silent.
Blood culture	If infection is suspected
Purified protein derivative (PPD)	If tuberculosis is suspected
HIV test	If risk factors for HIV infection are suspected

Rapid plasma reagin (RPR)	If risk factors for syphilis are present or physical findings suggest the presence of syphilis infection
Growth hormone	If endocrine deficiency is suspected
Testosterone level	If low testosterone level is suspected
Sigmoidoscopy or colonoscopy	If a colonic lesion is suspected
Computed tomography scanning	Low yield, but may be helpful in diagnosing malignancy, abscess, chronic pancreatitis, intestinal complications, and so on.
Serum pre-albumin, transferrin, and albumin	Not useful in determining the etiology of weight loss, but may be used to guide supplement selection

Further Reading

Alibhai SM, Greenwood C, Payette H. An approach to the management of unintentional weight loss in elderly people. *Can Med Assoc J.* 2005;172:773–780.

Bouras EP, Lange SM, Scolapio JS. Rational approach to patients with unintentional weight loss. *Mayo Clin Proc.* 2001;76:923–929.

Gaddey HL, Holder K. Unintentional weight loss in older adults. *Am Fam Physician.* 2014;89:718–722.

Gazewood JD, Mehr DR. Diagnosis and management of weight loss in the elderly. *J Fam Pract.* 1998;47:19–25.

Huffman GB. Evaluating and treating unintentional weight loss in the elderly. *Am Fam Physician.* 2002;65:640–650.

Robertson RG, Montagnini M. Geriatric failure to thrive. *Am Fam Physician.* 2004;70:343–350.

Index

Note: Page numbers followed by *f* indicate figures, and *t* indicate tables.